THE ESSENTIALS OF HEALTH CARE IN OLD AGE

SECOND EDITION

Gerald C J Bennett, MB BCh, FRCP

Senior Lecturer in Health Care of the Elderly, London Hospital Medical College, London, UK

and

Shah Ebrahim, DM, FRCP, FFPHM, MRCGP

Professor of Clinical Epidemiology, Royal Free Hospital School of Medicine, London, UK

Edward Arnold

A member of the Hodder Headline Group

LONDON   BOSTON   SYDNEY   AUCKLAND

First published in Great Britain 1992 by
Edward Arnold, a division of Hodder Headline PLC,
338 Euston Road, London NW1 3BH as
The Essentials of Health Care of the Elderly

Second edition 1995

Distributed in the Americas by Little, Brown and Company
34 Beacon Street, Boston, MA 02108

British Library Cataloguing in Publication Data
A catalogue record for this book is available from the British Library

Library of Congress Cataloging-in-Publication Data
A catalog record for this book is available from the Library of Congress

ISBN 0 340 61372 6 (pb)

1 2 3 4 5   95 96 97 98 99

Typeset in 10/11½pt Ehrhardt by
Phoenix Photosetting, Chatham, Kent
Printed and bound in Great Britain by
The Bath Press, Avon

THE ESSENTIALS OF HEALTH CARE
IN OLD AGE

We dedicate this book to our patients, their carers and the teams who look after them.

CONTENTS

PART THREE   SERVICES FOR ELDERLY PEOPLE

PREFACE TO THE SECOND EDITION

This new edition of *Essentials of Health Care of Old Age* builds on the first edition, *Essentials of Health Care of the Elderly*. The title has changed to reflect a growing concern with the stigmatizing and stereotyping effect of talking about 'the elderly'. Why a new edition? Principles and practice of health care in old age are moving quickly in the wake of the implementation of recent health and social service reforms in the UK. We were extremely encouraged by the positive reactions to the first edition from our students, our peers, and most surprisingly, many of our potential patients!

The book is divided into three sections: gerontology — the science of ageing; the medicine and psychiatry of old age; and the organization of health care for elderly people. The chapters are short and finish with key points to aid revision and suggested further reading.

Much of the content has changed. Advances in thinking about the biological nature of ageing are included in Chapter 1. New chapters have been included on diagnoses not to be missed, management of confusional states at home and in hospital, ethnic elders, ageing in developing countries, community care, psychological aspects of physical illness, and ethics of health care for older people. Other chapters have been updated in the light of health service reforms and advances in knowledge. Many new references to key articles and books are included.

The purpose of the book remains the same: undergraduates in medicine, nursing, and professions allied to medicine will find much of interest and value to them. Candidates studying for postgraduate examinations will find it a useful introduction to the principles and practice of health care in old age.

ACKNOWLEDGEMENTS

We are grateful to our colleagues at St George's Hospital Medical School, Nottingham University Medical School, The Royal Free Hospital School of Medicine, The Medical College of St Bartholomew's Hospital and the London Hospital Medical College who contributed greatly to the concepts contained in this book. We are also grateful for the many comments and suggestions made by colleagues following publication of the first edition which have helped us in preparing this second edition.

Our thanks also go to Miss Johannah McGowan for expert typing of the manuscript.

Gerald CJ Bennett
Shah Ebrahim
1995

PART ONE
ESSENTIALS OF AGEING

1 AGEING: POPULATIONS, ORGANISMS AND CELLS

- Ageing or disease?
- Medical care versus social care
- Impairments, disabilities and handicaps
- Population ageing
- Rectangularization of survival
- Individual ageing
- The mechanisms of human ageing
- Starvation and longevity
- Theories of ageing: so what?

Ageing is a reproducible and highly recognizable process. You only have to look at friends or TV and cinema stars and you can guess their age usually correctly to within a few years. But the process is very variable. Some people look much older than their years and others much younger. What is clear is that the same changes occur but at different rates.

An ageing population is defined epidemiologically as one in which there is an increase in age-specific death rates. Death rates start to increase remarkably early in life (Fig. 1.1), from about the early 20s. Medical and nursing students are already well into the ageing process by the time they have finished their courses! Male rates are higher than female rates but this is usually attributed to men's tendency to smoke, drink too much and take part in risky activities, like riding motorcycles.

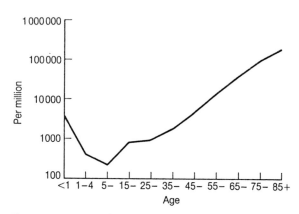

Figure 1.1 Age-specific death rates in men, England and Wales 1991

AGEING OR DISEASE?

What is ageing? Ageing is a developmental process, part of the cycle beginning at conception and ending with death. Ageing is not the same as disease, but diseases do become much more common among older people. This association between ageing and disease is the cause of much confusion about what is in store for us as we age. And it is a confusion that tends to affect doctors more than their patients. Patients complain to their doctors of pain and immobility only to be told that its due to their age — which is seldom true.

For example, a patient develops difficulty getting in and out of the bath. This may be due to ageing: a decline in the number of functioning muscle cells leading to weakness. It may be due to a disease affecting the peripheral nerves, a metabolic disease (e.g. diabetes or osteomalacia), or disease of large joints (e.g. osteoarthritis). This is demonstrated in Table 1.1.

Table 1.1 The relationships between ageing and disease

Ability to get in and out of bath	Disease process (e.g. osteomalacia)	
	Present	Absent
Unable	May be due to the disease	May be due to age-related decline in strength
Able	Occult disease	Healthy

MEDICAL CARE VERSUS SOCIAL CARE

In the example given, a social model of care would lead to assessment of the problem and provision of a bath board and rails around the bath. A medical model would sort out disease from ageing, and attempt to treat any underlying disease process. A collaborative approach would lead to both treatment (in its widest sense) of any disease underlying the disability and provision of any aids or lifestyle modifications to overcome the disability. Collaboration and teamwork are the hallmarks of health care for elderly people.

The medical model is often criticized for its preoccupation with diagnosis and drug treatment, for its focus on organ systems, and for its super-specialization. But the medical model has much to offer elderly people. Disease does become so much more common with increasing age and deserves to be diagnosed and treated. Despite much disease being chronic, degenerative and irreversible, a great deal can be done for its disabling and handicapping consequences. However, the doctor is seldom able to combat disease consequences single-handedly. Teamwork is necessary, and the concept of diagnosis has to be extended to assessment, treatment becomes management, and prognosis becomes monitoring and evaluation of achievement of goals.

An exclusively social model, bypassing the question

'Is this problem due to disease or not?', is just as inadequate for solving problems as a solely medical model. Collaboration is essential, and is best achieved through comprehensive services for elderly people.

IMPAIRMENTS, DISABILITIES AND HANDICAPS

Although these terms are often used interchangeably, they do have precise meanings that can help in understanding what comprehensive care means (Table 1.2).

Table 1.2 Definitions of impairment, disability and handicap

Impairment
   Damage caused to a cell, organ or system by a disease process

Disability
   Difficulty in carrying out tasks — such as activities of daily living, or driving a car — that are a consequence of the disease

Handicap
   Effect the disease has on the lifestyle of the patient — the disadvantage caused by the disease

Some treatment may reduce impairment. For example, exercise against progressively increased resistance may increase muscle strength and joint flexibility in an arthritic joint. The measurement of muscle strength and joint range of movement would be the best indicators of success and failure.

Other treatments may have no effect whatsoever on the impairment caused by disease. For example, no amount of physiotherapy will reduce the amount of brain damaged by a stroke. However, therapy may well reduce the time taken to get independently mobile again. In this case the correct measure of success is the measure of an aspect of disability — mobility.

For many diseases, neither the impairment nor the disability is affected by rehabilitation teamwork. This is not to say that useful management is impossible. It is this type of patient who is often viewed as a 'no-hoper' on an acute medical ward, but is transformed into a 'major rehabilitation challenge' on a health care of the elderly ward! There is no special magic in this, but simply a more realistic appraisal of the possibilities by the team, and a tendency to focus on handicap or lifestyle.

It is vital that services for elderly people understand their contribution to the overall picture, and do not attempt to demonstrate the supremacy of their particular skills over those of other equally needed and important skills. The impairments, disabilities and handicaps framework is a useful way of ensuring a comprehensive approach.

POPULATION AGEING

Most people know that we are living in an ageing society, indicated by such phenomena as the greying of America, the rise of the Grey Panthers, the growth of retirement and nursing homes. One of the major justifications for health care for elderly people is the increased number of them. This is highlighted by the tremendous increase in the number of centenarians in the UK who receive a birthday telegram from the Queen each year.

The spectacular population changes over the last century are due to two major factors: declines in fertility and decreases in death rates at all ages. Fertility declines because of a smaller number of babies born and increasing maternal age at first birth. These trends began with the industrial revolution and the associated socio-economic development which made large families less advantageous. Family planning has accelerated the process in many developing countries. A willingness to use family planning methods depends on culture, education and religion, but with increased economic wealth a move to smaller families is inevitable. Prosperity is no longer measured by the size of the family (see Chapter 34).

Death rates have also declined dramatically over the last century and the decline has affected the old and the young. The explanation for the decline is found in improved nutritional status, better social and economic conditions and the major public health reforms of clean water and sewage disposal. Medical care was not responsible for the changes. Over the last century, the world has — despite appearances — become a healthier place to live, and more of us are doing it for longer.

It is paradoxical that an ageing population is a consequence of living in a successful society that ensures that babies do not die, that promotes the autonomy of women to control their fertility, and that has reduced the chances of death over the entire lifespan. The large numbers of elderly people are our heritage, and the rewards of socio-economic development. Turning back the clock to the turn of the century when old age was not a 'problem' is impossible, and countries where high fertility and infant mortality rates occur do not wish to stay at that point in development. A better understanding of ageing, removing the myths and stereotypes, and

improving the health, social and economic lot of elderly people are keys to the solution.

RECTANGULARIZATION OF SURVIVAL

Survival curves have changed in shape over the last few hundred years (Fig. 1.2). This process has been called the 'rectangularization of survival'. One of the consequences of the increased chances of survival is that average life expectancy begins to approach maximum lifespan. The maximum lifespan is around 115 years, but the average expectation of life at birth is around 80 years for women in the most successful countries (Japan, USA). Deaths, instead of being spread across a fairly long part of the human lifespan, are now compressed into a shorter time. This should mean that people are sicker for a shorter time as well, and in essence will tend to be healthier for longer.

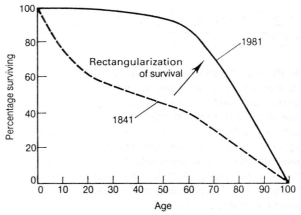

Figure 1.2 The rectangularization of survival: survival curves for 1841 and 1981

This optimistic scenario for the next century may come true, but for the foreseeable future it is more likely that increased survival will be associated with increased risk of non-life-threatening, but disabling chronic diseases. At present, the rectangularization of survival is associated with a far greater number of very old people, which is producing an explosion of morbidity, and an increased pressure on health and social care resources.

INDIVIDUAL AGEING

We have become used to hearing how things change, usually for the worse as we get older. Blood pressure goes up with age, hearing and vision get worse, bone density declines, intelligence declines, and so on. As humans grow and develop they reach a peak in physiological and anatomical capacity in their late teens, but subsequently capacity declines. It seems to matter little which type of capacity is considered: muscle strength, stamina, lung volume, kidney function, brain volume. All show age-related declines.

Cross-sectional and longitudinal studies

There is a large trap for the unwary here. Most of the studies of age-related declines are not really studies of ageing at all. In fact they are studies of a number of young people, a number of middle-aged people, and a number of old and very old people, all examined at the same point in time. None of the subjects has aged at all during the study, they are simply of different ages at the time of the study. Such studies are cross-sectional — snapshots — and we have to make some assumptions before we can accept that they are a good indication of true ageing changes.

The first assumption is that what is true for 60-year-olds now will be true for 50-year-olds in 10 years' time. We have to believe that the effects of belonging to a group — or cohort — of people born around the same time, and living through a unique set of life experiences, is not relevant to the factor (e.g. blood pressure, brain volume) under study. The effects of belonging to a cohort have been extremely important over the last century. For example, women born at the turn of the century had far fewer chances for marriage than those born later because of World War I. Men who went to fight in that war, if they survived, were subsequently much more likely to die of lung cancer because of smoking habits acquired during the war. Cohort effects can be powerful, and are impossible to detect in a simple cross-sectional study.

The second assumption to be made is that conducting the study at a particular point in time is irrelevant. It is unlikely that a cross-sectional study of changes in, say, muscle strength and age conducted in 1989 would come up with different results to one conducted in 1990. But over a period as short as five years, differences in the relationships between blood pressure and age have been found.

A third assumption is that older subjects are disease free. For example reductions in air flow with age may be due to changes in the elasticity of the lung, but inclusion of older people with chronic bronchitis will lead to much greater age-related reductions in air flow due to the combined effects of age and disease.

The reason that scientists continue to examine the effects of age by cross-sectional studies is because such studies are generally much cheaper than cohort — follow-up or longitudinal — studies. Provided such studies give more or less the same answer, no harm is done. However, in the few cases where comparisons can be made between cross-sectional and cohort studies, the answer can be strikingly different.

The best example of a discrepancy between cross-sectional and cohort effects are the changes in performances on intelligence tests at different ages. The general conclusion of cross-sectional studies is that intelligence declines with age, supporting stereotyped images of confused old people. The cohort changes are strikingly different: far from getting more stupid over the years, people tend to improve on some aspects of intelligence and remain more or less the same on others, and decline in only a few areas (Fig. 1.3).

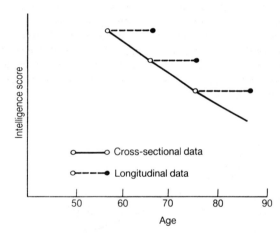

Figure 1.3 Changes in intelligence with age: cross-sectional and cohort studies compared

So why the difference? It probably arises out of a cohort effect. People born in 1920 had limited schooling and access to educational mass media like television and newspapers. People born in 1930 enjoyed better education. When studied cross-sectionally in 1990, those born in 1920 are 70 years old and will do worse on the intelligence tests than the 60-year-olds born in 1930.

Describing true ageing effects

Describing true age effects requires complicated studies of successive cohorts of people over long periods of time — so-called 'cohort-sequential' studies. This is because a single cohort invariably experiences a unique set of circumstances thrown up by the age they live through (e.g. wars, economic depression) — period effects that have an impact at all ages. The task is to separate the effects of ageing from the effects of the era in which people age. This can only be done by studying a succession of cohorts to determine whether age-related changes are consistent across each cohort. Very few studies like this have ever been set up, so we have to make do with the information from cross-sectional studies. However, never take such information at face value: always ask — could this be due to cohort or time period effects?

Statistically, ageing can be defined as facing an increased risk of death over time. What does this mean? If you take 1000 glasses and count how many 'survive' over a period of years you would not be surprised if many of them 'died'. The death rate of the glasses can be calculated as the number broken divided by the number at the outset. However, a small adjustment has to be made for the fact that once a glass is broken it cannot be broken again, and must be removed from the denominator of the calculation of the 'death' rate. If this is done, a glass survival curve can be drawn, giving the percentage of glasses surviving at the end of each year (Fig. 1.4).

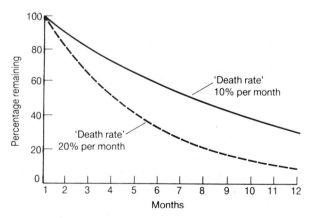

Figure 1.4 Theoretical survival curves for wine glasses

Now glasses do not age: their molecules contain no ability to replicate, they are inert. And yet a population of glasses appears to 'age', and has a survival curve. The key is that the rate of breakage of glasses is constant — there is a constant accident hazard that systematically removes glasses until they are all gone. Death rates of populations do not show a constant rate, but an ever-increasing rate with increasing chronological age. This gives population survival curves their characteristic rectangular shape. The point at which death rates start to rise can be viewed as the start of human ageing. It comes as a surprise to see how early in life this starts — late teens, early 20s!

Many factors change as people get older. Some people get richer, most get poorer. Their homes age with them, often becoming hazardous. Social contacts and status within the family alter. These factors are called 'extrinsic'.

THE MECHANISMS OF HUMAN AGEING

Ageing has fascinated scientists, philosophers and poets for centuries. What is ageing? Why do we age? What is ageing for? How can we slow down or stop the process? These are weighty questions and need unravelling into smaller questions that are more easily tackled. An inherent difficulty in the study of ageing is that the findings from easy-to-study animal species (bacteria, paramecium, mice) are not directly transferable to humans.

Strehler's framework of ageing states that, for a process to be truly due to ageing (rather than due to pathology), it must be universal, progressive, intrinsic and deleterious.

Cellular and molecular ageing

Cells get old and die just like the whole organism, but they do it at a more rapid rate. The cells of the epidermal layer of the skin shed themselves within a few days. The red blood cell lives for about four months. Theories of ageing have to accommodate the following observations about ageing.

Hayflick limit to cell division

The Hayflick limit is the number of cell divisions that human fibroblasts — connective tissue cells — grown in a cell culture can undergo before stopping. They stop after about 50 cell divisions. By contrast, many human cancer cells continue to replicate unchecked, and are called immortal.

Rate of DNA repair between species is linked to life expectation

DNA gets damaged in the rough and tumble of cellular life, so DNA repair enzymes spontaneously deal with the problems. Species that are long-lived, such as humans and elephants, tend to have better DNA repair efficiency than short-lived species.

Increased autoimmune damage and reduction in protective immune responses

As people get older they become more prone to infections, such as pneumonia, and cell-mediated immunity to diseases like tuberculosis may wane, leading to a greater risk of disease. The occurrence of auto-antibody diseases (e.g. thyroid disease, pernicious anaemia, collagen-vascular diseases) becomes more common with age.

Accelerated ageing syndromes (progeria, Down's syndrome, diabetes)

The very rare inherited premature ageing, or progeria, syndromes lead to early death with many of the characteristics of very old people. The fibroblast cells of affected people demonstrate a reduced ability to replicate.

Increased cross-linking in DNA, collagen, proteins

Collagen fibres start to form rigid cross-linked sulphur bonds which interfere with connective tissue functions. In DNA, cross-links may form which are difficult to break, leading to errors in replication.

Enzyme, second messenger, accumulation of lipofuscin changes

Many cellular functions appear to change with increasing age. It is difficult to know which are prime forces in ageing, and which are merely consequences of more fundamental changes.

Energy use per kilogram per lifetime

With the exception of humans, the rate at which different species use energy is roughly similar when allowance is made for body weight. In experiments on ageing it has been found that mice that are starved live longer than those fed at will.

Damage theories

The damage theories of cellular ageing are strongly supported by work on DNA repair enzymes and free radicals. Free radicals are oxidants — electron donors — produced as a byproduct of metabolism, and have an extra free electron. They are unstable, and when they combine with cell membranes this leads to damage, producing lipid peroxides and aldehydes which cause increased cross-linking in proteins and DNA. Many enzyme systems are devoted to combating the adverse effects of free radicals. Antioxidants include vitamins C and E and selenium, and are often included in proprietary 'anti-ageing' drugs. There is no evidence that these drugs work. The damage and toxic accumulation theories have been described as the 'clinker' theory, perhaps after the deposit that is found in the grate of an open fire or from its American usage as a term for a mistake or error. Somatic mutation caused by radiation exposure is another variant of the error theories, but is now discounted as the levels of radiation would have to be far too high to explain ageing changes.

Programmed ageing: genetic theories

Programme theories state that ageing is developmentally controlled and that the whole process from conception through differentiation and growth to senescence is under a regulatory gene complex. However, it is possible that longevity genes are linked with characteristics that make us more resistant to disease, or make us more ingenious, and that ageing is simply an unfortunate byproduct of advantages reaped earlier in life. As a species the advantages of elders for social organization and repositories of knowledge may have outweighed their physical disadvantages, allowing the older men continued access to women as the means for ensuring the survival of their genes.

The programmed ageing theories and the damage theories can be brought together. It is possible that the regulation of DNA repair mechanisms, of antioxidants and of immunological mechanisms is under programmed genetic control. There is evidence that the major histocompatability (MHC) system in the mouse is associated both with immunological competence and with longevity. The comparable human leucocyte antigen (HLA) system in humans is associated with several autoimmune disease processes and has also been shown to be linked with longevity.

If you know how old your grandparents and parents were when they died you may feel that you have a good idea of your own survival prospects. No so. The heritability of longevity is only small. Different species have different survival prospects, so clearly their genetic material must have some bearing on longevity. In general, big species live longer than small ones. However, some simple organisms — for example, hydra — do not appear to age at all and can regenerate themselves from tiny fragments. The key here is to do with the distinction between the germ line (i.e. those cells that are involved in reproduction) and the soma (i.e. those cells that have no capacity for reproduction). Inevitably very simple organisms are less differentiated than more complex ones and consequently appear immortal for the simple reason that the germ line is immortal. The soma is always a dead end and is simply a means of transporting the germ line.

Progeria syndromes provide further evidence of the genetic contribution to ageing although the effects of these disorders are not clearly the same as ageing in all organs. The fibroblasts of people with progeria have a limited capacity for division.

Evolutionary theories of ageing

It was once thought that ageing was an adaptive response to the threat of overcrowding and that it might be associated with accelerated evolutionary change and was essentially 'good' for the species. This is quite wrong. In the wild average life expectancies are very short compared with survival in a protected environment. Natural selection — the key evolutionary process — cannot therefore lead to the acquisition of ageing genes as none lives long enough in natural conditions. Furthermore, natural selection does not operate at a species level but at the level of individuals who survive with a greater chance of preserving their germ line.

Disposable soma theory

An organism has to achieve a balance between the energy it puts into reproduction and the energy it puts into maintenance. The degree of evolutionary fitness of a species is related to the energy investment in maintenance. If investment in maintenance is very high a species will effectively appear immortal — non-ageing — but this is at the expense of some evolutionary fitness (i.e. the responsiveness to change mediated via environmental hazards). If the investment in maintenance is very low, the species will age rapidly and have only a short lifespan, but this tends to be offset by a higher reproductive potential. There is likely to be an optimum

balance between maintenance and reproduction and this is struck by considering the degree of environmental hazard to which a species is exposed.

For example, birds are exposed to low risks of danger from other species and can therefore invest in maintenance of their bodies (soma). They have a relatively low reproductive rate and an associated long lifespan. On the other hand, species such as mice have a very high risk of hazard and must complete their reproduction as quickly as possible. They invest in very little maintenance and therefore have a short lifespan but a high reproductive rate. More primitive species such as hydra appear immortal because they can reproduce themselves from tiny fragments of themselves. They are relatively unfit in an evolutionary sense but have invested heavily in maintenance.

The disposable soma theory states that, for a given level of environmental hazard, the optimal level of maintenance is less than the minimum required for immortality or non-ageing. In other words, wear and tear are an inevitable part of being alive.

The costs of maintenance

The organism must spend energy on several activities:

1. intracellular DNA repair and protein turnover;
2. free-radical scavenging;
3. cell renewal; and
4. construction of non-renewing parts.

Random molecular damage occurs which leads to accumulation of defects which in turn leads to the age-related changes in organs and systems that we recognize as ageing.

The peak in evolutionary fitness related to investment in maintenance is broad and this leads to some latitude in where the optimum point actually occurs. This suggests that precise control of the balance between maintenance and reproduction is under polygenic control and the broadness of the balance point explains the innate variability of individuals as they age.

It is likely that there is a network of mechanisms under genetic control that all age at different rates but it is probable that the mechanisms that have the shortest life are those that determine the average lifespan of a species.

STARVATION AND LONGEVITY

Lean times are associated with longer survival. Some Americans routinely starve themselves in an attempt to live longer. With limited energy it is likely that any organism will put all available energy into maintenance. Cells will have to recycle proteins for re-use and this will require greater accuracy of repair enzymes and this in turn is the explanation for greater longevity.

THEORIES OF AGEING: SO WHAT?

Unravelling the mystery of why we age will inevitably preoccupy some scientists as an end in itself. Some of the theories are summarized in Table 1.3. The more exciting possibilities lie in understanding how to alter the expression of DNA, to reverse some of the adverse effects of ageing. At the individual level it may be possible to reduce the rate at which some organ systems decline by active interventions such as physical exercise. At the population level, the forecasting of changes in the future should allow us time to develop appropriate health and social policies. Such policies should allow us to alleviate some of the adverse consequences of an ageing population, and use some of the positive benefits of having large numbers of experienced senior citizens.

Table 1.3 Theories of ageing: a summary

Genetic–molecular theories
  Codon restriction: accuracy of DNA–mRNA impaired
  Error theories: accuracy of mRNA–proteins impaired
  Gene regulation: post-reproductive changes in gene expression
  Somatic mutation: radiation damage to DNA

Cellular theories
  Wear and tear: with use the body wears out and dies
  Age pigments: lipofuscin deposition as a primary cause of ageing
  Free-radicals: lead to cell damage and thus ageing
  Cross-linking: increased cross-linkage leading to irreversible damage to DNA and enzymes

Disposable soma theory

System level theories
  Neuro-endocrine control: a biological clock controls development through neural and hormonal mechanisms
  Immune control: thymus gland as an 'immunological clock', leading to cell destruction due to failure to recognize self

Key points

- Population ageing is the result of reductions in infant mortality and fertility, and reduction in mortality at older ages. These changes are consequences of successful societies with high levels of socio-economic development.
- Organ systems of individuals age at different rates, but all show declines starting in early adult life.
- Cross-sectional studies of the effects of ageing may hide changes associated with the cohort studied and the time period in which the study is conducted.
- Cellular ageing may be due to damage to DNA and cellular proteins which may be regulated genetically, bringing together the damage and genetic theories of ageing.

FURTHER READING

Clarke CA. Centenarians and the ultimate age attainable by man. *Nutrition Bulletin* 1984; **13**: 132–140.

Comfort A. *The Biology of Senescence*. 3rd edn. Elsevier, New York, 1979.

Coni N, Davison W, Webster S. *Ageing: The Facts*. Oxford University Press, Oxford, 1984.

Fries JF, Green LW, Levine S. Health promotion and the compression of morbidity. *Lancet* 1989; i: 481–483.

Strehler BL (ed.). *Advances in Gerontological Research*, vols 1 and 2. Academic Press, New York, 1964 and 1967.

Takata H, Suzuki M, Ishii T, Sekiguchi S, Iri H. Influence of major histocompatibility complex region genes on human longevity among Okinawan-Japanese centenarians and nonagenarians. *Lancet* 1987; ii: 824–826.

Timiras PS (ed.) *Physiological Basis of Aging and Geriatrics*. Macmillan, London, 1988.

2 AGEING SKIN

- Epidermis
- Dermis
- Ultraviolet light
- Transparent skin syndrome
- Senile purpura
- Hair
- Pruritus
- Growth factors
- Anti-ageing measures

The generally held view is that as skin ages it develops characteristic physiological signs (i.e. wrinkles, pigment alteration, thinning). It is now known that this is not normal ageing but pathological changes mainly due to ultraviolet light exposure. Obviously some conditions will occur from unavoidable environmental exposure, genetics and the effects of disease etc., but normal ageing produces surprisingly few skin changes. The exposure to sunlight, however, produces very deleterious effects with numerous pathological conditions including keratoses, squamous cell carcinoma, basal cell carcinoma and malignant melanoma. Less life-threatening effects include wrinkling and hyper- and hypopigmentation. Thus there is very little evidence that the skin 'ages' apart from the effects of genetics, environment and disease.

EPIDERMIS

The changes to the epidermis as a person gets older are minimal and subtle. The skin may become thinner,

especially where it has been exposed to sunlight, and oxygen consumption may be slightly decreased. Metabolic processes appear unchanged.

DERMIS

The changes in collagen are qualitative more than quantitative. There is some decrease in thickness, especially in light-exposed skin, but the main changes include increases in the cross-links on the collagen with some deterioration in fibre organization. The flexibility of the skin is due to the dermal collagen and there is minor deterioration with age. However, it is very marked in the pathological state known as the 'transparent skin syndrome' (Fig. 2.1). With respect to age and keratinocytes, it is clear that ageing skin epithelializes more slowly after injury and that the thinner epidermis (mainly due to UV light exposure) provides a diminished barrier function. There is an age-related reduction in the skin's immunosurveillance system:

keratinocytes, Langerhans cells, epidermotrophic lymphocytes, etc. In addition there is an age-related increased risk of photocarcinogenesis in habitually sun-exposed and photo-aged skin (see 'UV light', below). One must not forget, however, that wounds heal well in normal elderly people.

ULTRAVIOLET (UV) LIGHT

The dangerous components of UV light are the shorter wavelengths, the effects being initially erythema (sunburn), increased thickness of the stratum corneum and increased melanocytes (hence a sun tan). Repeated exposure, especially with 'burning', results in pathological effects including the skin cancers. This is important because advertising still tells us that 'brown is beautiful' and that sun tans are 'healthy'. The side-effects of accelerated skin ageing and the potential dangers are not mentioned as prominently.

Early pathological changes include yellowing and the formation of wrinkles (though excess wrinkles probably have a genetic component). A few people get depigmentation and obvious superficial 'broken' blood vessels — telangiectasia. The backs of the hands can develop keratotic nodules as well as the face. The skin around the eyes may show yellow plaques — Dubreuilh's elastoma. The thick, deeply lined 'crazy-paving' type skin on the back of sun-exposed necks has the wonderful name of cutis rhomboidalis nuchae of Jadassohn!

Other sun-induced changes include keratoacanthoma, basal cell carcinoma and squamous cell carcinoma. The most dangerous is the malignant melanoma which has now become so common in Australia that doctors have been doing 'rounds' on the beaches, examining people and giving advice.

Very little is known about skin changes and age in the black population.

TRANSPARENT SKIN SYNDROME

People with transparent skin syndrome have skin which looks and feels like tissue paper, especially on the backs of the hands and forearms (Fig 2.1). The skin is loose and wrinkled and the underlying structures are seen easily. This type of skin has very poor elastic (i.e. tensile) properties. Histologically there is a thin dermis.

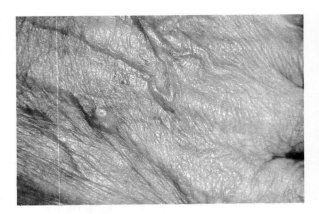

Figure 2.1 Transparent skin syndrome

This is probably a pathological condition and not an ageing process. Interestingly it is associated with osteoporosis and hence collagen abnormalities may be implicated. The skin 'tears' easily and is difficult to suture. It skin also bleeds and bruises easily. A similar finding is found in patients who have taken steroids ('steroid atrophy') and in patients with rheumatoid arthritis. The condition could possibly be related to other 'lax-skin' conditions which are increasingly being diagnosed in non-pure forms. Transparent skin may also have white pseudoscars (thought to be due to episodes of minor trauma) and has an increased tendency to senile purpura.

SENILE PURPURA

Many elderly people develop bruising, especially over the hands and arms, without having the full-blown transparent skin syndrome. It is presumed that they still have less elastic collagen and hence blood vessels are less well tethered and are more easily ruptured by minor trauma. The purpura stays longer because reabsorption is much slower. Other vascular changes include the appearance of a few spider naevi and an occasional splinter haemorrhage under the fingernails (traumatic in origin). The most common skin lesion noted is the small red Campbell de Morgan spot, a benign lesion seen most often on the trunk and abdomen.

HAIR

Grey hair is genetically determined (autosomal dominant) and is far less traumatic than the loss of hair (again genetically determined in men). Both men and women lose their hair with age, men simply lose it sooner, faster and more comprehensively! Male vanity and the media have determined that enormous sums are being spent to stop and reverse this most benign of ageing processes.

PRURITUS

This is so common in the elderly that the term 'senile pruritus' is well known. However, it is again pathology rather than normal ageing that is more important in the aetiology, diagnosis and treatment (Table 2.1).

Table 2.1 Common causes of pruritus in the elderly

Drugs
Blood disorders (e.g. polycythaemia rubra vera, anaemia)
Malignant disease (e.g. lymphomas)
Liver and kidney disease (esp. with jaundice and uraemia)
Dryness (exacerbated by washing, detergent residues in clothes, temperature)
Infestations (scabies, lice)
Skin disorders (eczema, lichen planus, pre-pemphigoid)
Incontinence (the effects of urine and faeces)

GROWTH FACTORS

Growth factors are peptides with mainly stimulating effects on cell proliferation. They are named after the target cell or source that led to their discovery (e.g. epidermal growth factor, EGF). Within this rapidly expanding field there are some areas of special interest. Donor age seems to influence the proliferative capacity and lifespan of cells in culture, and there is a diminished *in vitro* response and impaired growth factor processing by cells with increasing age. Age appears to influence growth factor production by cells.

The physical changes in skin associated with ageing (thinner epidermis, altered dermis with reduced amounts of extracellular matrix proteins, collagen and elastin) may have significance with growth factors. It has been suggested that there may be possible interaction and stabilization of growth factors in the extracellular matrix. The matrix may even protect growth factors from degradation or provide long-term storage.

ANTI-AGEING MEASURES

Because the superficial effects of 'ageing' are so visible it is not surprising — in a youth-obsessed culture — that a whole industry has developed to keep people looking younger. More could be achieved simply by avoiding sunlight. Most creams are useless apart from their camouflage effect. However isotretinoin (used to treat severe acne) does cause 'peeling' in normal skin, erasing the finest of the wrinkles. More dramatic is the use of plastic surgery, and 'face-lifts' are becoming increasingly popular. People should be warned, however, that repeat procedures may lead to the umbilicus becoming an unusual beauty-spot on the chin! Many manufacturers of facial skin creams and suntan lotions are now including anti-UVA (photo ageing) sun blocks. The economic if not health message is getting across.

There is increasing evidence that free radical damage is part of the ageing process (see Chapter 1, damage theories). The role of antioxidants including vitamins C and E, selenium and beta-carotene remain speculative.

Key points

- Normal physiological ageing produces few skin changes.
- Growth factors are peptides that stimulate cell proliferation.
- The pathological effects of ultraviolet light produce wrinkles, thin/transparent skin, pigmentation changes and benign and malignant tumours.
- Senile purpura is common and is due to poor blood vessel tethering.
- Grey hair and hair loss are genetically determined and occur to some degree in both sexes.
- To avoid 'ageing' changes and cosmetic surgeons — do not sunbathe!

FURTHER READING

Dalziel KL, Bickers DR. Skin aging. In: Brocklehurst JC, Tallis RC, Fillit HM (eds), *Textbook of Geriatric Medicine and Gerontology*, 4th edn. Churchill Livingstone, Edinburgh, 1992.

Fenske NA, Lober CW. Structural and functional changes of normal ageing skin. *J Am Acad Dermatol*; 1986; **15**: 571–585.

West MD. The cellular and molecular biology of skin ageing. *Arch Dermatol* 1994; **130**(1): 87–95.

3 THE AGEING EYE

- Anterior chamber
- Presbyopia
- Cataract
- Other ageing effects
- Acute and chronic visual loss
- Diabetic retinopathy

Apart from being the windows to the soul, the eyes of elderly people are interesting both in health and in disease. The transition from physiological (i.e. age-related) to pathological (i.e. disease-related) change can be indistinct. Most of the 'ageing' changes reported are in fact pathological. Characteristically the eyes are sunken due to loss of periorbital fat, which may be severe enough to cause ptosis (drooping of the upper lid) and redundant skin at the lateral borders. This loss of fat can cause the lower eyelid to curl in (entropion) and irritate the cornea, causing redness and watering (epiphora). A simple stop-gap measure is to apply tape just below the eyelid and pull it down slightly using the adhesive effect of the tape on the cheek. This will suffice until an expert opinion can be sought and a minor surgical procedure performed if necessary. This laxity also enables the eyelid to fall outwards slightly (ectropion), again this can lead to epiphora and subsequent inflammation and conjunctivitis.

A whitish circle around the iris (arcus senilis or gerontoxon) is seen commonly in some elderly people but as it is a lipid infiltrate in the periphery of the cornea it is probably not a true ageing process. It is initially comma-like at the top and bottom but eventually extends around until a dense white border results. A full arcus in a comparatively young person may indicate a lipid abnormality and premature ischaemic heart disease.

ANTERIOR CHAMBER

Numerous factors contribute to the anterior chamber of the eye becoming more shallow as we age. The lens especially becomes thicker and the size and shape of the eyeball change. This can be clinically significant in the condition angle-closure glaucoma (Fig. 3.1). In this state the iris blocks the fluid-filtering mechanism and the intraocular pressure rises acutely (far in excess of the normal upper limit of 21 mmHg), usually causing severe pain, vomiting and blurred vision. The condition can present, however, as an acute confusional state or even an 'acute abdomen' (due to vomiting and collapse). Urgent diagnosis and referral to a specialist is required, where treatment may be medical (the use of drugs, e.g. pilocarpine) or surgical.

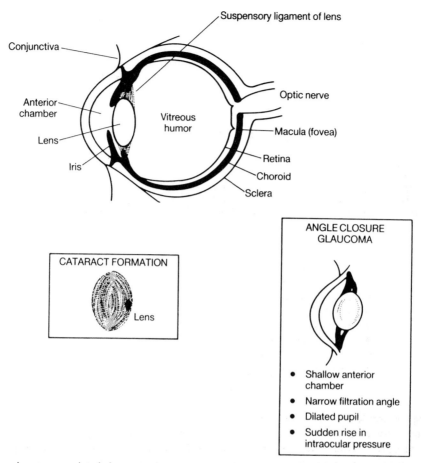

Figure 3.1 The eye and some age-related changes

In open–angle glaucoma there is a much slower rise in the intraocular pressure (secondary to abnormal drainage of aqueous humour). Vision is gradually lost, 'tunnel vision' results and help may only be sought when this too is compromised. Routine examination may pick up pathological cupping of the optic disc, abnormal field defects or raised intraocular pressures. Treatment is again either medical or surgical. This condition is familial and close relatives (including children) should be screened.

Pupillary diameter decreases with advancing age and the iris becomes more fibrous. There is thus a reduced response to accommodation and reduced light access. This means that because of slower dark adaptation additional illuminating light is needed and it has been estimated that the eye needs to double the illumination approximately every 13 years to maintain recognition in subdued light. Typical room lighting is around 150–200W, whereas for optimal vision, elderly people require around 400W.

PRESBYOPIA

The crystalline lens (Fig. 3.1) is unique in that as we age new lens fibres are laid down over the old (like layers of an onion skin). Not only does this result in the lens getting bigger but it also becomes more dense and rigid. Focusing is achieved by relaxation of the suspensory ligament by the action of the ciliary muscle. This increased rigidity, however, means that the lens can no longer alter its shape sufficiently to become convex enough to allow adequate focusing. The power of the lens also reduces with age so that clarity for near objects is only achieved by increasing the focal length, i.e. holding the object further away. Eventually one's arms are no longer long enough and corrective lenses are needed! This loss of power for accommodation of near vision is known as presbyopia.

CATARACT

The increase in the layers around the lens is progressive and eventually causes central compression, the middle becoming hard (nuclear sclerosis) and increasingly opaque. This phenomenon appears to be universal, making cataract formation a true ageing rather than pathological event. The posterior pole of the lens is a common site for this initial sclerosis and here it acts as a visual plug and, with the added problem of the smaller pupil, can cause an incapacitating loss of vision. Peripheral (cartwheel) cataracts may be initially less disabling but eventually cause light dispersal and can make vision impossible in bright light. Hence a lot of elderly people with these early cataracts wear peaked caps or shade bright lights to decrease this effect.

The metabolic changes within the lens are receiving considerable attention as possible markers of disease and also as preventive pathways. There is a general reduction in metabolic activity with age but in cataract sufferers there is also a marked decrease in the tripeptide glutathione (present in high concentrations in the normal lens). Soluble proteins are reduced and may have been changed into insoluble complexes or leaked out. Diabetics are extremely prone to cataract formation and in this condition the lens concentration and metabolism of sorbitol is markedly abnormal.

Much can be done to help in the management of the cataract-affected elderly person. It is preferable to arrange reading lights so that they shine over the shoulder on to the page, thus ensuring the pupils are somewhat shaded and hence more dilated. Myopia should be corrected and pressures checked which will permit the pupils to be dilated (by drugs) to get light around a central or polar opacity. The increased risk of retinal detachment and glaucoma means that unilateral or second eye cataracts are not usually removed. Cataracts are removed surgically when poor vision interferes with normal activities. The operation can be done under local anaesthetic in selected cases. Post-operative contact lenses are not too successful in the more frail patient and spectacles with corrective lenses are more commonly used. Unfortunately the corrective aphakic lenses produce spherical aberrations which cause

straight lines (such as the edges of a doorway) to appear curved. They also produce the 'jack-in-the-box' effect whereby on walking through doorways or confined spaces the edges suddenly disappear only to suddenly reappear in a startling effect. Increasingly, lens implantation at the time of surgery is used with benefit.

OTHER AGEING EFFECTS

Vitreous opacities (floaters) result from degeneration of the vitreous body. They are common and unimportant but a sudden 'shower' may herald a retinal detachment. Common fundal changes include drusen (pale patches) and senile macular degeneration (dark mottled appearance around the macula). Macular degeneration is accompanied by decreased visual acuity, the only help being lenses with increased magnification. The use of bifocal spectacles to correct lens abnormalities is becoming increasingly popular. One hidden danger, especially in the elderly, is that depth perception is altered and falls can result, especially on coming down stairs.

ACUTE AND CHRONIC VISUAL LOSS

Visual loss is a comparatively common symptom in elderly people. It can be conveniently subdivided into acute and chronic onset with corresponding causes (Table 3.1).

Table 3.1 Causes of loss of vision

Acute Onset
Retinal detachment
Vascular causes (central retinal artery/vein thrombosis)
Angle-closure glaucoma
Temporal arteritis
Chronic Onset
Cataract
Macular degeneration
Open-angle glaucoma
Diabetic retinopathy

Acute onset causes include retinal detachment (due to the formation of a retinal hole and accompanied by flashes of light prior to loss of vision) and vascular conditions. Temporary loss of vision (amaurosis fugax) is usually secondary to platelet emboli. Total loss of vision is due to central retinal artery occlusion and is usually permanent. The cause of amaurosis fugux (i.e. the origin of the emboli) should be sought and treated. Temporal (cranial) arteritis can cause sudden loss of vision in one eye. A typical history and elevated ESR plus a characteristic biopsy confirm the diagnosis; however, steroids should be given on presentation to prevent blindness in the other eye. Retinal vein occlusion is more common and clinical presentation is dependent on the nearness to the macula.

Chronic-onset loss of vision is most commonly caused by macular degeneration. In the 'atrophic' form there is a degenerative change affecting the photoreceptors. For most patients there is no treatment apart from the magnifying aids. In the 'exudative' form hyaline deposits (drusen) occur near Bruch's membrane, possibly causing adhesions, impaired blood supply with subretinal haemorrhage and loss of vision. In this form laser therapy may be helpful.

- Acute angle-closure glaucoma requires urgent medical attention.
- Open-angle glaucoma causes gradual visual loss and is familial.
- The crystalline nature of the lens causes it to become dense and rigid, affecting focusing.
- Central lens compression leads to opaqueness and hence cataract formation.
- Macular degeneration is accompanied by decreased visual acuity which can be helped by magnifying lenses.
- Visual loss may be of acute or chronic onset.
- Acute causes of visual loss include retinal detachment, central retinal artery thrombosis, temporal arteritis and acute-angle closure glaucoma.
- Chronic onset causes of visual loss include cataract, macular degeneration, open-angle glaucoma and diabetic retinopathy.

DIABETIC RETINOPATHY

Diabetic retinopathy occurs both in patients with type I diabetes and in those with type II diabetes. The retinal capillary circulation is affected, with leakage, oedema and exudates. The retina responds with a neovascular proliferation and these new vessels in turn can leak and haemorrhage. Treatment of this proliferative retinopathy includes laser photocoagulation.

Key points

- Altered fat distribution in the eyes can result in ptosis, entropion and ectropion.

FURTHER READING

Brodie SE. Aging and disorders of the eye. In: Brocklehurst JC, Tallis RC, Fillit HM (eds), *Textbook of Geriatric Medicine and Gerontology*, 4th edn. Churchill Livingstone, Edinburgh, 1992.

Graham P. The eye. In: Pathy MSJ (ed.), *Principles and Practice of Geriatric Medicine*. John Wiley & Sons, Chichester, 1985.

Nuzzi R, Schiavino R. Geriatric ophthalmology. *Panminerva Medica* 1993; **35**(1): 36–46.

Weale RA. *The Ageing Eye*. HK Lewis, London, 1963.

4 THE AGEING EAR

- Presbycusis
- Other changes
- Audiograms
- Hearing aids
- Communication with hearing-impaired people

Hearing impairment is extremely common in old age, with over half of those over 75 years old having some hearing problem. The commonest cause of hearing loss with age (presbycusis) is due to an age-related decline in the ability to perceive high tones, above 2000 Hz. Speech frequencies are in the range of 500–6000 Hz, with consonants tending to have higher frequencies than vowel sounds. Since much of the sense of speech is embodied in the consonants, high tone loss has a disproportionate effect on the ability to understand normal speech.

PRESBYCUSIS

Presbycusis is a sensori-neural form of deafness, meaning that it is caused by degeneration of the cochlea and its neurones, as opposed to conductive deafness which is due to problems with the middle or external ear (Fig. 4.1). Although the underlying reasons for presbycusis are not clear, it is known that the process is progressive, bilateral and starts from about the age of 40. It is likely that genetic factors are involved. Black men are less likely to suffer than white men, even if they have had heavy exposure to industrial noise.

OTHER CHANGES

The external ear is a frequent cause of problems due to ageing. The skin of the meatus contains sebaceous and cerumen glands, which secrete wax. With age, the number and activity of these glands decline leading to a reduction in skin moisture, and a tendency to produce dry, impacted ear wax. These changes may also lead to itchiness in the ear, another common complaint, which can be aggravated by attempts to relieve the itch with hairpins or cotton-wool buds, leading to an itch–scratch–itch cycle.

In the middle ear, the conduction of sound from the ear drum to the cochlea occurs through an intricate arrangement of three bones: the malleus, incus and stapes. With age, changes occur in the articular cartilage of these bones similar to those seen in larger arthritic joints (calcification in the joint capsule, reduction in the joint space, fraying of the joint cartilage). However, these changes do not seem to contribute to any conductive hearing loss.

In addition to presbycusis, the inner ear is affected by many disease processes that are commoner with age (vascular insufficiency, autoimmune diseases, neoplasms,

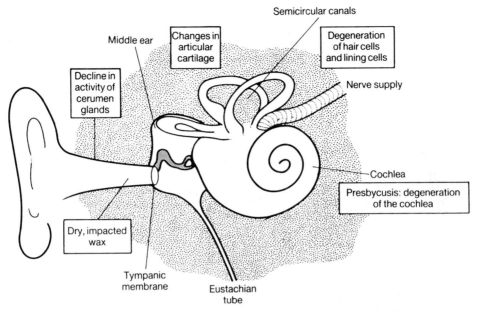

Figure 4.1 The ear and some age-related changes

Ménière's disease and drug-induced damage). The inner ear also serves in the control of balance, through the semicircular canals (the labyrinth). Tinnitus is a noise that occurs within the hearing system, and its effects range from mild to extremely disruptive. It occurs more frequently in older people, can be independent of hearing loss and its cause is usually elusive. Treatment (from masking devices to antidepressants) is usually unsuccessful. Like the cochlea, the labyrinth also suffers an age-related degeneration of its lining cells, its sensitive hair cells, and nerve fibres. While dizziness is a common symptom, it is seldom due to disease or ageing of the inner ear. Vertigo, the sensation of rotation, may be caused by many disease processes, but a condition called benign paroxysmal positional vertigo (in other words, vertigo occurring from time to time, and precipitated by the position of the head) may be caused by age-related degeneration of the labyrinth.

AUDIOGRAMS

The volume of noise is measured in decibels (dB). Speech ranges from less than 25 dB (a whisper), through 40–60 dB (normal speech), to 80+ dB (shouting).

A pure-tone audiogram presents sounds at a succession of given frequencies (250 Hz through to 8000 Hz).

For each frequency, sounds are made progressively louder until they are registered by the subject. Loss of up to 20 dB is considered within the normal range. Loss of hearing begins to become apparent when 30–40 dB are lost (Fig. 4.2).

In addition to measuring the response to pure tones, patients are asked to discriminate single syllable words at normal volumes and the effects of amplification are measured. Those who do better with amplification will usually benefit from a hearing aid.

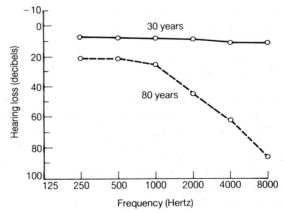

Figure 4.2 Presbycusis as demonstrated by two typical audiograms

HEARING AIDS

It is important that the patient with hearing loss is a full partner in discussing management. If the patient has unrealistic expectations of what a hearing aid will offer, disappointment will be inevitable, and the aid will not be used. For each patient — and their family — time will be required for counselling and review.

A hearing aid basically amplifies sound, but as technology improves, aids are becoming smaller and more specific for speech frequencies. Some also have noise-suppression units to aid speech discrimination in noisy environments. It is worth becoming familiar with the types of aid, their controls, and with simple maintenance: cleaning, changing batteries and reassembling (Fig. 4.3).

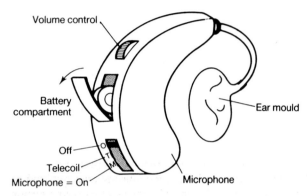

Figure 4.3 Behind-the-ear hearing aid

Trouble-shooting

1. Hearing aid batteries do not last long — about a week if used for most of the day.
2. Setting the volume too high results in a high-pitched whistle.
3. The switch settings are not intuitively obvious: 'O' means 'off' and not 'on'.
4. 'T' stands for 'telecoil' which can be used in cinemas, theatres and many other public places displaying the hard of hearing sign.
5. A paper clip can be used to extract wax blocking the mould.

COMMUNICATION WITH HEARING-IMPAIRED PEOPLE

Shouting does not help, and may reduce the ability of a deaf person to understand. However, increasing the volume of speech a little is useful, and widely practised. The other keys to better communication are shown in Table 4.1.

Table 4.1 Better communication with hearing-impaired people

1. Get the attention of the person
2. Ensure you face the person at the same level
3. Sit in a good light
4. Avoid eating or touching your mouth while speaking
5. Speak towards the better ear at a distance of up to 1 metre
6. Reduce background noise to the minimum
7. Speak slowly and clearly
8. If the person has an aid, switch it on
9. If the person does not have an aid, speak loudly or use a portable amplifier or speaking tube
10. Write important information down for the person to read

Hearing impairment has powerful psycho-social effects. It is a potent risk factor for depressive illness and also leads to withdrawal from social occasions. Early recognition and treatment of hearing problems is essential to reduce these all too common consequences.

Key points

- Loss of hearing in older people is most often due to presbycusis, a degeneration of the cochlea.
- Speech ranges from 25 dB (a whisper) to 80+ dB (shouting). Loss of hearing is apparent when 30–40 dB are lost.
- Provision of a hearing aid (which is simply an amplifier) requires careful counselling and review.
- Communication is aided by raising your voice (but not shouting), obtaining attention, sitting face to face, reducing background noise, and speaking slowly and clearly.
- Hearing impairment has powerful psycho-social effects, leading to isolation and depression, particularly if left untreated.

FURTHER READING

Fisch L, Brooks DN. Disorders of hearing. In: Brocklehurst JC, Tallis RC, Fillit HM (eds), *Textbook of Geriatric Medicine and Gerontology*, 4th edn. Churchill Livingstone, Edinburgh, 1992, pp. 480–493.

Han SS, Coons DH (eds). *Special Senses in Ageing*. Institute of Gerontology, University of Michigan, Ann Arbor, 1979.

Hinchcliffe R. *Hearing and Balance in the Elderly*. Churchill Livingstone, Edinburgh, 1983.

5 THE AGEING KIDNEY

- Age changes
- Impaired homeostasis
- Abnormalities of urea and electrolytes
- Problems with drugs

The kidney consists of millions of nephrons, divided into the glomerulus (a filter with pores too small to let through simple proteins like albumen), the proximal tubule, the loop of Henle and the distal tubule (Fig. 5.1). The tubules and loop are responsible for the control of salt, water and acid–base balance. The proximal tubule carries out most of the active reabsorption and excretion processes that are energy and enzyme dependent. The loop of Henle and distal tubule produce the countercurrent multiplier effect that leads to urine concentration, regulated by the effects of antidiuretic hormone (ADH) and aldosterone.

AGE CHANGES

With increasing age renal size and function decline. The kidney in adult life weighs about 400 g, but by the age of 90 it has shrunk to less than 300 g. Even more dramatic is the fall in the number of nephrons, half of which are lost between the ages of 40 and 70 years. The rate at which the glomeruli filter fluid — the glomerular filtration rate — also falls from 140 ml/min/ 1.73 m² in mid-adult life by 8 ml/min/1.73 m² for each decade. This rate of reduction in glomerular filtration is accelerated in people with high blood pressure.

However, simply losing nephrons does not lead to any problems, as is shown by the fact that young people are capable of surviving perfectly well with only a single kidney. Indeed, a lone young kidney will hypertrophy as a compensatory change, although this does not occur in old age.

Renal blood flow also falls disproportionately to the reduction in renal size (from approx. 600 ml/min in an adult to approx. 300 ml/min at age 80, a 10 per cent decrease per decade), and is most marked in the renal cortex. The glomerular basement membrane also changes, becoming more permeable, and more likely to let proteins through. In some glomeruli degenerative changes occur, leading to sclerosis. These changes contribute to the reduction in surface area available for filtration, and explain the reduced glomerular filtration rate.

IMPAIRED HOMEOSTASIS

The renal changes are of no great significance in themselves, but they dramatically alter the ability of the body to compensate for external changes — to maintain

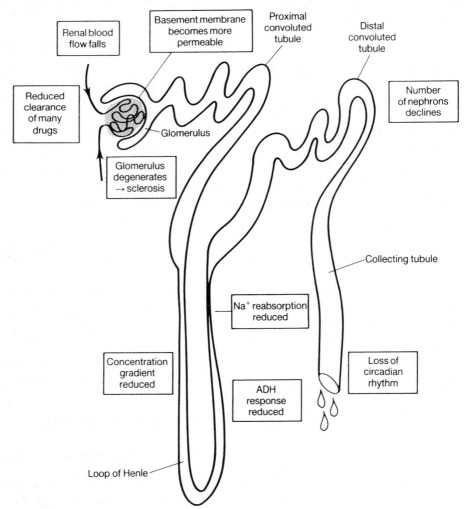

Figure 5.1 A nephron and some age-related changes

homeostasis. For example, if salt is removed from the diet, the kidney will compensate by removing as much sodium as possible from the urine to achieve sodium balance. In young people this takes place twice as fast as it does in older people. The problem for older people is probably in the ascending limb of the loop of Henle where the ability to reabsorb sodium is greatly reduced. This in turn reduces the efficiency of the countercurrent multiplier system that concentrates urine, leading to a less efficient response to water depletion.

When faced with lack of water elderly people tend to produce more urine and less concentrated urine than younger people. It is probable that elderly people, like patients with chronic renal failure, have to produce a finite volume of urine to ensure that the reduced number of nephrons are capable of dealing with the solute load. The renal blood flow to the medulla of the kidney is well preserved with age, whereas cortical supply falls. It is possible that this relatively greater medullary flow washes away the normal concentration gradient.

The release of antidiuretic hormone (ADH) is affected by ageing. If hypertonic saline is infused into a healthy elderly person, the expected increase in plasma ADH which normally leads to conservation of water is exaggerated. However, the effects of dehydration and moving from lying to standing, which also provoke an ADH response, are blunted in many elderly people. Recent studies have demonstrated a loss of the circadian rhythms of urine excretion in elderly people, which may explain the need to get up at night to urinate.

ABNORMALITIES OF UREA AND ELECTROLYTES

It is common for 'routine' blood chemistry results to be reported as abnormal. It is as well to remember that the laboratory 'normal range' is usually based on data from young adults. It is also a statistical normal range; in other words, 95 per cent of normal subjects will lie within the upper and lower limits. This means that 5 per cent of normal subjects will be outside the normal range.

Blood urea concentrations are often raised, particularly among hospital inpatients. This is usually due to dehydration, or diuretic therapy, or both. The serum creatinine is usually normal, because muscle mass falls with increasing age.

Low plasma sodium concentrations (hyponatraemia) are often a source of worry. Up to a quarter of all elderly patients admitted to hospital are hyponatraemic. The mechanisms to consider are the decreased ability to excrete water, water intoxication with concurrent diuretic therapy, and increased (inappropriate) ADH secretion. It is essential to measure the plasma osmolality to decide whether the patient is truly short of sodium, and therefore hypo-osmolar. If the patient has high levels of plasma lipids or proteins, a pseudo-hyponatraemia may result. It is necessary to decide next whether the patient is volume-depleted, volume-expanded or about normal. Volume depletion is common in patients on too aggressive diuretic therapy. Volume expansion occurs typically in congestive cardiac failure.

High plasma sodium concentrations occur because of loss of body water (at a greater rate than loss of sodium), inadequate water intake or increased sodium intake. In elderly people, thirst may not be recognized, leading to severe dehydration and hypernatraemia. This is very common amongst demented institutionalized patients.

PROBLEMS WITH DRUGS

Many drugs are excreted by the kidney, of which digoxin is the best example. Reduced renal clearance of such drugs means that doses have to be reduced to avoid toxicity. Diuretics are amongst the most commonly prescribed medications for elderly people, but given the precarious state of the ageing kidney, they are often the cause of admissions to hospital with iatrogenic severe dehydration and electrolyte imbalance. Tetracyclines should also be avoided in old people as they have a catabolic effect which raises blood urea, and they may be nephrotoxic.

| Key points |

- Renal function declines with age. Approximately half the nephrons are lost between the ages of 30 and 70 years.
- Reduction in renal function leads to impaired homeostasis, making older people much more vulnerable to the effects of dehydration and water overload.
- Circadian rhythms of water excretion are lost, leading to nocturia.
- Many drugs are excreted by the kidney and usual adult doses may lead to drug toxicity.

FURTHER READING

Fillit H, Rove J, The aging kidney. In: Brocklehurst JC, Tallis RC, Fillit HM (eds), *Textbook of Geriatric Medicine and Gerontology*, 4th edn. Churchill Livingstone, Edinburgh, 1992, pp. 612–628.

Kirkland JL, Lye M, Levy DW, Banerjee AK. Patterns of urine flow and electrolyte excretion in healthy elderly people. *Br Med J* 1983; **287**: 1665–1667.

Lindman RD, Tobin J, Chock NW. Longitudinal studies on the rate of decline in renal function with age. *J Am Geriatr Soc* 1985; **33**: 278-285.

Phillips TL, Rolls RJ, Ledingham JGG *et al*. Reduced thirst after water deprivation in healthy elderly men. *N Engl J Med* 1984; **311**: 753–759.

6 AGEING BONE, MUSCLES AND JOINTS

- The endosteal envelope phenomenon
- Bone collagen
- Osteoporosis
- Vitamin D
- Osteomalacia
- Muscles and joints
- Thresholds for independent life

Bone comes in two forms: cortical and trabecular (or cancellous). The cortical bone forms the dense outer shell of the long bones and the trabecular bone is the network of thin sheets of bone between the cortical shell.

Bone is composed of living cells and a bone matrix, principally collagen, upon which bone salts are deposited. Throughout life, even after cessation of longitudinal growth, cancellous and cortical bone are constantly being replaced. Changes in the balance between formation and resorption underlie disease affecting the adult skeleton. In both sexes, the amount of bone in the body increases until the fourth decade, and then starts to decline. The quantity of bone present at maturity depends upon sex, race, height, body build, posture, exercise and the supply of calcium, protein and vitamin D during growth and development.

THE ENDOSTEAL ENVELOPE PHENOMENON

Bony material lies outside the bone cells and remodelling takes place from the surfaces upon which the cells active in remodelling reside. Three surfaces or envelopes have been defined: the periosteal which lines the outside of all bones, the endosteal which lines the marrow cavities and covers the trabeculae of cancellous bone, and the intracortical or Haversian which lines the Haversian canals. In the normal adult, most bones are inactive.

Remodelling is a local phenomenon and proceeds in a uniform sequence (Fig. 6.1). First, a localized area of the mesenchyme is activated and osteoclasts are formed which resorb or remove the adjacent bone surface. After about a month the osteoclasts disappear and are replaced by osteoblasts formed from mesenchymal precursors. Osteoblasts deposit new bone on the previously resorbed surface until finally a resting stage is established. Remodelling units are activated by parathormone (PTH). The time required to complete the sequence is estimated to be from 3 to 4 months.

The periosteal surface is predominantly a bone-forming surface, so the external diameters of bones increase with age. The endosteal surface is predominantly a resorbing surface, so the marrow cavity also enlarges with age.

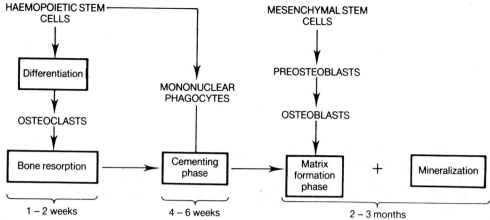

Figure 6.1 Bone remodelling

BONE COLLAGEN

The function of collagen is mainly mechanical. Throughout the body, collagen fibres are stabilized by a system of covalent interchain cross-links. Both intramolecular and intermolecular cross-links increase with age. The proportions of both soluble collagen in human bone and dihydroxylysinonorleucine (DiOH-LNL) decrease markedly with age. It is not known whether the increasing cross-linkages which strengthen the bone are eventually deleterious, nor whether the change in solubility of collagen affects bone loss. Changes in the cross-linkages are responsible for the type of fractures: few cross-linkages are associated with greenstick fractures seen in children.

OSTEOPOROSIS

There are two groups of old people with the clinical syndrome of osteoporosis — too little bone of normal composition. First, there are those who, having a small bone mass in adult life, have gradually lost sufficient with advancing years to develop clinical osteoporosis. The second group are those with a precipitating cause such as hyperthyroidism, neoplastic disease, scurvy, malabsorption (e.g. following partial gastrectomy), or spontaneous or iatrogenic Cushing's syndrome.

Approximately 90 per cent of bone is fibrous collagen protein, the remainder being mainly calcium and phosphorus. A loss of 30–50 per cent of bone must occur (by excessive resorption over formation) in order to produce osteoporosis. This means an average loss in the skeleton of 50 mg calcium per day for 20–30 years. No significant changes occur in bone composition with increasing age.

Prolonged immobilization can cause bone loss at any age. Significant bone loss has been demonstrated in a hemiplegic limb as soon as nine weeks after the onset of disability but this is not found in the presence of active motion of the limb.

Osteoporosis classically presents at the time of fracture, either of a vertebral body or of a long bone. A collapse fracture of a vertebral body may present with sudden onset of knife-like back pain, often encircling the girdle. The pain itself is self-limiting and usually lasts about six weeks. Assessment of osteoporosis in the vertebral column is difficult. Radiographs of the spine can be misleading, but points to look for are anterior wedging of the vertebrae and accentuation of the vertical trabeculation of the vertebral body. There is a close correlation between osteoporosis and backache but not between backache and X-ray findings. Chronic bone pain almost certainly indicates some other disorder.

Mobilization remains the mainstay of treatment and prevention. The effects of immobilization and the benefit of exercise were dramatically demonstrated in astronauts. In the early flights significant loss of calcium from bone was demonstrated during a four-day flight. The bone loss was regained by 47 days after the flight. Institution of an exercise regime for later flights prevented such loss. Precipitating causes must be identified and if possible treated. More aggressive approaches include the use of hormone replacement therapy, cyclical biphosphonates, calcium and human growth hormone as well as preventative regimes of exercise.

VITAMIN D

Vitamin D is the name given to a group of fat-soluble secosteroids which act by attaching themselves to macromolecules and thus alter their structure. Vitamin D is found in fish oils, margarine and, in small amounts, in eggs and milk. Dietary vitamin D is absorbed from the small intestine, mostly in the form of vitamin D_2 in the presence of bile salts which are needed for the formation of micelles. There is an enterohepatic circulation, vitamin D being secreted in the bile as glucuronides and reabsorbed through the intestinal mucosa. The main source of vitamin D is the conversion in the skin of 7-dehydrocholesterol into vitamin D_3 by the action of ultraviolet light. Some authorities consider that only at times of lack of exposure to sunlight is dietary vitamin D_2 required.

25-Hydroxylation occurs on the endoplasmic reticulum of the liver cells, converting vitamin D_3 to 25-hydroxycholecalciferol (25-OH-D_3) under the influence of the enzyme vitamin D_3 25-hydroxylase. 25-Hydroxy vitamin D_3 then undergoes 1-hydroxylation in the mitochondria of the renal tubular cells. The compound thus formed is 1,25-dihydroxycholecalciferol (1,25-OH$_2$-D_3). 1,25-Dihydroxy vitamin D_3 increases intestinal absorption of calcium and also acts at the renal tubular level to enable reabsorption of calcium from the tubular lumen.

Hypocalcaemia is recognized by the parathyroid glands which in response secrete parathormone. In the kidney parathormone facilitates the reabsorption of calcium and stimulates the release of 1,25-dihydroxy vitamin D_3 which acts alone to increase calcium absorption from the small intestine and together with parathormone to mobilize calcium from bone, thus causing a rise in serum calcium. When serum calcium has reached its normal level the stimulus to parathormone secretion is cut off and the process is stopped. In hypercalcaemia, the processes are reversed. Calcitonin is secreted from parafollicular C cells in the thyroid gland in response to a raised serum calcium and restores the level to normal. Calcitonin produces its effect by an action on the bone cells, osteoclasts, osteocytes and osteoblasts.

These actions of vitamin D are shown diagrammatically in Fig. 6.2.

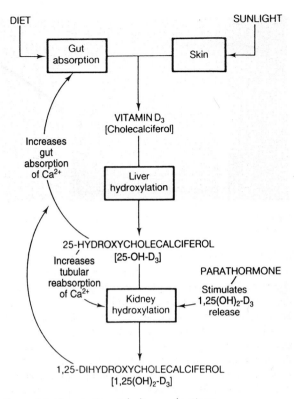

Figure 6.2 Vitamin D metabolism and actions

OSTEOMALACIA

Lack of vitamin D in elderly people is responsible for the clinical syndrome of osteomalacia. Symptoms include recurrent fractures, difficulty in walking (especially climbing stairs) and a constant low back pain.

Signs are generalized bone tenderness and a waddling gait, associated with proximal myopathy. The presence of Looser's zones (pseudo-fractures) on X-ray over the lateral border of the scapula, first rib, greater trochanter or pubic rami is pathognomonic. Figure 6.3 shows a Looser's zone in the right inferior pubic ramus. Serum biochemistry may be normal or show a low or normal calcium, a low phosphorus and raised alkaline phosphatase. Iliac crest bone biopsy demonstrates widening of the osteoid seams.

The incidence has been put as high as 4 per cent of admissions to geriatric units. Some evidence of osteomalacia has been found in 20–30 per cent of women and in about 40 per cent of men with fractures of the proximal femur. Elderly people tend to expose only their hands and faces to sunlight and the presence of

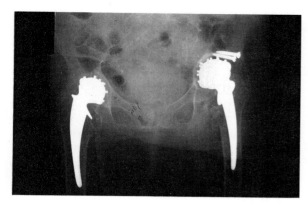

Figure 6.3 Looser's zone in right pubic ramus arising from osteomalacia

cataracts may necessitate the wearing of a wide-brimmed hat, thus reducing sunlight exposure to the face. Atmospheric pollution also cuts down ultraviolet irradiation. The housebound elderly are particularly at risk since window glass absorbs ultraviolet irradiation. A vicious circle is set up with lack of exposure to the sun causing deficient vitamin D production, development of back pain and the myopathic gait which makes getting out of chairs and climbing stairs increasingly difficult. Osteomalacia should be suspected in all housebound people.

In addition, elderly people have reduced vitamin D intake. Vitamin D is fat-soluble and needs bile salts for its absorption. Chronic liver disease can lead to bone disease because of a defect in 25-hydroxylation or interference with the entero-hepatic circulation. Any cause of malabsorption in the elderly may lead to the development of osteomalacia because of the entero-hepatic circulation of vitamin D and its fat solubility.

The renal tubule is the site of the 1-hydroxylation and this is the explanation for the early occurrence of bone disease in disorders affecting the renal tubule rather than the glomerulus. It has been suggested that mitochondrial enzyme induction in the liver might be the reason why epileptic patients on therapy with anticonvulsant drugs develop osteomalacia, cholecalciferol being metabolized to inactive metabolites. Patients with epilepsy who remain on anticonvulsant treatment despite symptoms of osteomalacia have been treated with vitamin D in doses of 4000 units per day.

Prevention and treatment

Exposure to ultraviolet light encourages vitamin D formation. Supplementation of dietary intake by switching from butter to margarine which is fortified is sensible. Treatment with vitamin D is necessary in the frank case of osteomalacia, and in people with neither renal impairment nor malabsorption there are no benefits in using the expensive 'one-alpha' preparation. Prolonged daily usage or too high a dose can lead to hypercalcaemia. Bone pain and tenderness may become worse about two days after starting treatment but tend to improve after one week. Maintenance therapy should be titrated according to the clinical response to treatment.

MUSCLES AND JOINTS

Muscle strength declines with age, from its peak values in the early 20s to 40s. Strength in some muscles may decline by as much as 5–7 per cent per year from the age of 70. These declines are associated with parallel reductions in muscle mass. There are changes in both the numbers and size of muscle fibres, affecting predominantly type II fibres. These changes are probably due to reductions in the numbers of anterior horn cells in the spinal cord that innervate skeletal muscles, leading to progressive loss of muscle mass and weakness.

Such reductions in muscle strength are paralleled by similar changes in physical capacity, including maximal oxygen consumption, airways resistance and joint flexibility. Reduced range of movement across a joint may also lead to further wasting and weakness, as will any damage within a joint.

Osteoarthritis is so common with increasing age (up to 85 per cent of people at ages 75–79 have this condition) that it is tempting to assume that it is part of 'normal' ageing. However, the changes that occur in the cartilage of osteoarthritic joints are not the same as those that occur in old joints. Cartilage consists of chondrocytes, collagen, proteoglycans (chondroitin sulphate and keratan sulphate) and water. Adult cartilage contains less water, and its proteoglycan structure and content changes, although the total level remains the same. The number of chondrocytes also falls.

By contrast, in osteoarthritis the water content of cartilage is higher because the collagen becomes disrupted, and less densely woven together, and drinks in water like a sponge. As the cartilage gets more damaged, chondrocytes start to divide and become much more active, producing a wide range of destructive enzymes, including collagenase, as well as attempting to repair damage by production of more collagen, proteoglycans and hyaluronic acid. Microfractures occur in the bone around the joint and lead to cysts and sclerosis. Erosions in the cartilage are associated with proliferation of bone and osteophyte formation at the joint margins. The underlying aetiological factors are not known, although genetic factors, occupation and trauma are probably implicated.

THRESHOLDS FOR INDEPENDENT LIFE

Age-related declines in physical capacity are of no significance in themselves until they prevent a person from carrying out necessary tasks (Fig. 6.4). Many very elderly people find it almost impossible to get out of a low chair without arms. This is because their muscles cannot generate sufficient force to overcome their body weight. An acute illness or a spell of bed-rest may accelerate the loss of strength and this explains why an apparently mild illness can have quite devastating effects on a person who is on the threshold of being unable to carry out activities of daily living. Much of the rehabilitation required by elderly people during and after acute illnesses is essentially aimed at improving muscle strength, flexibility and stamina.

Even in old age, improvements in muscle strength and joint flexibility can be achieved of similar scale to those experienced by younger people. For example, regular use of the legs to lift weights by people in their 80s and 90s can lead to about 15 per cent improvement in muscle strength. More importantly, it enables some chair-fast subjects to get up without help. Regular exercise can therefore help overcome some of the age-associated changes, and raises the question of whether such changes are truly due to ageing, or more correctly attributed to lack of activity.

Key points

- Bone collagen cross-linkages increase with age. The significance of these changes in determining bone strength is not known. Greenstick fractures are common in young children who have few cross-linkages.
- Osteoporosis is defined as too little bone of normal composition. Bone mass reaches a peak in early adult life and then falls, rapidly after the female menopause.
- Osteomalacia is due to vitamin D deficiency which is often the result of poor dietary intake and inadequate sunlight exposure. Malabsorption, chronic liver disease and chronic renal failure are rarer causes.
- Muscle strength reaches a peak during the young adult years and then declines, probably because of reductions in the numbers of anterior horn cells in the spinal cord.
- Osteoarthritis is not due to ageing changes in joints. Osteoarthritis is associated with thinning of articular cartilage, whereas cartilage tends to increase in thickness with age.
- Physical exercise may ameliorate some of the adverse changes in muscle strength and joint flexibility.

FURTHER READING

Aniansson A, Grimby G, Rungren A, Svanborg A, Olander J. Physical training in old men. *Age and Ageing*, 1980; **9**: 186–187.

Fentem PH, Bassey EJ, Turnbull NB. *The New Case for Exercise*. Health Education Authority, London, 1988.

Kay MMB, Galpin J, Makinodan T (eds). *Aging, Immunity and Arthritic Disease*. Raven Press, New York, 1980.

Smith EL, Serfass RC (eds). *Exercise and Aging: The Scientific Basis*. Enslow Publishers, Hillside, NJ, 1981.

Shepherd R. *Physical Activity and Ageing*, 2nd edn. Croom Helm, London, 1987.

Smith R. Osteoporosis causes and management. *Br Med J* 1987; **294**: 329–332.

Young A. Exercise physiology in geriatric practice. *Acta Med Scand* (suppl) 1986; **711**: 227–232.

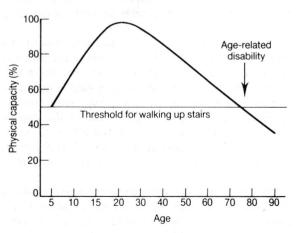

Figure 6.4 Age-related changes in muscle strength: a threshold for independent life

7 THE AGEING BRAIN

- Brain structure
- Brain function
- Forgetfulness and intelligence
- Dementia
- Other ageing changes

The human brain has developed to a remarkable extent, giving us huge cerebral hemispheres that sit on top of the more primitive mid- and hindbrain structures that control basic life processes.

BRAIN STRUCTURE

During embryonic development the brain surface is smooth up to 4 months, but then becomes irregular, producing the characteristic ridges and troughs (gyri and sulci) of the brain surface. These undulations increase the surface area of the brain to around 30 times that of the skull size, thus packing in much more grey matter. The grey matter is made up of nerve cells and the white matter is made up of nerve fibres streaming from the cells. Each nerve cell has a fibre (axon) transmitting impulses away from the cell and many more connections (dendrites) connecting the brain cell with other cells.

With age, the brain volume gets smaller by about 10 per cent of young adult volume, the gyri become more prominent and the sulci deeper, and the ventricles get larger. It is likely that old brains contain fewer nerve cells, although since there are many millions of brain cells no one has ever counted them to prove whether this really is so. The difficulty of studying true ageing changes, rather than the effects of pathological processes must be borne in mind. In dementia syndromes dramatic loss of neurones is typical and it is impossible to be sure that human brains studied post-mortem were not affected by early stages of a dementia syndrome.

It appears that cells are lost at different rates in different parts of the brain. Neuronal loss in the cortex is estimated to be about 1 per cent per year, but much faster rates of loss occur in the basal ganglia and cerebellum. The locus ceruleus, which has a large number of catecholaminergic cells, loses cells at the rate of about 44 per cent per year after the age of 60 years. Animal studies have demonstrated very little change in the numbers of neurones with age and an increase in glial cells.

The number of dendrites decreases with age, which may be due to a reduction in the rate at which they are renewed, or may be a genuine loss. The loss of dendrites is associated with a reduction in synaptic activity, and presumably communication and information processing is reduced. The changes seen in Alzheimer's disease are severe, but the significance of the much milder changes in normal aged brains is not known.

BRAIN FUNCTION

Various areas of the brain perform specific functions (Fig. 7.1). For example, in the motor area of the cortex that controls movement, the body is represented from the foot at the midline to the hand at the lateral edge of the motor area. A comparable sensory area of the cortex receives information from the body. These motor and sensory areas are interconnected with other parts of the brain through the branching network of dendrites. This permits the fine control of movement and the coordination between eye and hand.

The pathways that the axons follow from cortical neurones cross over in the brainstem. As a result, the left motor cortex controls movement of the right side of the body and vice versa.

The parietal lobe is located between the back of the brain — the occipital cortex where vision resides — and the sensory cortex. It is concerned with recognition of objects and spatial awareness. Damage to this part of the brain was the cause of the symptoms that gave the title to Oliver Sacks' celebrated book (and opera and film) *The Man who Mistook his Wife for a Hat*.

The frontal lobes of the brain are large and were formerly considered to be 'silent'. Large amounts of frontal cortex can be destroyed and the person can live on quite normally. However, the frontal lobe has an important role in the control of behaviour, attention and emotion. Damage to the frontal lobes can give rise to a characteristic syndrome of disinhibited, crude behaviour. Surgical damage (pre-frontal lobotomy) is still used as a treatment for severe, and otherwise untreatable, depression.

The temporal lobes and adjacent deep stuctures (hippocampus, nucleus of Meynert, etc.) are concerned with memory. Study of the pathology of Alzheimer's disease has shown that the disease appears to strike these areas most severely. Ideas about the structure of memory are expanding rapidly. Short-term memory is probably stored in the form of electrical potential differences between neurones for a matter of a few minutes. These electrical changes then lead to the laying down of memory by protein synthesis for a period of a few hours. Finally, long-term memory is held by changes in the dendrites and their interconnections.

Acute loss of memory — amnestic syndromes — are associated with damage to the hippocampus, thalamus and limbic system. No impairment of thinking, personality, attention or concentration occurs, and it is usual for very remote memory to be unaffected, suggesting that this sort of memory is laid down very widely. A common cause of an apparent complete loss of memory, without any other evidence of brain damage, is hysteria.

Right- and left-handedness are indicators of which

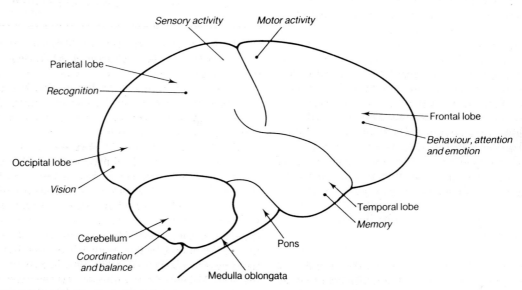

Figure 7.1 Lobes of the brain and their functions

side of the brain is dominant. In right-handed people, the left side is dominant, but a proportion of left-handed people also have left-sided brain dominance. Speech is a complex function, with the speech areas located in the dominant hemisphere in the frontal, temporal and parietal regions. Interestingly, while speech may be lost if the left side of the brain is damaged by a stroke, the ability to sing may not be affected. Second languages may also be unimpaired.

The mid- and hindbrain are concerned with basic life-supporting functions (breathing, arousal, maintenance of circulation) and with control of posture and movement. These parts of the brain are also extensively connected with cortical areas.

FORGETFULNESS AND INTELLIGENCE

Forgetting things is a normal everyday behaviour. A young child forgetting to take an exercise book to school is considered quite normal, whereas an elderly person forgetting to take money on a shopping trip may think this indicates early dementia. It is often necessary to reassure elderly people that such forgetfulness is normal, and the term 'benign senile forgetfulness' has been coined for this problem.

Both young and old forget things at similar rates, but in older people the ability to remember strings of numbers or items on a list is less. This may be due to true ageing changes, but more probably reflects a cohort effect. People born in 1900 had less schooling, less exposure to modern media, and less need to remember strings of numbers for the telephone. Their performance on such 'intelligence' tests is therefore less good than people born a generation later. In fact there is good evidence that many aspects of intelligence do not deteriorate with increasing age in longitudinal studies. Speed of response, which is a factor in some intelligence tests, does decline with age and may also make elderly people appear to do less well in tests. Some of the tests themselves are rather childish and may irritate elderly subjects, thus leading to poor performance.

DEMENTIA

For normal brain function, adequate supplies of energy, oxygen, vitamins and hormones are required. Interference with these basic needs will lead to global functional deterioration (confusion) which, provided the interference is only temporary, can recover. By contrast, the damage caused by dementing diseases is permanent and progressive.

The typical findings in Alzheimer's dementia are of diffuse cortical atrophy with loss of neurones. Neurofibrillary tangles and vacuoles (holes) are found inside the neurones, together with plaques of amyloid deposits. These changes are most marked in the hippocampus, the temporal–parietal–occipital junction, and in the nucleus basalis of Meynert. In addition to these changes, the interconnections between neurones wither away. Alzheimer's disease also leads to reductions in neurotransmitters, particularly acetylcholine, and corresponding reductions in enzymes such as choline acetyltransferase. Attempts to simply substitute the deficient neurotransmitter (in the same way as L-dopa is used to substitute for low levels of dopamine in Parkinson's disease) have not proved successful, demonstrating that the fundamental nature of the disease is not fully understood (Table 7.1).

Table 7.1 Pathological changes in Alzheimer's disease

Senile plaques
    These are granular fragments surrounded by astrocytes, often containing microglia, and amyloid

Neurofibrillary tangles
    These are thickened neurofibrils which swing around the cell nucleus and form a circular shape in the cytoplasm

Granulo-vacuolar degeneration
    Affected neurones show clusters of intracytoplasmic vacuoles, each of which has a dense, round central granule

The brains of normal old people are not immune from similar changes: plaques of amyloid deposition, intraneuronal tangles and vacuoles all occur. The difference is in their numbers and distribution. It is generally accepted that dementia is due to structural and irreversible damage to the brain, rather than an acceleration of a normal ageing process.

Alzheimer's can run in families and when it does, around 50 per cent of all children are affected, suggesting an autosomal dominant mode of inheritance. When the gene for familial Alzheimer's disease was found to be on chromosome 21, this led to great excitement because Down's syndrome (trisomy 21) is associated with a dementia and with very similar pathological changes in the brain. The trail went very cold when it was found that the gene responsible was not the same in different families with Alzheimer's disease, nor was the gene implicated in the much more common non-familial disease.

OTHER AGEING CHANGES

In addition to the cortical changes, the peripheral nervous system declines with age. Awareness of pain, touch, temperature, joint position and vibration sense all get worse with age. Indeed it is quite normal for vibration sense to be absent at the ankles in elderly people. Some of these changes may be due to reductions in nerve conduction velocity.

The control of posture and balance also declines, making old people more prone to falls, and to adopt a broader-based walking pattern. Indeed, it is unusual to see a very old person who does not walk with a gait reminiscent of early Parkinsonism. The mechanisms for changes in gait, posture and balance are not understood. It is likely that many different but interrelated mechanisms are involved. These may include neuronal loss in the basal ganglia and cortex, reduction in reaction times, muscle atrophy, changes in labyrinthine and visual perception, and reductions in proprioception.

Key points

- Brain weight, volume, cell numbers and dendrites decline with age, although there are marked regional variations within the brain.
- Brain functions are localized. There are the motor and sensory cortices; the parietal lobe concerned with recognition; the frontal lobes with control of behaviour, attention and emotion; the temporal lobes, hippocampus and nucleus of Meynert with memory. Speech is complex, with multiple association areas in the temporal, parietal and frontal regions.

- Not all forgetfulness heralds the onset of dementia. Old and young people suffer with forgetfulness to a similar extent.
- Alzheimer's disease is characterized by senile plaques, neurofibrillary tangles and granulo-vacuolar degeneration. Normal old brains show the same kind of changes, but in Alzheimer's disease the amount of change is far greater and the distribution of changes is most marked in the hippocampus, the temporal–parietal–occipital junction, and in the nucleus basalis of Meynert.
- The characteristic neurotransmitter deficit in Alzheimer's disease is of acetylcholine with reductions in the enzyme choline acetyltransferase.

FURTHER READING

Brayne C, Calloway P. Normal ageing, impaired cognitive function, and senile dementia of the Alzheimer's type: a continuum? *Lancet* 1988; **i**: 1265–1267.

Jarvik LF. Thoughts on the psychology of ageing. *Am Psychol* 1975, May: 576–583.

Jorm AF. *The Epidemiology of Alzheimer's Disease and Related Disorders*. Chapman & Hall, London, 1990.

Prusiner SB. Some speculations about prions, amyloid and Alzheimer's disease. *N Engl J Med* 1984; **310**: 661–663.

Rinn WE. Mental decline in normal ageing: a review. *J Geriatr Psychiat Neurol* 1988; **1**: 144–158.

Tanzi RE, Gusella JF, Watkins PC *et al*. Amyloid B protein gene: cDNA, mRNA distribution, and genetic linkage near the Alzheimer locus. *Science*, 1987; **235**: 880–884.

8 THE AGEING CARDIOVASCULAR SYSTEM

- Structural changes
- Heart rate and cardiac output
- Blood pressure
- Other points

Ageing of the cardiovascular system has long been thought of as the basis for the general physiological decline attributed to ageing. Leonardo da Vinci wrote that the cause of ageing was 'veins which by the thickening of their tunics in the old, restricts the passage of their blood and by this lack of nourishment destroys the life of the aged without any fever, the old coming to fail little by little in slow death'. The aged cardiovascular system exemplifies the dilemma of physiology versus pathology in the normal ageing process. It is now evident that the physiological changes associated with age are comparatively minor and amount to slightly poorer function whereas the pathological changes (especially those of atherosclerotic coronary artery disease) are severe, extremely damaging, and often life-threatening.

STRUCTURAL CHANGES

Cardiovascular structural changes with age are well documented. Aortic elasticity declines (due to changes in the media, not the intimal changes of atherosclerosis) and the aorta commonly widens (seen clinically on chest X-rays as a widened aortic arch). The elasticity changes mean that systolic blood pressure may thus rise slightly with age. Heart valves (especially the aortic) can become less mobile in a proportion of elderly people (exacerbated by atheromatous disease and calcification) and cause the commonly heard ejection systolic murmur. Degeneration and calcification of the mitral valve can result in either apical ejection murmurs or the more common pansystolic mitral incompetence/regurgitant murmur. Age changes in the myocardium result in the accumulation of the 'waste product' lipofuscin and the so-called 'brown atrophy'.

HEART RATE AND CARDIAC OUTPUT

The effect of age on the resting heart rate is equivocal but it appears that the heart rate increase in response to stress is probably less effective in advanced old age.

Cardiac output falls slightly with advancing age (about 1 per cent per year) and with the slight rise in systolic blood pressure means that the systemic peripheral resistance is somewhat increased. The changes in cardiac output are probably related to the small decreases in body size that occur and also to the fact that slightly less blood is pumped per heart beat per unit body size.

There is evidence for an age-related loss of the pacing myocytes (P cells) in the sinoatrial node and some increase in fibrous tissue, but very little effect on the atrioventricular node. This decrease in the number of conducting cells is probably potentiated by diseases such as hypertension or ischaemic heart disease, making the clinical finding of atrial fibrillation more common in elderly people.

BLOOD PRESSURE

Systolic and diastolic blood pressures rise with age in most Western populations but as it is not universal it is unlikely to be a true ageing process (neither is it always progressive or irreversible). Even though vascular ageing changes may occur that predispose to hypertension, other compensating factors may be important (diet, physical fitness, etc.). Hypertension in the elderly, its definition and its possible treatment is still a highly contentious area. Blood pressures need to be measured accurately and over a period of time, bearing in mind that they can be labile and that readings can change with posture — hence lying and standing measurements should be made.

Although 'hypertension' must be seen in the context of the individual, it may be thought that biological rather than chronological age is a better guide to possible intervention measures. Evidence from clinical trials suggests that treatment is beneficial up to the age of 80 years, and for levels above 160/100 (phase V). The end-organ effects of sustained hypertension (angina, left ventricular failure, etc.) may obviously influence the management. If hypertension is found to be part of a generalized atheromatous state, thought should be given to the issue of whether, in that particular person, the physiological parameters have been set at a new 'higher' level determined by the disease process and necessary for function. Changing this may result in more, rather than less, damage being inflicted. The side-effects of drug management in the very old must be weighed against the expected benefits (morbidity and mortality reduction) and should be carefully examined.

Hypotension is a common finding in elderly people, especially posturally related hypotension. This usually results from either the use of drugs with a hypotensive effect (e.g. diuretics, major tranquillizers, L-dopa, alcohol, etc.) or more rarely, impairment in the baroreceptor reflex mechanism (diabetic neuropathy, tabes dorsalis, Parkinson's disease, Shy–Drager syndrome, etc.).

OTHER POINTS

Cardiovascular disease is a very common finding in an ageing population (depending on the definition of cardiovascular disease and the completeness of the physical and laboratory investigations). A large subpopulation of the elderly have enlarged hearts but as hypertrophy (increase in size due to increased workload over long periods) is not inevitable in all elderly individuals it cannot be considered an ageing process.

Organ perfusion decreases with age, indicated by data from peripheral resistance to blood flow and clearance of certain substances. These changes in organ perfusion may be secondary to either less blood being supplied to the capillaries due to atheroma of the large vessels or reductions in cardiac output (not a major influence). Organ perfusion can also be altered secondary to changes in tissue (metabolic demands or loss of compliance). Peripheral resistance increases with age and this probably plays a role in decreasing blood flow.

The efficiency of the oxygen transport system declines with age as does, to a small extent, thermoregulation which in part depends on heat conduction by cutaneous blood flow which becomes more sluggish. A change in one part of the cardiovascular system influences every other and it is difficult to distinguish primary from secondary age changes. However, most of the changes with age are probably due to a small number of factors which are intrinsic.

Normal cardiovascular ageing may be hard to find in Western societies but we must not let the common pathological changes found in elderly patients influence the fact that normal ageing means slight and sometimes subtle changes in measurements. Clinical findings may include a slight rise in blood pressure and possibly atrial fibrillation and ejection systolic 'flow' murmurs.

Key points

- Cardiovascular physiological changes with age are minor; pathological changes severe.
- Structural changes often include a widening aortic arch and ejection systolic murmurs.

- The heart rate increase in response to stress is less effective.
- Cardiac output falls slightly with advancing age (about 1 per cent per year).
- There is an age-related loss of P cells but atrial fibrillation is potentiated by disease processes.
- Systolic and diastolic blood pressures rise with age in Western populations (though it is not universal).
- Blood pressures need to be measured accurately and over a period of time.
- Treatment of hypertension in the elderly needs to take into account 'biological' age, end-organ damage and potential side-effects.
- Postural hypotension is a common finding in elderly people.

FURTHER READING

Finch CE, Schneider EL (eds). *Handbook of the Biology of Ageing*. Van Nostrand Reinhold, New York, 1985.

Wei JY. Age and the cardiovascular system. *N Engl J Med* 1992; **327**(24): 1735–1739.

9 THE AGEING RESPIRATORY SYSTEM

- Structural changes
- Functional changes
- Examining the elderly chest
- Chest X-ray

The respiratory system comprises airways that transport inspired air to the alveoli where transfer of gases takes place, and the supporting structures of the chest wall. All of these are affected by ageing, and many of the age changes are accelerated by smoking.

The large airways are kept open by rings of cartilage. As the airways branch out and narrow the support that keeps them open is provided by the elastic recoil of the lung parenchymal tissue, and cartilage is not present in these very small-diameter airways.

STRUCTURAL CHANGES

(Table 9.1)

With ageing, the elasticity of the lungs declines. This leads to early closure of the very small airways on breathing out, resulting in the trapping of air. In addition, the reduction in parenchymal support to the airways tends to reduce their overall size and makes the lung more compliant — or distensible.

This combination of loss of elasticity and increased distensibility makes the lungs occupy a bigger space and on chest X-rays it may look as if the lungs are

Table 9.1 Changes in the chest wall and lung

Chest wall
  Stiff costovertebral and costochondral joints
  Increased AP diameter due to kyphosis
  Wasting of respiratory muscles
  Increased use of diaphragm

Lung
  Alveoli support diminished
  Increased mucous glands
  Reduced elasticity
  Increased physiological dead space
  Reduced surface area for gas exchange
  Reduced capillary circulation

overinflated. The diaphragm is flat and the ribs become more horizontal. The X-ray chest appearances are similar to those seen in emphysema, and indeed the loss of elasticity, and the air-trapping lead to a progressive dilation of the alveoli and a form of emphysema, very similar to that seen in patients with alpha-1 antitrypsin deficiency, in which the lung parenchyma is 'digested' away. In smokers, these changes are aggravated and are associated with mucous cell hypertrophy and inflammatory changes as well.

In addition to the ageing changes within the lung, the chest wall ages. Perhaps the most dramatic change is the kyphosis that is common in many elderly people which is due to degeneration in intervertebral discs, and may be aggravated by osteoporosis with thoracic vertebral collapse. Kyphosis reduces the diameter of the chest, and, with calcification of costal cartilages, makes the chest wall more rigid. The respiratory muscles, along with other skeletal muscle, also become weaker with age.

FUNCTIONAL CHANGES

The ageing changes in structure lead to predictable functional effects. The volume of air that can be expired in one second (FEV_1) falls because of the reduction in elasticity and air-trapping, and also because of weakness of respiratory muscles. The declines in FEV_1, peak flow rate and forced vital capacity can be predicted from standard equations. It is necessary to take into account sex, height and smoking habits, all of which will affect lung ventilation.

The relative proportions of lung volumes change with age (Fig. 9.1). The tidal volume remains about the same at about 0.5 litre, but the inspiratory reserve and expiratory reserve volumes both decline and the residual volume increases quite markedly (Fig. 9.1).

Although data from cross-sectional studies show an apparently linear decline, small studies of very elderly people suggest that the rate of decline increases in the very old. If data from younger subjects are extrapolated to the very old, this will lead to predicted values being too high, and the assumption that the elderly person has lower than expected lung function.

Cross-sectional studies also tend to overestimate the loss of lung function with age. The longitudinal rates of decline found are smaller than those obtained from cross-sectional studies. This may be due to a form of selection bias. To remain in a longitudinal study, a subject must survive, and survival is associated with better lung function.

Gas exchange is also affected by ageing. Ventilation of the lung is matched by blood flow. Areas of the lung with less ventilation automatically receive less blood, and vice versa. When sitting upright, the ventilation to the lung bases is higher than to the upper parts of the lung. This is matched by increased blood flow to the bases. The tendency to early closure of airways, with air-trapping, reduces the ventilation of the bases, and leads to a mismatch between ventilation and perfusion. The result of this is an age-related reduction in the arterial oxygen saturation.

On exertion, the respiratory system is stressed and the functional reserve capacity has to be used. With age, the reserve capacity is much more limited. In particular, the weakness of respiratory muscles contributes to the exertional breathlessness seen in elderly people. It is likely that training can improve respiratory efficiency, even in the very old, and thus reduce some of the adverse consquences of ageing on the respiratory system.

It is often forgotten that the lung is also an immunological organ coping with the challenges of many different potential allergens and pathogens with each lung full of air. With age, the lung defence mechanisms — mucus production, local antibodies and cell-mediated immunity — wane, making elderly people much more susceptible to infection.

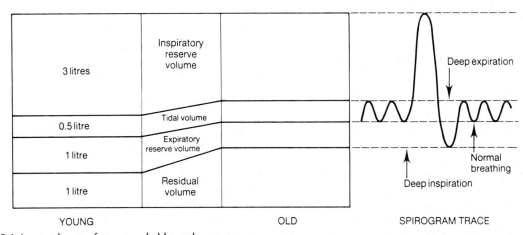

Figure 9.1 Lung volumes of young and old people

EXAMINING THE ELDERLY CHEST

Examination of the chest comprises a ritual of assessing the chest wall, checking whether the trachea is central, gauging expansion by eye and hand (but seldom tape-measure), followed by percussion, tactile and vocal fremitus, and listening for abnormal sounds. Much of this has been demonstrated to be of virtually no value at all, with very poor agreement between doctors on the presence or absence of signs, and low validity when compared with the gold standards of chest X-ray and CT scanning. However, some parts of the examination are worth carrying out.

Respiratory rate

Counting the respiratory rate is one of the most useful screening examinations for elderly people. At rest the normal respiratory rate will be around 15 breaths per minute. The anxiety of a clinical examination may push this up to 20 per minute. With respiratory distress caused by heart failure, pneumonia, pulmonary embolus, asthma, etc., one of the first mechanisms brought into action to maintain gas transfer and avoid hypoxia is an increase in respiratory rate. It is not until rates increase to 35–40 per minute that a person looks obviously short of breath, so it is necessary to count the rate over at least half a minute to pick up less severe problems.

Chest movement

In normal elderly people the chest wall does not move as much as in young people. It may be difficult to decide if expansion is symmetrical because the chest wall moves so little. Abdominal respiration is not affected, and it is obvious that anything that limits abdominal respiration (e.g. abdominal surgery, abdominal pain, tight corsets, gross obesity) will have a disproportionate effect on respiratory efficiency, and lead to hypoxia.

Breath sounds

Doctors are taught to listen for crackles in the lung bases as a sign of heart failure. These crackles are probably caused by the opening and closing of very small airways. In elderly people, the increased fine crackles of heart failure are masked by much coarser noises produced by the air-trapping caused by loss of lung elasticity. Such noises should not be assumed to be pathological.

THE CHEST X-RAY

In a sick elderly person a chest X-ray is an essential investigation, regardless of the presence or absence of signs or symptoms. The elderly person's chest X-ray may tell a story, and the best way to understand the story is to make the effort to get hold of old films which may help in interpretation.

Common changes are apical shadowing from tuberculosis, calcification in chondral cartilages, pleural calcification from past pneumonia, old rib fractures, and more rarely occupational dust exposures.

A major problem for elderly people is to adopt the required posture for a good-quality PA erect chest X-ray. All too often a supine film is done, usually not in full inspiration, and with a degree of rotation. This makes it impossible to determine whether effusions are present, and makes heart size and the mediastinum impossible to assess. Sick elderly people are not easy to X-ray well, and a sympathetic and experienced radiographer is essential.

Key points

- The elasticity of the lungs declines with age, leading to early closure of very small airways and air-trapping. Parenchymal support also declines, reducing the size of the lungs and making them more compliant.
- The chest wall becomes more rigid with age (due to kyphosis and calcification of costal cartilage), increasing the work of respiration.
- The structural changes lead to reductions in FEV_1 and other indicators of lung function. The rate of reduction is markedly affected by smoking.
- Arterial oxygen saturation falls with age because of ventilation–perfusion mismatching occurring at the lung bases.
- Counting the respiratory rate is one of the most useful parts of chest examination. Basal crepitations are almost universal in the chests of older smokers.
- Always try to obtain a good-quality PA chest X-ray, and any previous old films for comparison.

FURTHER READING

Edge JR, Millard FJC, Reid L, Simon G. The radiographic appearance of the chest in persons of advanced age. *Br J Radiol* 1964; 37: 769–774.

Milne JS. *Clinical Effects of Ageing. A Longitudinal Study*. Croom Helm, London, 1985.

Mittman C, Edelman NH, Norris AH, Shock NW. Relationship between chest wall and pulmonary compliance and age. *J Appl Physiol* 1965; 20: 1211–1216.

Spiteri MA, Cook DG, Clarke SW. Reliability of eliciting physical signs in the examination of the chest. *Lancet* 1988; i: 873–875.

Thurlbeck WM, Angus GE. Growth and ageing of normal human lung. *Chest* 1975; 67: 3s–7s.

10 THE AGEING ENDOCRINE SYSTEM

- Women
- Men
- Sexuality
- Other endocrine organs

The changes that occur in the endocrine system with age were once thought to be the sole cause of the generalized ageing process and hence that this process could be reversed by the replacement of numerous hormones. 'Ageing' is now seen to be far more complex but replacement of some of the previously thought non-essential hormonal loss is gaining importance.

WOMEN

The menopause is defined as the cessation of menstrual periods but is associated with numerous other bodily changes. Menstruation usually becomes irregular before finally stopping and some women suffer severe physical and mental symptoms associated with the hormonal changes. These include flushing/sweating attacks, altered libido, mucosal changes in the vagina with some dryness and periods of melancholy or even frank depression. During this time the levels of circulating and urinary gonadotrophins — follicle-stimulating hormone (FSH) and luteinizing hormone (LH) — are raised, probably reflecting the lowered levels of circulating oestrogens causing a negative feedback on the hypothalamus. With increasing age the oestrogen found in the urine decreases to very low levels. In elderly women oestrone is the main circulating hormone, derived by conversion of plasma androstenedione of adrenal cortical origin, and this conversion increases with age. In addition to producing less hormones the production of germ cells by the ovaries is also affected by age. The quality of the oocytes declines, as evidenced by an increase in chromosomal abnormalities in older women, the most notable result being trisomy of chromosome 21 resulting in Down's syndrome. It has been theorized that oocytes that have spent longer in the ovary are more prone to damage by radiation, infection, autoantibody effects, etc. Eventually, the postmenopausal ovary fails to respond to the gonadotrophic hormones and it becomes increasingly fibrotic.

For a few years prior to the menopause the uterus increasingly fails to support pregnancy, probably due to the physical changes in the uterus and altered hormonal balance. Following the menopause the uterus slowly atrophies. In postmenopausal women the vagina contracts, shortening the organ and gradually decreasing the size of the lumen. There is loss of elasticity and the epithelium becomes thin, pale and dry. These changes usually occur slowly and imperceptibly and should not interfere with sexual intercourse even in the very elderly. However, the hormonal changes that especially affect the epithelium (causing dryness) can be clinically significant, cause discomfort and distress and need to be recognized and treated urgently.

With ageing there is a gradual replacement of glandular breast tissue with fat. Breast carcinoma is the leading malignant cause of death amongst women, and the risk increases with age. Particular attention should be paid to education, self-examining techniques and screening with mammography.

Hormone replacement therapy (HRT)

This topic remains controversial despite an increasing demand from older women and an increasing awareness amongst doctors as to its benefits. HRT lessens and even avoids the unpleasant sequelae of the menopause in many women. There is the protective effect from post-menopausal osteoporosis with its devastating resultant morbidity and mortality from fractures. The common fracture sites are wrist, neck of femur and vertebral body, and 50 per cent of women will have sustained such a fracture by the age of 75.

In young women oestrogens protect against cardiovascular disease via lipoprotein metabolism. This protection is gradually lost post menopause but the reintroduction of oestrogens causes a rise in the cardioprotective high-density lipoproteins and this is being further evaluated.

In addition there is the added value of increased psychological well-being (feeling better) as well as the effects of HRT on collagen, improving skin texture and tone (looking better). Oestrogen can be given orally, transvaginally, transdermally (patch) or subcutaneously. Progesterone is also needed if a woman has not had a hysterectomy (i.e. uterus is in place) to prevent unopposed oestrogen endometrial hyperplasia and adenocarcinoma.

Contraindications to HRT include hormone-dependent breast or endometrial cancer but not controlled hypertension or susceptibility to thromboembolism. Therapy can continue indefinitely. As menopausal symptoms are temporary, many clinicians favour shorter courses but the long-term treatment lobby cite the bone and heart protection effects and the wishes of older women. Long-term therapy necessitates regular blood pressure and breast examination checks (especially if there is a positive family history). There is a regular withdrawal bleed after progesterone, perpetuating 'menstruation' into old age.

MEN

The ageing of the male reproductive system is a gradual process. It probably has a variable period of onset and although devotees of Woody Allen movies would feel there is a lot of evidence for a 'male menopause' or 'andropause' it usually passes without major physical side-effects or psychological trauma. There is no decline in the size or weight of the testes and spermatozoa continue to be produced into old age and are viable. The secretion of testosterone decreases in elderly men. There is fibrous change in the trabeculae of the corpus spongiosum, followed by sclerosis of the arteries and veins. Similar changes occur in the corpora cavernosa.

After the fifth decade the prostate shows less secretory activity and degenerative changes begin which further lessen secretions. Nodular hyperplasia, benign prostate hyperplasia (BPH) within the stroma of the prostate gland becomes very common in Caucasians (but not other races) after the age of 50. This gives rise to the symptoms of prostatism: difficulty in initiation of flow, poor stream and postmicturition dribbling. A digital examination of the prostate gland is mandatory. It can give a crude indication of prostate size, help detect carcinoma and check the rectal mucosa at the same time. Prostatic outflow obstruction can be helped by the use of alpha-1-adrenoreceptor blocking drugs (instead of or pre-prostatectomy). Most prostate operations are via the paraurethral route.

Prostatic cancer becomes increasingly common in old age (again predominantly in Caucasian men). Rectal examination reveals a hard, often craggy prostate.

Prostate-specific antigen (PSA) is a specific marker for prostatic acinar epithelium and although it can be slightly raised in BPH, values > 10 mg/ml are highly suggestive of carcinoma. PSA measurement should be undertaken in all cases of prostatism (as well as rectal examination). Unfortunately, at presentation 20 per cent of men already have a positive isotope bone scan (before any skeletal X-ray changes.) PSA measurement and a subsequent bone scan should form the basis of assessment in most cases.

SEXUALITY

Sex drive (libido) is said to decline with age and ejaculation time lengthens. There is, however, considerable variation and numerous other factors have to be taken into account such as the general health of the person plus that of their partner, their sexual needs and wishes viewed over time. The influence of 'society's' views should not be underestimated. Currently sex in old age is seen in some way as being perverse (imagine and witness the 'difficulty' if two residents in an old people's home wanted to have sex and needed a degree of privacy and even help to achieve it). There are no norms for adults: sex should be mutually enjoyable and desired by both partners, at any frequency and at any age. Homosexual relationships are as valid as heterosexual and this aspect of sexuality should not be overlooked or devalued in elderly people.

OTHER ENDOCRINE ORGANS

The endocrine response to stress declines somewhat with age yet there is no evidence to show that this is due to a deficiency in the pituitary–adrenal axis. Underactivity of the adrenals (Addison's disease) does occur in the elderly whereas overactivity (Cushing's disease) is extremely rare over 70. Insulin deficiency appears to be strongly age-related. In glucose tolerance tests the ability to utilize the glucose load declines with increasing age. The deterioration is so large that many elderly lie in the 'diabetic' category. Whether or not these people are suffering from diabetes mellitus is debatable, although progressively higher blood glucose levels are associated with increased mortality, especially from cardiovascular disease and strokes. It is not clear whether this change is due to ageing or disease.

The thyroid gland of even very elderly people maintains adequate function. The secretion rate of T_4 decreases with age, whilst plasma T_4 levels do not. The TSH response is unchanged. Thyroid function tests may be altered during illness — the 'sick euthyroid' syndrome with a low T_4 but also a low TSH (hypopituitarism being excluded). There are lower levels of plasma T_3 circulating in elderly people. It has been theorized that since this is the active hormone there may be a decrease in the effective hormone with ageing. However TSH levels do not rise, so there would also have to be a deficiency in the negative feedback mechanism.

Diagnostic problems are often encountered in thyroid disease. Hypofunction (hypothyroidism) is a condition that can be diagnosed late because the symptoms and signs are subtle (constipation, dry skin and hair, lethargy, puffy features) and slow onset (deeper voice,

tendency to cold intolerance, etc.). The symptoms are also accepted as normal age changes by the patient (and often by the doctor as well) and as constipation, dry skin, tiredness and cold intolerance occur commonly in normal elderly people then a high index of suspicion is necessary. It is said that patients who are seen regularly (by carers and doctor) are the ones that are missed, the 'classic' case with a pulse of 40 and slow relaxing ankle jerks being a doctor's mother!

Similarly, hyperfunction (hyperthyroidism, thyrotoxicosis) can also be difficult to diagnose. Patients may present classically but the 'masked' or 'apathetic' presentation (with general debility and inability to cope) with few of the usual symptoms and signs is not uncommon. Thyroid function tests are a useful screening tool in unusual cases of ill-health.

In normal old age the endocrine glands perform their function and few specific changes are evident (some prostatic enlargement in men, altered breast tissue in women). Other findings often accepted as 'ageing' and hence normal should be viewed as pathological and investigated.

Key points

- The female menopause may be associated with marked physical and mental symptoms.
- Circulating FSH and LH levels are raised via negative feedback of lowered oestrogen levels on the hypothalamus.
- Clinical symptoms of hormonal loss (e.g. vaginal dryness) may need treatment.
- Breast carcinoma risk increases with age.
- Hormone replacement therapy (HRT) decreases menopausal symptoms and protects against osteoporosis and cardiovascular disease.
- In HRT oestrogen and progesterone must be given together to protect against endometrial hyperplasia and carcinoma.
- The male menopause (andropause) usually passes without major comment.
- Benign prostatic hyperplasia (BPH) is common and gives rise to the symptoms of prostatism.
- Assessment of prostatic carcinoma includes digital rectal examination, prostate-specific antigen (PSA) measurement and, where indicated, an isotope bone scan.
- All aspects of sexuality may continue into extreme old age.
- The ability to utilize a glucose load declines with increasing age.

- Thyroid function may be altered during illness — the 'sick euthyroid' syndrome.
- Thyroid function tests are a useful screening tool in unusual cases of ill-health.

FURTHER READING

Bancroft J. *Human Sexuality and its Problems*, 2nd edn. Churchill Livingstone, Edinburgh, 1989.

Belchetz PE. Hormonal treatment of postmenopausal women. *N Engl J Med* 1994; **330**(15): 1062–1071.

Gosden RG. *Biology of the Menopause: The Causes and Consequences of Ovarian Ageing*. Academic Press, London, 1985.

Korenman SG (ed.). *Endocrine Aspects of Ageing*. Elsevier, New York, 1982.

Levy EG. Thyroid disease in the elderly. *Med Clin North Am* 1991; **75**(1): 151–167.

Miller M. Disorders of the thyroid. In: Brocklehurst JC, Tallis RC, Fillit HM (eds), *Textbook of Geriatric Medicine and Gerontology*, 4th edn. Churchill Livingstone, Edinburgh, 1992.

Mooradian AD, Greiff V. Sexuality in older women. *Arch Intern Med* 1990; **75**(5): 881–883.

Sarrel PM. Sexuality and menopause. *Obstet Gynaecol* 1990; **75**(4 suppl.): 265–305; discussion 315–355.

Schiavi RC, Schreiner-Engel P, Mandeli J, Schanzer H, Cohen E. Healthy aging and male sexual function *Am J Psychiat* 1990; **147**(6): 766–771.

Vermeuler A. Clinical review 24: androgens in the aging male. *J Clin Endocrinol Metab* 1991; **73**(2): 221–224.

11 THE AGEING ALIMENTARY SYSTEM

- Teeth
- Mucosa
- Oesophagus
- Stomach
- Small bowel
- Large bowel
- Motility
- Appetite and nutrition

Age-related changes occur in the gastrointestinal tract but function is usually maintained at a more than adequate level.

TEETH

Dental caries is responsible for the majority of tooth extractions in young people. In elderly people, however, periodontal disease is the main factor. Periodontal disease is accelerated by:

1. poor oral hygiene;
2. decreased production of saliva due to age changes in the salivary glands;
3. age atrophy of the alveolar bone with progressive exposure of the root surfaces and loosening of the teeth; and
4. epithelial atrophy of the mucous membranes giving easily friable and traumatized surfaces.

Other serious problems include loss of teeth, oral mucosal lesions and root surface caries.

Improved oral hygiene in the younger population should eventually lead to less dental problems. However, currently the majority of elderly people are edentulous. In the edentulous the alveolar bone is resorbed and lower dentures especially will become loose. The use of dentures can pose significant problems, especially in institutions. Dentures should be marked and cleaned regularly. Problems with fit (poor speech or eating difficulties) should be referred early. A simple adjustment may be all that is necessary; however, some problems may need specialist attention by either a general dental practitioner or one who has undergone postgraduate training specifically in the field of dentistry for older people. There is an unmet need for dental treatment for elderly people; for specific groups, e.g. the mentally frail or institutionalized, the need is even greater.

MUCOSA

Leucoplakia appears as small white patches on the oral mucosa. It is associated with repeated mucosal trauma and may become malignant. Varicosities on the under-surface of the tongue (caviar lesions) are seen in 40 per cent of elderly people. Their significance is unknown but attempts have been made to implicate vitamin C deficiency. In some cases they may indicate vascular abnormalities elsewhere in the gastrointestinal tract.

Reduced saliva production predisposes to oral infections, especially ascending infection of the parotid gland producing septic parotitis. A dry mouth (decreased saliva production) is a common side-effect of many medications, including anticholinergics and antidepressants.

Candidiasis (caused by the fungus *Candida albicans*) causes soft white plaques on the mucosa and tongue. The background mucosa is usually quite reddened and attempts to remove the plaques cause discomfort and slight bleeding. Mucosal candidiasis usually occurs in older people secondary to antibiotic use or during chemotherapy. Treatment is with a suitable topical (lozenge or suspension) anti-fungal agent.

OESOPHAGUS

This conveys food from mouth to stomach helped by peristaltic contractions. Primary peristaltic waves occur after swallowing and secondary waves arise when the upper oesophagus is distended by food. Sometimes a localized series of ring-like non-peristaltic contractions occur spontaneously. These tertiary contractions occur more frequently in the elderly and can produce symptoms of dysphagia (difficulty in swallowing).

In presbyoesophagus the normal swallow is not followed by a primary peristaltic wave. Instead non-propulsive contractions occur and there is incoordination in the lower oesophageal sphincter-relaxing mechanism.

Clinically, diverticula (pharyngeal pouches) can occur at the upper end of the oesophagus (more common in men and thought to be secondary to high pressure). Food may be aspirated from the pouch and hence patients may present with dysphagia, coughing or repeated chest infections. Herniation of the lower oesophagus and upper part of the stomach (hiatus hernia) occurs in up to two-thirds of elderly people. The cause is probably muscular weakness around the diaphragmatic hiatus but constipation, straining, obesity and the wearing of corsets have all been implicated. Benign and malignant strictures are comparatively common.

Dysphagia is a common but late symptom of oesophageal carcinoma. A progressive dysphagia (first large solids, then small pieces through softer foods to liquids) is the characteristic presentation of a carcinoma. Strictures can occur, however, from a variety of causes and a barium swallow/gastroscopy is needed to establish a diagnosis.

STOMACH

Atrophic gastritis becomes more common in the elderly. The histological findings include decreased thickness of the gastric wall due to atrophy of the mucosa and muscularis mucosae; infiltration with leucocytes; and loss of gastric glands. It is associated with an increased risk of pernicious anaemia (vitamin B_{12} deficiency) and gastric carcinoma. Gastric atrophy may produce achlorhydria. Pepsin activity is reduced whilst gastrin levels increase (correlated to the presence of antibodies to parietal cells). Gastric emptying appears delayed for fats but not for carbohydrates.

Gastric ulcers are more common in elderly people, especially the benign giant ulcer. Complications include haemorrhage, perforation and pyloric obstruction with higher mortality rates. Gastric carcinoma is also more common, possibly because its predisposing conditions (e.g. pernicious anaemia) are more frequent. Atypical 'silent' presentation of gastric ulcers includes general debility, anorexia and weight loss.

SMALL BOWEL

The changes that occur here in normal ageing are quite subtle. Of clinical significance is that duodenal diverticula occur and bacterial colonization can cause steatorrhoea (fatty stools). This is due to bile salt deconjugation by the bacteria leading to malabsorption (especially of iron, calcium, folate and B_{12}). The appendix gradually becomes involuted with age and appendicitis is rare. Age changes in the small intestine are small and their significance doubtful.

LARGE BOWEL

The large bowel and its nerve and blood supply is probably the part of the gut most affected by 'ageing'. The pathological consequences carry considerable mortality, morbidity and misery in elderly people. The colon receives liquid ileal contents, absorbs water, sodium and chloride, secretes potassium, bicarbonate and mucus and then stores faeces until evacuation.

Histological changes include an increase in connective tissue, atrophy of the muscle layer and arteriosclerosis. Colonic diverticula increase with age in some populations (but not those eating high-fibre diets).

MOTILITY

Eating food normally stimulates gut motility (the gastro-colic reflex) which is thought to be hormonal in nature. The response is increased by physical activity and there is poor gut motility in an immobile person whatever the age. This relationship between gut motility and physical activity is one of the main factors affecting constipation in elderly people. Using radiopaque markers or dyes, elderly people have been shown to have a slower gut transit time. Constipation is a term used frequently yet it can mean different things such as a decreased frequency of bowel actions, the difficult passage of hard faeces or the increased retention of faecal material in the colon.

Causes of constipation

In elderly people there may be a combination of causes (Table 11.1). The main complication of constipation is faecal impaction which can lead to:

- faecal incontinence — impacted faeces act as a ball valve and liquid stool from higher up leaks around the faecal mass producing spurious diarrhoea;
- intestinal obstruction (rarely perforation and peritonitis);
- restlessness and agitation in the confused (but never causes confusion);
- retention of urine which may progress to overflow incontinence; and
- rectal bleeding due to mucosal ulceration.

Carcinomas of the colon and rectum are common in the elderly, a rectal examination being mandatory as part of the routine examination. Benign polyps of the large bowel, familial polyposis coli and ulcerative colitis are recognized as premalignant conditions. Ischaemic colitis is common in elderly people but because of good anastomotic channels atheroma of the mesenteric vessels causes less problems than in the brain and peripheral circulation.

Table 11.1 Causes of constipation

Primary
Slow transit time aggravated by immobility
Incomplete emptying of the bowel due to poor muscle tone, unsatisfactory toilet arrangements or mental confusion
Diminished awareness of a loaded rectum as in neurological disease
Ignoring the urge to defaecate due to immobility, pain, confusion, poor toilet arrangements
Low bulk content due to poor dentition or inadequate diet
Inadequate fluid intake

Secondary
Gastrointestinal disease, e.g. diverticular disease, carcinoma of colon or rectum, anorectal lesions such as fissures or haemorrhoids
Hypothyroidism, hypercalcaemia
Drugs, e.g. morphine derivatives, iron and anticholinergics

APPETITE AND NUTRITION IN ELDERLY PEOPLE

Appetite was thought to decline with age, yet studies have shown that in those who reach extreme old age without impairment of physical and mental capabilities food intake is unchanged. Most reduction in appetite is secondary to acute or chronic disease processes compounded by social factors such as isolation, poor housing and poverty. Control of appetite (satiety and hunger) can be viewed as conditioned reflexes which are learned early in life and are continuously modified by external (environmental) and internal (homeostatic) mechanisms. There is only a small but continuous decline in basal metabolic rate after age 60. Hungry rats and humans prefer carbohydrate-rich foods as these are often readily absorbed and satisfy quickly. The elderly person living alone existing on a diet of sweet tea, jam sandwiches and chocolate is the classic example for the development of widespread deficiencies. Beliefs about the likely wholesomeness of food on the basis of its appearance, colour, texture, smell and temperature are important in influencing appetite.

Meals are also social events and apart from health problems and medication etc. the ambience of a meal may to some extent determine appetite and actual amounts of food eaten — hence the value of luncheon clubs and day centres for the isolated, lonely, recently bereaved and mildly confused.

The flavour of food is a combination of taste, texture, smell and temperature, but perception of taste and smell decline with age (and smoking). Sweet, sour and to a lesser extent bitter are gradually lost, though salt perception is only impaired much later. These facts may to some extent explain age differences in meal flavours and 'the young sweet tooth'. The elderly also take longer to eat a meal and this is particularly important in institutions where food may be taken away before a person has finished and suboptimal nutrition result. Anorexia is commonly seen as an acute symptom with infections, malignant disease, depression and alcohol abuse, and as a side-effect of medication. It is also seen in severe dementia and post-stroke.

Table 11.2 Major factors which influence nutrition

Ignorance
Elderly women of today learnt their cooking skills in a time of poverty and shortages
Elderly men may have never had to cook for themselves, hence the term 'widower's scurvy'

Social isolation
The buying, preparing and eating of food is a social event (developed into an art in France), those living alone having a much poorer dietary intake

Physical disability
This may prevent people shopping, preparing and even eating food, e.g. rheumatoid arthritis, stroke

Mental disturbance
Depression and confusional states can markedly affect nutrition

Iatrogenic
Special diets ('gastric diet') are still being followed 40 years after a doctor advised them

Poverty
Existing on a state pension alone is equivalent to living on the poverty line. The elderly who can supplement their pension have been shown to have a better diet. In cold weather the choice may be between food or fuel and there is a close association between malnutrition and hypothermia

Impairment of appetite
By both emotional and physical causes

Dentition
Poor or absent dentition will alter a person's choice of diet (necessitating soft and mainly starchy foods)

Malabsorption
From whatever cause will affect nutritional state. Common causes of malabsorption in the elderly are post-gastric surgery, adult coeliac disease, pancreatic disease and bacterial overgrowth

Alcohol and drugs
With alcohol look for thiamine and folic acid deficiency

Increased requirements
Illness, pressure sores, infections and stress will all increase the requirements

Malnutrition is common in vulnerable sections of the population and studies have shown that about 7 per cent of the people show clinical signs of malnutrition. There is undoubtedly a further group with subclinical malnutrition, only diagnosed when disease or stress causes their condition to become overt. A dietary history is therefore an integral part of the assessment of an elderly person. The major factors that influence nutrition in the elderly are shown in Table 11.2.

Diagnosis

The diagnosis of nutritional deficiency states in elderly people is made more difficult by the usual symptoms and signs being masked by disease. Biochemical and haematological investigations can be helpful but caution is needed in that the quoted normal values are mainly from studies performed on medical students some years ago (they were not usually of retirement age and mostly male!).

It is necessary to be vigilant about the following more common deficiency states:

1. the anaemias
   —microcytic (iron deficiency/nutritional)
   —macrocytic (B_{12}, folate, hypothyroid etc.)
   —normocytic (chronic disease);
2. B complex deficiencies (riboflavin, niacin and pyridoxine);
3. vitamin C (ascorbic acid, resulting in scurvy, subclinical forms common);
4. vitamin D (osteomalacia).

Key points

- Periodontal disease is the main cause of teeth extraction.
- Currently the majority of elderly people are edentulous.
- Oesophageal problems (tertiary contractions, presbyoesophagus, phalangeal pouches, benign and malignant strictures) are common.
- Gastric ulcer may be symptomatic (haemorrhage, pain) or 'silent' producing general debility, anorexia and weight loss.
- Constipation is usually due to primary causes (decreased mobility, fluid intake and fibre) but can be due to secondary factors, e.g. hypothyroidism.
- Constipation never causes confusion.
- Appetite is unaffected in normal ageing.

- The flavour of food is a combination of taste, texture, smell and temperature but perceptions of taste and smell decline with age.
- Seven per cent of elderly people show clinical signs of malnutrition.
- Major factors which influence nutrition include ignorance, social isolation, physical and mental disability, poverty and illness.

FURTHER READING

Brocklehurst JC. The large bowel. In: Brocklehurst JC, Tallis RC, Fillit HM (eds), *Textbook of Geriatric Medicine and Gerontology*, 4th edn. Churchill Livingstone, Edinburgh, 1992.

Durrin JVGA, Lean MEJ. Nutrition — considerations for the elderly. In: Brocklehurst JC, Tallis RC, Fillit HM (eds), *Textbook of Geriatric Medicine and Gerontology*, 4th edn. Churchill Livingstone, Edinburgh, 1992.

Ferguson MWJ, Devlin H. Aging and the oro-facial tissues. In: Brocklehurst JC, Tallis RC, Fillit HM (eds), *Textbook of Geriatric Medicine and Gerontology*, 4th edn. Churchill Livingstone, Edinburgh, 1992.

Hellmans J, Vantrappen G (eds). *Gastrointestinal Tract Disorders in the Elderly*. Churchill Livingstone, London, 1984.

Reinus JF, Brandt LJ. The upper gastrointestinal tract. In: Brocklehurst JC, Tallis RC, Fillit HM (eds), *Textbook of Geriatric Medicine and Gerontology*, 4th edn. Churchill Livingstone, Edinburgh, 1992.

Texter EC (ed.). *The Ageing Gut*. Masson, New York, 1983.

12 THE AGEING IMMUNE SYSTEM

- Humoral immunity
- Thymus
- Cellular immunity
- Autoimmune disease
- Tissue grafts
- Cancer
- Diagnosis of infection
- Immunodeficiency in old age

The age-related changes that occur in the immune system have been described as 'dramatic'. The subsequent immune dysfunction increases our susceptibility to infections, cancer and autoimmune disease. To function adequately the immune system is dependent upon numerous factors including histocompatibility genes, hormonal changes, age, nutrition, antigen exposure and even psychological state.

The immune system has numerous component parts: bone marrow, lymph nodes, lymphatic vessels, reticuloendothelial system, spleen and thymus. The cell types and secretory factors are listed in Table 12.1.

Table 12.1 Cell types and secretory factors

B lymphocytes
T lymphocytes
Monocytes
Granulocytes
Natural killer cells
Thymic factors
Lymphokines

HUMORAL IMMUNITY

Once the first two defence systems in the body are breached (skin/mucosa and phagocytic digestion by macrophages) the third line of defence against an infecting organism is the humoral response. This involves an attack by specific antibodies secreted by mature B cells. Levels of natural antibody and isoantibody appear to decline with age, indicating deterioration in the B cell system (this is probably qualitative rather than quantitative). The primary antibody response, however, is also reduced in old age and this may have clinical implications — there is an age-related rise in common infectious diseases.

THYMUS

Following puberty the thymus declines both anatomically and functionally until middle-age thymic hormone levels are negligible or absent and the gland is vestigial. The thymus matures T cells giving them suppressor and helper characteristics. It is not clear whether there are changes of clinical significance associated with this decline.

CELLULAR IMMUNITY

There is no obvious decrease in circulating lymphocyte numbers with age; however, it is probable that T lymphocyte function deteriorates. It is well known that acquired delayed hypersensitivity reactions are reduced with age (anergy) as assessed by skin testing. The reaction should activate T-helper cells to release lymphokines, eventually causing localized tissue inflammation and destruction of the antigen. Anergy may have clinical significance in the reactivation of such diseases as tuberculosis and herpes zoster and in the clinical response to infections.

Macrophages appear to function normally in elderly people. Neutrophil function may be less good (seen clinically in the problem of severe staphylococcal infections in old age).

AUTOIMMUNE DISEASE

Some of the more common autoimmune diseases are listed in Table 12.2. A few appear to be related to age, for example rheumatoid arthritis and autoimmune thyroiditis. In these conditions antibodies and/or T lymphocytes attack self-antigens. It appears that there is a genetic predisposition (via histocompatibility genes) and hence some people will develop autoimmune disorders as they grow older.

Table 12.2 Autoimmune diseases

Addison's disease
Hashimoto's thyroiditis
Haemolytic anaemia
Myasthenia gravis
Pemphigus vulgaris
Rheumatoid arthritis

Although antibody production declines, auto-antibody production increases (nuclear antigens, immunoglobulin and gastric parietal cell) with the aforementioned rise in autoimmune disease.

TISSUE GRAFTS

Generally there is less immune rejection of tissue grafts in elderly people (including organ transplants).

CANCER

As we age there is an increase in the number of cells that 'escape' normal growth and become cancer cells. At younger ages these abnormal cells are detected (probably via surface antigens) and are destroyed by macrophages, antibodies, T cells and natural killer cells. In old age two things occur which probably account for the increase in clinical cancer: (a) there is an increase in cancer cell numbers and (b) surface antigens may be absent.

The thymus has a maturing effect on T lymphocytes in middle age and this declines with advancing years. Other lymphoid organs (gut lymphoid tissue, tonsils and appendix) get smaller with age. Stem cells (the precursors of lymphocytes) still replicate in old age but their function is impaired.

DIAGNOSIS OF INFECTION

The above changes have specific clinical features but also more general implications. Some elderly people do not mount either a pyrexial response or a leucocytosis in the face of obvious infection. This may not be 'normal' ageing but is common enough to warrant mention. Studies have shown that if rectal rather than oral temperatures are taken, more patients show a pyrexia indicating that the site of temperature measurement may be more important than the underlying immune changes. It does mean, however, that treatment may need to be given if infection is suspected on clinical grounds before bacteriological confirmation and in the absence of some of the more common physical signs.

IMMUNODEFICIENCY IN OLD AGE

It has been pointed out that there are many similarities between elderly people with age-related immunodeficiency states and those whose acquired immunodeficiency is due to HIV. In old age the clinical presentation includes:

1. frequent and prolonged infections;
2. failure to respond to normal therapy;
3. infections due to unusual organisms;
4. reactivation of tuberculosis or herpes zoster; and
5. lack of fever, leucocytosis, few chest X-ray changes with pneumonia, poor rebound tenderness with peritonitis.

In older people this acquired immunodeficiency can have many causes, including malnutrition, drugs (e.g. steroids, NSAIDs, antidepressants, etc.), intercurrent disease (e.g. acute and chronic infections), cancer and stress. Treatment of these causes can thus have a significant impact on the immune response. It is also important to remember HIV as a potential secondary cause. An increasing number of elderly people are HIV positive (due to earlier transfusions during surgery or sexual activity).

Secondary causes of immunodeficiency should be sought and where possible treated. Primary (idiopathic) immunodeficiency is an area currently undergoing extensive research involving thymic hormone replacement and other immuno-enhancing agents. Protection against disease in old age includes adequate immunization. The clinical implications of acquired immunodeficiency in particular groups, e.g. the institutionalized and physically frail, mean that single-dose vaccines will sometimes fail to achieve sufficiently high antibody titres and repeat vaccinations may become necessary (pneumococcal pneumonia, influenza, tetanus toxoid).

Key points

- The thymus gland declines both anatomically and functionally after puberty.

- To function adequately the immune system is dependent upon numerous factors including histocompatibility genes, age, nutrition and antigen exposure.
- Levels of natural antibody decline with age because of a deterioration in the B cell system.
- T lymphocyte function deteriorates.
- Autoimmune diseases increase with age; there is a genetic predisposition via histocompatibility genes.
- There is less immune rejection of tissue grafts.
- The immune system is less effective in destroying cancer cells with advancing age.
- Some elderly people do not mount a pyrexial response or a leucocytosis in the face of obvious infection — treatment should be given on clinical grounds before bacteriological confirmation.
- The concept of an age-related acquired immunodeficiency state is a useful one.
- Secondary causes of acquired immunodeficiency should be sought and where possible treated.
- The changes in the immune system mean that in the chronically ill repeat vaccinations may be necessary.

FURTHER READING

Fillit H, Meyer L, Bana C. Immunology of aging. In: Brocklehurst JC, Tallis RC, Fillit HM (eds), *Textbook of Geriatric Medicine and Gerontology,* 4th edn. Churchill Livingstone, Edinburgh, 1992.

Sternberg H. Ageing of the immune system. In: Timiras P (ed.), *Physiological Basis of Ageing and Geriatrics.* Macmillan, New York, 1988.

13 THE AGEING PSYCHE

- Disengagement
- Use-it-or-lose-it
- Denial
- Losses
- Successful ageing

Psychological changes in old age are difficult to research because most studies are cross-sectional, comparing the attitudes and behaviour of people of different ages at the same point in time. When differences are found it is tempting to put them down to ageing, but it is clear that generational, or cohort, effects may be the cause. For example, it is well known that as we get older we become more preoccupied with our bowel function and more likely to take laxatives. However, middle-aged people are very concerned about indigestion and frequently take antacids, and young people subscribe to the value of fibre and vitamins to remain vital. These anxieties and behaviours reflect the eras in which successive generations grew up, and the prevalent medical concerns and advice given at different times.

Some of the cross-sectional data reinforce stereotypes and enter into the dogma of the psychology of ageing. People stop having sex as they get older — true or false? The Kinsey Report, a cross-sectional study, found that 20 per cent of males were impotent at 65 years and 50 per cent at 75 years. However, a longitudinal study which followed men for six years (admittedly only a short time) found only a small decline in activity.

It is likely that if you start out sexually active, you will keep it up.

DISENGAGEMENT

One of the most popular theories of the psychology of ageing is disengagement. This theory grew out of the Duke University longitudinal studies of ageing. Investigators observed that those subjects with the highest life satisfaction (contentment, happiness) were those who had withdrawn from active engagement in social activities — the 'rocking chair' syndrome. It is unlikely that this method of growing old gracefully would suit everyone, and probably reflects biases in the sample of volunteers studied; perhaps they were the only ones who were not too busy to answer the interviewers' questions.

USE-IT-OR-LOSE-IT

In contrast to disengagement, the 'use-it-or-lose-it' approach to ageing has great popular acclaim, and is a guiding principle in promoting a positive attitude to ageing. Evidence that physical capacity is maintained by regular activity is abundant. Whether psychological and other abilities are maintained by regular practice is uncertain, but it seems a reasonable assumption. Maintaining social engagement, learning new skills, making new friends, going on holidays are all things that a large number of better-off old people do, and obtain great satisfaction in the process. Such approaches to encouraging involvement with others have to be tempered with a realization that the hearty 'joining in' spirit is not shared by everyone.

DENIAL

A mild denial of ageing is commonplace, and is promoted by the media in their 'keep young and beautiful if you want to be loved' youth image. Denial of some of the problems (e.g. financial, illness, bereavement) that accompany ageing can lead to an unwillingness to seek help, and to a tendency for problems to get worse. People who adopt the denial strategy may battle on to maintain independence in the face of falling standards. In extreme cases they may fall into the Diogenes syndrome (see Chapter 28) with awful self-neglect.

LOSSES

Old age is a time of multiple losses; of job, status, partner, health, wealth and so on. This gloomy picture of old age is central to the view of old age as a time of reflection on previous achievements to counterbalance the losses experienced. Surviving friends and relatives, coping with life's tragedies and experiencing its joys may be a source of inspiration, but with time, may be a cause of great unhappiness. Increasingly, older people become concerned about the need to leave something for their children and grandchildren, or to leave some record of their lives as part of the preparation for death. Death is one of the last taboos in Western society, and many elderly people do not have opportunities to talk about those who have died ('Don't go on about him, you'll only upset yourself'), or indeed their own deaths. Many elderly people will talk very freely about death, even to comparative strangers.

The specific illness behaviours of older people are largely to do with impending death, and associated dependency on others. Older people may become overly health conscious, wanting every symptom checked out and becoming over-reliant on their doctors. Women who have been traditional care givers may find it much harder to accept a dependent role than men who have always 'suffered' with learned, socially sanctioned dependency on women!

SUCCESSFUL AGEING

A recent arrival on the psychology of ageing scene is the concept of achieving successful ageing through selection, adaptation and optimization of ability. An elderly person may be unable to carry out all the activities of daily living and social engagement of a younger person. Doctors, nurses, therapists and social workers have relatively stereotyped views of how old people should invest their energy and time. For example, maintaining continence is viewed as a worthwhile objective for the expenditure of energy. However, if a person has only a finite amount of energy (perhaps because of physical ill-health) it may make better sense to exhaust that energy through some other preferable activity; perhaps going to the pub. Consequently we should expect elderly people to select activities for themselves and not impose our own ideas on them.

Next a person may require help with achieving their goals. This may require adaptation of the person's method of carrying out a task, or of the environment, or adaptation of the goal itself to make it more feasible. For example, the pub may have to come to the patient in hospital, rather than the patient to the pub. Optimization of ability refers to the practice required to achieve an adequate level of performance, and thus achieve the set goal.

The value of this theory of ageing is its wide applicability to the young old, the old old, and the oldest old. It also points a way for partners, relatives, friends and professionals to aid the process of successful ageing by emphasizing choices, the need to make priorities and to avoid stereotyped, repetitive lifestyles, particularly in institutions.

Perhaps the only certainty about the ageing psyche is that generalizations are imprecise, and heterogeneity is the rule.

| Key points |

- Cross-sectional studies are of very limited relevance in examining psychological aspects of ageing as the effects of both cohort and time period are likely to be marked. Such studies will tend to overestimate the true age-related changes: sexual activity is much less common in old men (from cross-sectional data), but sexually active old men are likely to remain active (longitudinal data).

- Disengagement theory states that elderly people gain contentment from withdrawing from active engagement — the 'rocking chair' syndrome.
- Use-it-or-lose-it theory is a more positive approach, suggesting that old people will gain most enjoyment (and feel better) if they keep up activities and learn new ones.
- Denial of ageing is a common defence mechanism, and may lead to failure to seek help when problems arise.
- Losses are a commonplace in old age, and none the less a source of much sorrow. Many elderly people find comfort in talking about their losses, particularly of intimate partners.
- Successful ageing is the latest theory emphasizing the need to select activities, adapt to circumstances and optimize ability in the chosen activities.

- Psychological ageing is very variable and no single theory is adequate, but each may help explain the responses of some elderly people.

FURTHER READING

Baltes P, Baltes M. *Successful Ageing*. Cambridge University Press, Cambridge, 1990.

Kinsey AC, Pomeroy WB, Martin CE *et al. Sexual Behaviour in the Human Male.* Saunders, Philadelphia, 1948.

Martin CE. Factors affecting sexual functioning in 60–79 year old married males. *Arch Sex Behav* 1981; **10**: 399–420.

Murphy E, Brown G. Life events, psychiatric disturbance and physical illness. *Br J Psychiat* 1980; **136**: 326–338.

Neugarten BN. Time, age and the life cycle. *Am J Psychiat* 1979; **136**: 887–893.

PART TWO
ESSENTIAL MEDICINE
OF OLD AGE

14 THE HISTORY OF GERIATRIC MEDICINE

- The Poor Laws
- Workhouse life
- The birth of modern geriatric medicine
- Social or medical care?
- Types of service
- The future

Since the beginning of recorded medicine doctors have been interested in old age and its diseases. Pythagoras recorded the ages of man as childhood, youth, manhood and old age and the most important of these was old age or the Gerocomice. Hippocrates (400 BC) wrote: 'old men suffer from difficulty in breathing, catarrh accompanied by coughing, strangury, difficult micturition, pains at the joints, kidney disease, dizziness, apoplexy, cachexia, pruritus of the whole body, sleeplessness, watery discharges from the bowels, eyes and nostrils, dullness of sight, cataract, hardness of hearing.' In Roman times units for the care of old people were called 'Gerocomia'. By AD 1000 the Arabian Avicenna (called the 'Prince of Physicians') outlined the care of the aged in his Canon of Medicine.

THE POOR LAWS

In medieval times the care of the sick (if it occurred at all) was based in religious institutions — mainly monasteries. Some religious orders in large premises (e.g. Tintern Abbey) built hospital wings and some monks became specialists in medical and nursing care.

Later, convents took on the caring/nursing role which in some centres continues to this day. Henry VIII, however, dissolved many of the monasteries in the sixteenth century, and later under Elizabeth I new laws were created to try to bridge the gap between alms/charity and vagrancy. The Elizabethan 'Poor Laws' were two Acts of Parliament passed in 1597 and 1601 specifically to keep the 'poor' off the streets and hence to discourage vagrancy (and its assumed concomitant lawlessness).

The Act of 1601 established a system of parish relief of the poor financed by compulsory 'poor rates' levied on property. The migrant poor remained a problem so in 1662 an Act of Settlement defined that after 40 days residency the parish was liable for such a resident. The parish was chosen as the basic unit because the essential charitable nature of the law was meant to come from the community. This may have worked in rural areas but in towns and cities rich parishes often had the smallest dependent population and labour mobility ensured that work and home parishes were different. Initially the routine work (collecting rates and distributing relief) was carried out by churchwardens. This was supervised via the vestry meeting (an assembly of ratepayers), and at the county level by magistrates.

The Poor Law system designed for temporary unemployment and short-term sickness became the provider of care for the old, chronic sick, single-parent families (widows, deserted wives and unmarried mothers) and orphans. The infamous workhouses began appearing in the 1630s because the laws stated that the poor had to work in order to obtain relief. In 1722 Knatchbull's Act of Parliament was passed enabling all parishes to voluntarily form into unions to build workhouses and limit the amounts of relief given out. The aim was to encourage hard work, thriftiness and possibly limit family size, concepts born in the age of Adam Smith, only to be rediscovered in the 1980s. Not surprisingly, a number of devices were tried to deter or uncover the potential fraudster, including legislation requiring 'paupers' to wear a badge with the letter 'p' and also published lists of relief receivers.

WORKHOUSE LIFE

By 1782 workhouses were renamed poorhouses and acknowledged as asylums for the old and infirm. A few years later the ruling classes felt the ripples of fear from the French Revolution as discontent spread to the UK. Bread famines occurred and unemployment soared, resulting in numerous measures to keep order yet still provide meagre relief. The industrial revolution was beginning and with it more rural unemployment. Following the Napoleonic War reform was long overdue. A Royal Commission was set up and in 1834 the Poor Law Amendment Act was passed. It deliberately set out to stigmatize the poor and its catchphrase was 'less eligibility'. The regimen of the workhouse was harshened, with men, women and children strictly segregated (exceptions being made for elderly couples of good character). Food was meagre (though presumably less awful than the diet of the destitute outside). The sick and elderly were given better rations. Work involved either laundry, cooking, stoking the boilers or tending the sick. Stonebreaking and oakum picking (separating the fibres of old ropes) were also part of this regime. The giving out of alms continued (out-relief) so that only about 20 per cent of Victorian paupers saw the inside of the poorhouse. However, the aged and chronic sick provided the majority of the inmates.

Most workhouses developed an infirmary initially for the people who became ill suddenly but the beds quickly became filled with the chronic sick and the disabled. Medical and nursing care were appalling and they soon developed a terrible reputation. The ill rich were visited in their own homes. Victims of accidents or those able to get 'sponsorship' via a wealthy subscriber were admitted to the voluntary hospitals (most of the major teaching hospitals in England came under this category). However, they were disinclined to take anything 'chronic' for fear of blocking the beds (and hence revenue) and would refuse admission of dubious cases. The parallel with some US practice and this re-emerging ethos in the UK health service is striking. By far the worst were the workhouse infirmaries (and their sister institutions the poor law infirmaries). Conditions were so bad that campaigns were organized by the *Lancet* and Florence Nightingale and things gradually improved. Poverty surveys concerning the elderly by Booth and Rowntree helped educate and sway public opinion but it was still necessary to wait for the Liberal reforms after the turn of the twentieth century before the provision of state pensions as a way out of poverty for the old became a reality.

THE BIRTH OF MODERN GERIATRIC MEDICINE

In France the term 'gerocomie' was used to describe the need for a separate facility for elderly people. In America, Nascher in 1907 coined the word 'geriatrics' (literally, 'old physician') to denote that branch of medicine dealing with the care of the aged. To live to be old, however, one must not die young and at the turn of the century improvements in public health measures and better housing led to a dramatic decline in childhood mortality. The unequal access to medical care (financial and due to age) continued and the plight of the ill elderly was appalling. Within the midst of this degradation and sickness dedicated doctors taking an interest in the care of elderly people began to emerge. These luminaries founded what was later to be called geriatric medicine. Marjorie Warren as a newly qualified consultant in 1935 wrote powerful descriptions of the dreadful conditions awaiting her in the workhouse wards of the West Middlesex Hospital:

> having lost all hope of recovery with the knowledge that independence has gone, and with a feeling of helplessness and frustration, the patient rapidly loses morale and self-respect and develops an apathetic or peevish, irritable, sullen,

morose and aggressive temperament which leads to laziness and faulty habits, with or without incontinence. Lack of interest in the surroundings, confinement to bed and a tendency to incontinence soon produce pressure sores, with the necessity for more nursing, of a kind that is appreciated by the patient. An increase of weight, especially the anterior abdominal wall, and an inevitable loss of muscle tone make for a complete bed-ridden state. Soon the well-known disuse atrophy of the lower limbs, with postural deformities, stiffness of joints and contractures completes the unhappy picture of human forms who are not only heavy nursing cases and a drag on society, but also are no pleasure to themselves and a source of acute distress to their friends.

The low status of the elderly became apparent during World War II when civilian casualties and wounded soldiers caused the aged sick to be evacuated into the workhouse wards. Complaints of neglect and under-treatment caused the Ministry of Health to set up an investigation which revealed a prevailing air of apathy about the care of the old. In contrast Dr Marjorie Warren and a friend, Dr Trevor Howell, outlined a new basis for care indicating that the frail elderly and chronic sick could only be properly treated after a thorough history had been taken and a full examination performed, followed by what is now seen as the rudiments of the art/science of 'rehabilitation'. Treatable conditions were corrected and movement and muscle tone helped by standing exercises using the rails at the end of the bed. Wards were redecorated and painted and a system of remedial exercises for stroke patients was instituted in an atmosphere of hope, activity and cheerfulness. Patients with fractured femurs were operated upon and then mobilized early. The slogan 'bed is bad' became one of the basic mottoes of geriatric medicine. Geriatricians with long waiting lists started visiting those patients at home to assess and pre-empt complications — another milestone in care. Trevor Howell, dealing with the Chelsea pensioners, began research into the normal phenomena associated with ageing. This marked the start of clinical gerontology, the scientific study of ageing and disease.

SOCIAL OR MEDICAL CARE?

Lord Amulree at the Ministry of Health (responsible for the aged and chronic sick) was impressed and saw the future — the new NHS taking responsibility not only for the chronic sick but also the frail elderly, managed by a new and developing breed of doctors — geriatricians. The argument that frailty in old age was often due to illness impressed him and when the 1948 National Assistance Act was debated in Parliament he argued that the frail elderly should form part of the responsibility of the NHS not of local government. He lost the vote and hence the frail old became (under Part 3 of the Act) the responsibility of local government via the social services to be housed in 'Part 3' homes. This was a poor outcome because he and the geriatricians were right and the difficulty remains to this day. Local authority residential homes are full of people placed there because of a perceived frailty; this has led to recent surveys showing that at least 50 per cent of residents are incontinent of urine and up to 75 per cent mentally confused. Frail? probably; sick? definitely. In the community and in hospitals are elderly people unable to find places in Part 3 homes, yet the homes are full of people who with earlier treatment might have continued to manage in their own home.

In 1947 Dr Howell and Lord Amulree founded the Medical Society for the Care of the Elderly, later to become the British Geriatrics Society. Through the Society and their personal teaching of interested doctors the specialty blossomed with national and international repercussions. Teaching hospitals founded chairs in the subject, bringing in the first wave of teaching excellence to undergraduates — Professors Williamson, Exton-Smith, Isaacs and Brocklehurst to mention but a few. Their inspired revolution in the medical, social and environmental aspects of health care led to enormous changes in bed, ward and even hospital management. Medical and nursing practices were challenged; for example, the use of tilt-back chairs and cot-sides were banned.

One area, the long-stay/continuing-care sector, remained a difficult backwater. The patients remained in poor accommodation with little or no medical and therapy input. The change in this state of affairs was largely helped by one man, Professor Peter Millard. His constant fight to improve the quality of care, indeed the quality of life, for this group has led to this area of care being considered to have its own separate expertise and knowledge base, especially within the nursing and paramedical fields. His unit led the way in showing what was possible with dedication, imagination and humanity.

TYPES OF SERVICE

Health care of the elderly/medicine of old age now has hundreds of consultants working closely with their counterparts in the psychiatry of old age and with multidisciplinary teams. Different types of practice have emerged. In the age-related service admission usually depends on being over a chronological point (occasionally over 65 but usually over 75 or even 85). Integrated services range from close integration with consultant physicians in general medicine (a physician and geriatrician being on-take together or the geriatrician being one of the physicians on the on-call rota) to a cooperation model with physicians but rotas stay separate. This is the case in appropriate-care/needs-related services which operate broadly on the needs of the patient, concentrating especially on rehabilitation, and hence do not admit all elderly people. Age-related and fully integrated services have attracted many other specialists (e.g. gastroenterologists, chest physicians) into the field via posts which combine their speciality with 'an interest' in elderly people. The advantages and disadvantages of the various services are still being debated, the issues and arguments being complex. The service, however, must respond to local needs and be locally responsive. The purchasers of health care thus have a view and an input into the local debate via the placing of contracts and insisting on a cost-effective service.

THE FUTURE

A new era is in prospect. Hospital-based continuing care (free to the user and family) is a diminishing resource. The Conservative government's decade of sponsoring the expansion of the private sector (and its financial penalizing of the NHS sector currently providing the care) spells its contraction and possible extinction. The starting point of the speciality of geriatric medicine may cease to exist.

NHS continuing care is only (in the government's view) for the complex patient needing specialized nursing and medical care. The corollary of this is that the majority of elderly people who previously 'qualified' for continuing care are now expected to receive this care in nursing homes. The very name 'nursing home' implies that a degree of professional expertise is offered, and the dilemma to the individual is that it is the doctor who decides (hopefully via a continuing care panel) who is deemed complex enough to receive free hospital care. Nursing home care is means-tested until one's last £8000 of savings are reached. This means that all savings/monies and property will be used to pay for care despite lifelong tax contributions. Social continuing care (rest homes and Part 3 homes) have always been means-tested. The cradle to grave motto of the NHS has proved to be too expensive to honour. As more and more elderly people and their carers and families realize the implications of this policy shift true hardship and anger materialize.

Geriatric medicine arose from the appalling neglect of the elderly people in workhouses; one hopes it will not be rediscovered in the nursing and residential homes in the future.

Key points

- Elderly people have interested doctors since the science of medicine began.
- The Elizabethan 'Poor Law' system became the provider of care for the old and chronic sick.
- The workhouse and poorhouse infirmary developed terrible reputations. This institutional 'stigma' remains with elderly people to this day.
- The term 'geriatrics' was coined in the US by Nascher and literally means 'old physician'.
- Dr Marjorie Warren and Dr Trevor Howell helped found the speciality of geriatric medicine in this country.
- The 1948 National Assistance Act irrevocably split the 'sick' elderly (NHS) from the 'frail' (social services) — a split opposed by Lord Amulree on the advice of geriatricians.
- Standards of teaching, research and care rose with the appointment of the first 'wave' of academic specialists in geriatric medicine. Many medical schools now have Chairs in the speciality.
- The types of service provision into which elderly people are admitted are usually either age-related or a form of integrated care.
- NHS continuing care is a diminishing resource but remains free to the user and their family.
- Nursing home care is means-tested and will involve the use of all an elderly person's resources down to a set figure.
- Continuing care (long-stay care) requires the greatest skills and a high input of resources from the various professionals.

FURTHER READING

Nascher IL. Geriatrics. *NY Med J* 1909; xx Aug 21: 358–359.

Oxley GW. *Poor Relief in England and Wales 1601–1834*. David & Charles, London, 1974.

Rose ME. *The English Poor Law*. David & Charles, London, 1971.

Warren MW. Care of the chronic aged sick. *Lancet* 1946; i: 841–843.

15 ELDERLY PEOPLE IN SOCIETY

- Stereotypes and ageism
- Demography
- Heterogeneity of elderly people
- Care in the community
- Institutional care

STEREOTYPES AND AGEISM

The very phrase 'the elderly' provokes an image in the mind: frail, confused, little old ladies, some of them nice like your granny, some of them not. Many other social groups experience stereotyping in society — ethnic minorities, homosexuals and lesbians, professional groups, trade unionists — partly because this is a means for people to cope with their ignorance, and deal with people they may fear. Stereotyping helps people to make sense of society, and their place in it. The phenomenon will not disappear, and advocates of elderly people (which includes elderly people themselves, as well as professionals) have a duty to ensure that some of the adverse consequences of stereotyping are reduced. Stereotypes lead to prejudice; this is ageism (Table 15.1).

The last four decades have been a period of growth and reconstruction following World War II. The major emphasis has been on young people — our future — often at the expense of the other end of the age spectrum. Society has become well-geared to the needs of young people because they are a major economic force,

Table 15.1 The stereotyped view of old people

Old people:
  need similar services
  are of little value
  are a burden on society
  are slow to accept change
  cannot look after themselves
  are deaf and need to be shouted at
  are sweet
  are like children

spending large amounts of money. Moreover youth culture, young looks and ideals have often been promoted by advertising agencies and the mass media.

The 1990s have seen a dawning of realization that young people are getting scarcer: school rolls are falling in many parts of the UK; the demand for young people in the workplace (particularly in health and social services) far exceeds supply. By contrast, there are more old people around, and some of them have relatively large amounts of money to spend — they are now an economic force to be considered by the market. This is now reflected in recent Paris fashion shows which featured many male and female models over 60 years old.

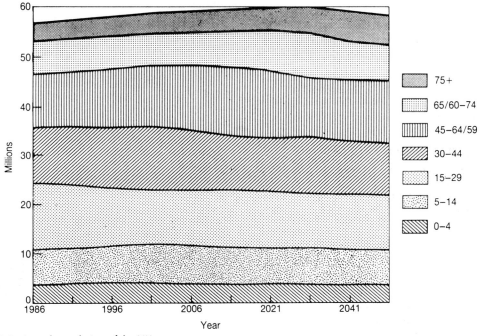

Millions

Figure 15.1 Projected population of the UK

Legend:
- 75+
- 65/60–74
- 45–64/59
- 30–44
- 15–29
- 5–14
- 0–4

In the USA, the 'greying of America' has been associated with a new wave of militancy amongst elderly people — The Grey Panthers! Elderly people have campaigned vigorously to ensure that politicians do not ignore the fact that they have needs that should be met by society and that they have paid taxes longer than most. From the political standpoint a key issue is that they have a lot of votes to contribute during elections.

DEMOGRAPHY

Remarkable changes in the age structure of the population have occurred over the last century which have been caused by two major forces: reductions in fertility and declines in infant mortality (not from better health care but from socio-economic development). These forces are discussed in Chapter 1.

The numbers of old people have risen from about 2 million in 1901 to around 10 million in 1991. Census figures and projections since 1971 are shown in Table 15.2.

Table 15.2 Pensioners* in Britain (millions)

	1971	1981	1991	2001
Population	54.4	54.8	55.2	56.0
60+/65+	8.9	9.8	10.1	9.9
Percentage	16.4	17.9	18.3	17.7

*Women 60+, Men 65+

But what do we mean by 'old people'. Old age is a long time — many people now survive into their high 80s, or even 90s. So it may last as long as 20–30 years. As long as many reading this text have been alive! It is necessary to split the elderly up into smaller age-groups to see what has been happening to them over the last few decades.

Census figures are also used to predict what will happen in the future (Fig. 15.1). Population prediction is a risky business, but provided there are no world wars or life-threatening epidemics, and we are not too ambitious in predicting the future too far ahead, predictions have given good guidance to what will happen. On the other hand, planners have been less good at doing anything about the demographic predictions.

HETEROGENEITY OF ELDERLY PEOPLE

Heterogeneity is made up of two Greek words: *heteros* meaning 'other', and *genos* meaning 'kind'. We use the term to mean 'made up of diverse kinds of people'. Old people are simply young people who have lived for a longer time than others. The idea of being a pensioner has led to chronological age (the number of years lived) being used to define 'old age'. We tend to think of the elderly as those people over 60 or 65 years. Such a definition is, of course, arbitrary.

It is useful to think of old people in three distinct groups: the young old (65–74), the old old (75–84), and the oldest old (85+). The social and biological characteristics of people in each of these age groups is sufficiently distinct to make these categories meaningful. For example, the young old are recently retired, tend to be wealthier than other elderly people, and often provide much of the care for the oldest old. By contrast the oldest old were born at the turn of the century, many of the women never married, or lost husbands in one of the World Wars. They went through the economic slump of the 1930s, and have tended to be poor, and live in old, unmodernized houses. They are much more likely to be disabled by physical and mental illness, and to live alone (Fig. 15.2).

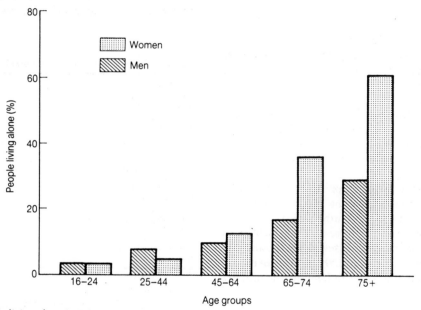

Figure 15.2 People living alone in Britain in 1988

CARE IN THE COMMUNITY

Most old people want to live in their own homes and fortunately the vast majority do. The present community care legislation in the UK (National Health Service & Community Care Act 1990) tends to make us think that community care is something new. It is not, and services to allow elderly people to live in their own homes have been around for a very long time (Fig. 15.3).

The services that are offered fall into six main categories: relatives and friends (informal carers); local authority social services; local health services; 'independent' (i.e. private and voluntary) sector services; local housing department services; and the central government department of social security. The characteristics of each of the services is very different, as is the range of services on offer. Informal carers are always available and will inevitably have to carry out whatever task needs doing, regardless of time of day, or skill required to do the job properly. By contrast,

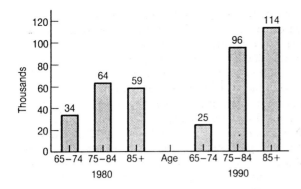

Figure 15.3 People living in institutional care in England, 1980 and 1990 (Department of Health estimates)

statutory services tend to provide much more circumscribed services, and disputes over who does what are increasingly common as services come under increased pressure.

Table 15.3 shows the main services provided by different agencies. No wonder that with so many providers of services it is sometimes difficult to work out who should do what, and who will pay for what. In part, this is what the community care legislation hopes to simplify.

For example, the dispute over who should bathe an elderly person — district nursing services or local authority home care services — has led to no baths at all in some areas. The task has now been redefined as 'social bathing' to put it firmly into the hands of the local authority services. Furthermore, many statutory services have to be paid for directly by the user.

COMMUNITY CARE LEGISLATION

The Act was due to come into effect in 1991, but was only implemented in 1993. The major change is that local authority social service departments now have lead responsibility for assessment of the individual needs of dependent elderly people, defining and managing the services provided and overall planning and monitoring of care for elderly (and disabled) people. Local authorities are also major providers of

services to elderly people (Table 15.3), but it is intended that the independent sector should take a much greater part in providing basic services like meals, home helps, respite care in future. This is being encouraged by central government limits on the amount of money local authorities can spend on services provided directly by themselves.

It is still too early to know whether these changes have had the desired effects of ensuring that individual clients no longer get a 'take it or leave it' package of services. Preliminary work suggests that the situation is very patchy, with some areas doing well and others, particularly inner cities, doing worse. Common problems are the delay involved in obtaining an assessment by local social services, disagreements between relatives and social services on need for services, and insufficient resources to meet needs.

Table 15.3 Some of the services provided for elderly people

Informal carers
Personal hygiene
Domestic tasks
Nursing tasks
Financial help
Counselling
Almost anything!

Local authority social services
Home helps
Meals on wheels
Part 3 homes
Social worker
Good neighbour schemes
Adult fostering
Respite care
Occupational therapy
Day centres
Lunch clubs

Local health services
Family doctor: treatment, 75+ screening
Hospital beds
Home nursing
Outpatients
Pharmacist
Therapists
Chiropody
Dietician

Private services
Institutional beds
Private nursing
Limited home care services

Voluntary services
Crossroads
Age Concern projects
Good neighbour schemes
Lunch clubs
Day centres
Residential homes

INSTITUTIONAL CARE

Institutional care is provided in three main settings: the local authority Part 3 (of the National Assistance Act, 1948) residential homes; the hospital long-stay wards; and the 'independent' sector — private residential and nursing homes, and 'not-for-profit' housing association residential homes (Fig. 15.4). A small number of specialist homes exist, for example, homes for elderly actors, elderly seamen, Jewish homes. These are usually run on a charitable basis.

These institutions have certain informal rules for selection of appropriate clients. In general, Part 3 and residential homes will take clients who are independently mobile (with or without aids), can dress themselves, and are continent of urine and faeces. Some will not take patients with dementia syndromes if there are associated behaviour problems (e.g. wandering, biting). Residential homes are not staffed by nurses, but by care attendants, and do not have sufficient staff or equipment to look after very dependent people. Nursing homes must have at least one trained nurse on the staff, but in practice the bulk of the care is provided by untrained care assistants. Nursing homes have variable selection criteria, and there is increasing evidence that private homes are taking less severely disabled patients than the hospital long-stay wards. This is not surprising since disabled people cost more to manage well, which eats into profit margins.

A major difference between long-stay hospital care and other institutional care is that the former is free! Consequently there can be conflict in deciding who should have a free hospital long-stay bed, and who should have to use their own resources to be looked after in other institutions. Escalating costs in the private sector preclude all but the relatively wealthy from going into a private nursing home. This has led to terrible disputes between hospitals who wish to discharge dependent elderly people to private sector care and patients and their relatives. In the private and local authority sector payment is determined by ability to pay (means tested). Central government guidance is contradictory: on the one hand, hospitals have an obligation to provide free NHS long-term care for those who need it; but on the other hand, the government wants to see the majority of people paying for their own long-term care.

It might be argued that the uncontrolled growth of private residential and nursing homes subsidized by the public purse was one of the main forces leading to the change in community care organization. It is a good example of how 'free markets' can lead to growth that is neither desirable — most people don't want to be in institutions — nor cost-effective. Of course, 'the market' was not really a free one. Central government funds were available to people wishing to go into private residential and nursing home care. The cost rose from £10 million in 1979 to £1 billion in 1989 and by the time of implementation of community care policy in 1993, had reached over £2 billion!

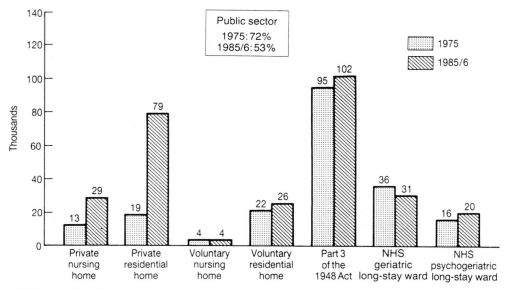

Figure 15.4 Elderly people in long-term care in England, 1975 to 1985/86 (Laing, 1988)

No amount of community care will stop some elderly people requiring institutional care, particularly the oldest old, living alone. A society that does not provide for such needs has ceased to care.

Key points

- Stereotypes of old age and old people are common and may disadvantage old people.
- The demographic changes are best classified into age bands: young old (65–74), old old (75–84), and oldest old (85+). The numbers of the oldest old will increase dramatically over the next 30 years.
- Care in the community is provided by many different agencies: informal carers; social services; health services; housing departments; independent sector. Each agency has a different range of services, operates under different constraints, and with a different philosophy.
- However much community care is provided for elderly people a small number will require institutional care. Without this back-up community care will not work.
- The growth in private sector nursing and residential homes has been extraordinary; the social security bill has grown from £10 million in 1979 to over £2 billion in 1993.

FURTHER READING

Caring for People. Community Care in the Next Decade and Beyond. HMSO, London, 1989.

Chappell NL. Living arrangements and sources of caregiving. *J Gerontol* 1991; 46(1): S1–8.

Fennel G, Phillipson C, Evers H. *The Sociology of Old Age*. Open University Press, Milton Keynes, 1988.

Gallo JJ. The effect of social support on depression in caregivers of the elderly. *J Family Practice* 1990; 30(4): 430–436; discussion 437–440.

Groves T. *Countdown to Community Care*. BMJ Publications, London, 1993.

Laing W. Living environment for the elderly: the mixed economy in long-term care. In: Wells N, Freer C (eds), *An Ageing Population: Burden or Challenge*. Macmillan Press, London, 1988.

Speare A Jr, Avery R. Who helps whom in older parent–child families. *J Gerontol* 1993; 48(2): S64–73.

Wells N, Freer C (eds). *An Ageing Population: Burden or Challenge*. Macmillan Press, London, 1988.

16 ELDERLY PEOPLE AND THEIR SOCIAL NETWORKS

- Social networks
- Requirements for a successful support system
- Anatomy of social networks
- Psychology of the members of the social network

The emphasis in the training of health care workers, and medical students in particular, is upon disease, for the detection, investigation, treatment and prevention of disease is the justification for medicine, its one specific function. Much of the teaching is inevitably in large hospitals where staff and facilities can be readily available and deployed to greatest advantage but it is important, given the nature of the diseases prevalent in the industrial countries in the 1990s and the state of medicine there, that students should see disease from a wider perspective. Even when detected and treated, disease often leaves disabilities. The majority of frail and disabled people including those with severe functional impairments live in private households. To do so they depend to a greater or lesser extent upon those who constitute their social networks — informal and formal. A knowledge of the anatomy and psychology of social networks is important.

SOCIAL NETWORKS

Any person can be regarded as being at the centre of and interacting with a series of subsystems of people.

These subsystems usually operate independently of one another but they occasionally intersect and this is particularly the case when there is disability and at a time of crisis.

The Informal Network

The informal network of support consists of kin (nuclear and extended family), friends and neighbours. The informal primary group is usually small in size and has a long history of contact with the old person, contact which may have been rewarding, hostile or mixed. There may have been emotional bonds and a more or less pronounced sense of commitment. It may have less skill than the formal network but it has the great advantage of availability at all times (usually), of being able to deal with unexpected events and emergencies, of being flexible and unencumbered by professional and other demarcation boundaries. Finally there are the virtues of familiarity and continuity. In contrast, the formal agencies can draw on a potentially larger pool of people and they possess a range of technical expertise, skill and resources which may be essential for the patient.

The formal network

The formal network of support consists firstly of the basic financial entitlements available to elderly people (e.g. retirement and supplementary pensions, attendance allowance). Then there are the statutory agencies which carry out the economic and social policies of central and local government, but actually provide the services: the National Health Service (general practitioner, district nurse, health visitor, etc.) and the local authority social services department (social worker, home help, meals on wheels, day centre). Finally there are the voluntary or quasi formal organizations independent of government but often encouraged and supported financially by it (e.g. Age Concern, Help the Aged, MIND, etc.).

REQUIREMENTS FOR A SUCCESSFUL SUPPORT SYSTEM

There are three major requirements for a social network to act as a successful support system:

1. socialization;
2. the carrying out of tasks needed in everyday living; and
3. assistance in illness or crisis.

To a considerable extent the informal network is sufficient for those needs. In a survey of elderly people living in a large inner city it was concluded that kin are clearly considered the primary source of help, regardless of the task. Only when family, particularly children, are not available do friends, neighbours and formal organizations become important in the provision of social support.

ANATOMY OF SOCIAL NETWORKS

No assessment of an older person with even slight disability is complete without a description of those people available to help. The enumeration must be systematic and should include the following particulars.

Informal networks

Names, addresses, telephone numbers and frequency of contacts with relatives, neighbours and friends should be noted and the nature of tasks undertaken for or on behalf of the patient listed.

Formal networks

Specific enquiry should be made about contact with the people and services listed in Table 16.1. The tasks undertaken and the frequency of involvement should be specified in detail. In practice it is surprising how much input rather than how little there is in the care of an elderly person. Much of it, however, is often unco-ordinated and unplanned. Part of the art of medicine is to visualize the person in their world rather than *in vacuo* or only in relation to one's own agency and then, as far as possible, to plan care jointly. The people partaking have their own attitudes and needs in relation to the patient and these views must be obtained. If necessary a case conference should be convened inviting all concerned in the person's care.

Table 16.1 Anatomy of the formal network

Domiciliary services
The primary health care team:
    General practitioner
    District nurse
    Health visitor
    Community psychiatric nurse
Social services:
    Social worker
    Home help/home care
    Meals on wheels
Voluntary groups:
    Sitting services
    Visiting schemes

Institutional services
NHS:
    Hospitals
    Day hospitals (medical or psychiatric)
Social services and independent residential and day care:
    Day centres
    Luncheon clubs
    Old people's homes

PSYCHOLOGY OF THE MEMBERS OF THE SOCIAL NETWORK

There are a great variety of feelings, attitudes and views held about frail and disabled old people, not solely by their families, friends and neighbours but also by professionals. In the assessment of what can be done to help the person these feelings may count for much more than marginal abnormalities in physical test results and may be as important as specific treatment. They must be recognized and channelled in support of the patient. For example, by helping the carer directly the patient may be helped indirectly.

Anxiety in the network may be constructive in moderate degrees but destructive if unjustified or excessive. It may be the latter because of:

1. ignorance of the facts surrounding the patient's illness as a result of communication barriers;
2. the patient being viewed as a burden which is unshared;
3. difficulty in accepting the lowered standards which may be inevitable with disability;
4. concern over risk; or
5. the fear of threat or criticism towards a carer should the patient come to harm.

Much can be done to reduce anxiety by listening, by allowing 'ventilation' to take place, by explanation and by jointly considering the possible steps to be taken. All too often barriers are erected by professionals where what is required is a sense of partnership between them and the supporters for the client's benefit. Depression can be alleviated by reducing the burden through partial relief from total care, by psychological support and sometimes by medication. Guilt may be a major problem. The person's behaviour may cause irritation, leading to outright hostility, rejection or even violence. Occasionally it can lead to a mixture of emotions (ambivalence) in which the negative features may be masked by intense compensations or reaction formation in which there is apparent excessive devotion concealing the resentment. The point to bear in mind is that such so-called psychodynamic factors always exist in relation to disabled people, whatever the disability and whatever the age of the patient. They must be understood and then they can be handled constructively by those with empathy, counselling skills and the willingness and ability to spend time. Many carers and patients would benefit from the support of more skilled counselling were it available. Self-help groups and large organiza-

tions such as the Alzheimer's Disease Society and the Parkinson's Disease Society can give invaluable support.

People under stress turn first to their nearest and dearest who provide most of the care for disabled people. It is never enough to view a person in isolation, let alone to be concerned only with the disease. Illness in one person inevitably has repercussions on those in their social environment. To help the client most, once everything possible has been done for the disease process, management must be planned for the carers as well as for the person.

Key points

- The majority of frail and disabled people (including those functionally impaired) live in their own homes.
- Support subsystems can be classified into formal and informal.
- Formal networks include financial entitlements, and the statutory agencies (health — GP and district nurse; and social services — social worker, day care). It also includes the voluntary sector.
- Informal networks include family/relatives, friends and other close carers.
- Successful support systems must help carry out the tasks needed in daily living, assist in illness or crisis and help in socialization.
- No assessment is complete without a full description of informal and formal networks.
- In times of crisis people turn to their nearest and dearest.

FURTHER READING

Abrams M. *Beyond Three Score and Ten. A Second Report on a Survey of the Elderly.* Age Concern, London, 1980.

Stevenson O. *Age and Vulnerability (a Guide to Better Care).* Age Concern, London, 1989.

Townsend P. *The Last Refuge.* Routledge & Kegan Paul, London, 1962.

Townsend P. *The Family Life of Old People.* Routledge & Kegan Paul, London, 1987.

17 PRESENTATION OF DISEASE

- Delay
- Atypical presentation
- Multiple pathology
- Social presentation of disease
- Teamwork
- Social networks
- The environmental revolution

Even for the lay person there are some disease processes that are immediately recognizable by their presentation. An adult complaining of crushing central chest pain that goes down his left arm, leaving him sweating, breathless and nauseated is likely to provoke the alarm bells of 'heart attack' and get the appropriate response. This pattern recognition of symptoms and signs is obviously enhanced to a fine art during medical training so that less common conditions than myocardial infarction result in the same process, history, examination and diagnosis. Thus there is a traditional pattern of disease presentation in younger people that even if not articulated well results in an 'I am sick — help me' scenario. Two major factors influence the recognition of disease processes in elderly people: acceptance of ill-health with subsequent delay in seeking help and the atypical presentation of disease processes.

DELAY

Acceptance of ill-health as 'ageing' and the resulting disabilities mean that many elderly people expect to be frail and rarely complain or seek help at an early stage. Dramatic complaints (severe pain, vomiting blood, etc.) may still elicit the traditional response but less life-threatening episodes can be accepted as change and part of the ageing process. This picture is especially noticeable in inner city areas with their history of poor primary health care and where health expectations (especially amongst older people) are low. Coming to terms with some disability/change is necessary at all ages and acceptance is part of successful survival. However, the tacit acceptance of deterioration in, for example, eyesight, hearing, teeth and feet as part of the inevitable ageing process may lead to treatable conditions being ignored and independence being lost.

ATYPICAL PRESENTATION

The pioneers in the field of health care of the elderly outlined some fundamental differences in disease presentation, simple in themselves and yet laying the foundation to one of the most complex branches of medicine. This fact of atypical presentation, understanding the concept and acting on it, is so profound as to border on being one of the most essential elements for a student and practitioner to comprehend. It is the starting point for good health care for elderly people.

The term 'geriatric giants' (Fig. 17.1) was coined by Professor Isaacs to describe the 'pattern recognition' set of symptoms and signs in old age that may have as their cause any disease process. Diseases as different in aetiology as pneumonia, myocardial infarction, urinary

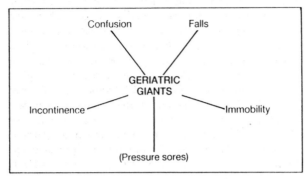

Figure 17.1 The 'geriatric giants' — symptoms and signs that occur in elderly people as a consequence of many disease processes

tract infection or drug toxicity can present classically or as one of the four 'giants' — confusion, immobility, falls and incontinence (many add a fifth — pressure sores). This pattern of presentation has been refined and expanded into another *aide mémoire* — the 'I's of old age (Fig. 17.2). A useful analogy is a 'fit' in a child. This is only a symptom and does not imply a diagnosis, which could be a febrile illness, epilepsy, meningitis, drugs, etc. Doctors would never dream of labelling fits

as 'childhood events'. In the same way neither should falls or incontinence be treated as an 'ageing process'. Look beyond the presenting symptom and find the disease behind.

In most cases alleviation of symptoms and treatment of disease will be possible. In some the disease process will not be cured but these will be a minority. Not responding correctly to the atypical presentation is not only an intellectual failure but is also profoundly detrimental to the patient and an enormous waste of resources.

There are two other important aspects concerning the altered presentation of disease in old age. One is the concept of multiple pathology being present in many elderly people and the other is the recognition of 'social' presentation of disease and the response that subsequently occurs.

MULTIPLE PATHOLOGY

The altered presentation of disease in elderly people is often secondary to more than one disease process in the individual. They may be causally linked, e.g. confusion secondary to hypoxia due to heart failure caused by ischaemic heart disease. Typically they are not and it is common to have a medical 'problem list' consisting of falls secondary to osteoarthrosis of the knees plus a contribution from onychogryphosis, hypothyroidism, hiatus hernia, and macular degeneration giving poor vision (making self-medicating and drug compliance a further problem). The art is in trying to identify and treat the most significant underlying diagnosis, and using a multidisciplinary approach, find ways of compensating for as many of the deficits as possible.

SOCIAL PRESENTATION OF DISEASE

It has been widely thought (since the Poor Laws of the sixteenth century) that medicine has nothing to do with social problems. This is manifestly untrue, for disease at any age leads to concomitant social and psychological upheaval. The holistic approach in the health care of elderly people recognizes this; indeed, 'social admission' should be the sixth basic geriatric giant. 'Social admission' is currently a pejorative term in a hospital setting, implying a lack of history-taking and examination that should have uncovered a disease process resulting in the

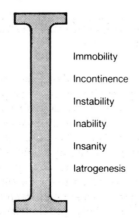

Figure 17.2 The 'I's of old age

'social' response. The response may be that of exhausted relatives leaving a person in Casualty or neighbours calling a social worker or police to 'do something'. Many patients are actually barred admission and referred to social services for 'appropriate' admission to an old people's home and the inappropriate cycle is established. This results in ill elderly people in social care (when they should be in hospital) and those in need of 'care' in hospital or at home denied access.

The recognition of the social presentation of disease means that some doctors have now been trained to rush towards rather than away from social problems. The traditional medical behaviour of history-taking and examination then leads to the identification of multiple problems. Investigation of and solutions to these problems require modern investigatory techniques and treatments. Departments of Health Care for Elderly People/Medicine of Old Age with beds in district general hospitals have access to these facilities and can provide a diagnostic and treatment service. The problem of limited resources means that conflict with professional colleagues can develop. Manifestations of this discord include the use of the term 'bed blocker' and the refusal to admit 'social problems' by some clinicians, and on the other hand the development of a strict age-related discipline by some geriatricians.

The learning curve of the pioneers in the field incorporated the problems of delay in diagnosis, atypical presentation, the role of multiple pathology and 'social' presentation. They developed a framework to cope with these problems and set the basis for the holistic nature that is the hallmark of health care for elderly people in the UK. Elements of this framework were the development of teamwork, the recognition of social networks and the environmental revolution.

TEAMWORK

Multiple problems require staff trained to deal with them or teamwork by staff trained to deal with individual problems. The range of people and their skill mix brought together to help solve client/patient problems is considerable (see Chapter 47). No one model of multidisciplinary working has achieved prominence and the practice is not always straightforward or without criticism. Inherent in teamwork is some form of conflict, for when faced with a difficult task each member of the team will suggest a different solution. Successful teamwork therefore requires leadership if anything is to be achieved.

If the team objective is set as rehabilitation and discharge then the team will consider it has failed if it does not resettle people at home or elsewhere. Such resettlement requires the development of methods of aftercare to ensure successful discharge.

SOCIAL NETWORKS

There is no such thing as independence because everyone is dependent upon others to some extent. Rather there is relative acceptance and tolerance. There are some general patterns to the social network around each individual but each network is different and to understand disease in old age it is essential that the social network is studied. This network can be simplistically divided into formal and informal (see Chapter 16). The formal consists of the statutory services, which are comprehensive but somewhat inflexible in timing and frequency. Informal networks (family, friends, carers and neighbours) are not 'professional' but are flexible and usually infinitely more available at unsocial hours.

Each social network is unique to an individual. Requests come to others for help when the tolerance levels of the networks change and acceptance changes to rejection. The point at which rejection occurs is dependent upon inherent strengths and weaknesses of the individuals or systems in the network. Some want help early, some too late and some not at all. An outline of a person's social network prior to admission and after discharge is an important ingredient of our knowledge concerning them. A comprehensive view of social networks is provided in Chapter 16.

THE ENVIRONMENTAL REVOLUTION

The fundamental new knowledge base of a consultant caring for elderly people is an attack on prolonged bed-rest. This has led to the refurnishing of wards with adjustable height beds without cot-sides (for they are not necessary if the bed is low) and chairs of variable height to suit people of varying height. Not all changes have been beneficial, with the unacceptable restraint of bed-rest having been swapped for the tilt-back chair or chair with restraining table or restraining belt. In the modern ward for elderly people, patients are now nursed in bed when sick, and up and dressed in their own clothes in the stage of rehabilitation. An environmental revolution has taken place that needs to be recognized and understood.

Key points

- Many elderly people accept ill-health as normal ageing and delay in seeking help.
- Disease processes in old age usually present atypically.
- The 'geriatric giants' consist of confusion, falls, immobility, incontinence and pressure sores.
- Older people often have more than one disease process — multiple pathology.
- The atypical presentation of illness often leads to an erroneous label of 'social problem'.

- Multidisciplinary teamwork is an essential element to the holistic approach to care of elderly people.
- Social networks consist of formal and informal groupings.
- Hospital environments have to be 'user-friendly' if rehabilitative results are to be achieved — the concept of the environmental revolution.

FURTHER READING

Abrams M. *Beyond Three Score and Ten. A Second Report on a Survey of the Elderly*. Age Concern, London, 1980.

Isaacs B, Livingstone M, Neville Y. *Survival of the Unfittest*. Routledge & Kegan Paul, London, 1972.

18 HELPING YOUR ELDERLY PATIENT TO HELP YOU: HISTORY AND EXAMINATION

- The GP consultation
- Meeting a patient for the first time
- Positioning, vision and hearing
- The environment
- Getting the story
- The confused patient
- Activities of daily living
- A drug history
- Corroboration of the evidence
- Examination
- 'Extras' for the elderly patient
- Explanation and reassurance
- Follow-up

Whether you are a doctor, a nurse, a therapist, a social worker, a student or a carer you will sometimes have to obtain information from an elderly person. Sources of difficulty can come from the information giver, the information taker, and the environment in which this is done. It is all too easy to blame the elderly person, and it is commonplace to see comments like 'Rambling old buffer', or 'Difficult, vague historian'. Such remarks written in case notes (and they are usually doctors' notes rather than any other professional group) tell us more about the attitudes and behaviour of the history-taker than the patient.

THE GP CONSULTATION

Much of what follows assumes a hospital or outpatient setting, but is just as relevant in the GP's surgery. A major problem for the assessment of elderly patients in general practice is familiarity. In general practice, history-taking is spread over months and even years as a mutual process of 'getting to know you' occurs. This is one of the strengths of general practice because it allows the doctor to interpret the patient's present symptoms in the light of previous encounters. The ability to do this is greatly improved by a structured case record with a problem list and a prescribing card. These should be reviewed prior to any consultation so that the present problem can be fitted rapidly into an overall picture of the patient.

The nature of the patient's presenting complaint must be sorted into potentially serious (e.g. chest pain, breathlessness, vomiting); might be serious (e.g. general aches and pains, weakness, a fall); probably not serious (e.g. a dizzy spell, feeling 'out of sorts', sore throat). Action may be decided at this stage for the potentially serious category. However, for most patients the key point to be established at the outset is whether there has been any deterioration in the patient's functional ability. Has she stopped doing the shopping? Is she unable to do the heavy housework? Has she lost interest in things generally? Further enquiry should be about the other 'geriatric giants' — incontinence, falls, confusion and iatrogenesis (see Chapter 17). If there has been no change in performance of activities of daily living and none of the common presentations of occult disease, then the GP can use time to make the diagnosis. This means reviewing the patient in a week or so to decide whether the symptoms are progressing or not, and whether new problems have arisen.

It is worth remembering that about 70 per cent of people aged over 80 years have some degree of disability, and in 20 per cent this will be severe. Age is quite a useful yardstick to determine how intensively to treat a problem. Very old people are much more vulnerable to sudden deteriorations. A 'mild' chest infection in an 85-year-old can rapidly turn into a fall with associated hip fracture, whereas in a 70-year-old this is much less likely. In general, early and aggressive treatment is likely to be rewarded by fewer complications.

To provide adequate assessments of elderly people in general practice is not easy. It requires a willingness to commit sufficient time to history-taking and examination — usually best done by seeing those patients who appear, during a short appointment, to have a potentially serious problem again for a fuller assessment of at least 30 minutes. Unless this is done the familiarity that is such a useful tool in general practice can become the enemy of older patients. It is worth remembering that it is no sign of incompetence or idleness to refer patients for a comprehensive assessment to the local Department of Health Care for Elderly People/Medicine of Old Age. Consultants have more time to spend with patients, and also have the resources of other professionals to draw upon. All too often problems of incontinence (both urinary and faecal), depres-sion, Parkinsonism, myxoedema, episodes of left ventricular failure, and many more have been going on for months or years before they are recognized and treated.

MEETING A PATIENT FOR THE FIRST TIME (Fig. 18.1)

The introduction is crucial to what follows. A cheerful 'How are you doing, grandpa?' is unlikely to be greeted with much enthusiasm by a retired bank manager you have never met before. Introductions should be straightforward, relatively formal, and should respect the dignity of the person. Eye contact, a greeting, an outstretched hand (expecting a returned handshake), your name, and the purpose of your visit are all that are required to get started.

Eye contact is the first step. Can the person see you, do they smile in response to your smile, do they look perplexed, do they recognize you? Depressed patients may avoid eye contact.

The hand contact is useful. Some patients who are delirious or have dementia may not respond — they do not recognize the social gesture. This alerts you to the fact that all may not be well with the brain. Furthermore, the hand contact is of social significance

---

TAKING A MEDICAL HISTORY

- The introduction

- Timing, interest

- Position and comfort

- Vision, hearing, cognition

- Environment

- Use of multiple sources

- Interview versus interrogation

Figure 18.1 Taking a medical history

for most of us. Frightened elderly patients may clutch, and maintain hand contact long after the formal handshake. Rarely, you may be surprised by the patient's unwillingness to let go; this may be a positive grasp reflex (a primitive reflex usually indicating damage to the frontal lobe of the brain, and not uncommon in people with dementia). The hand contact is the first step to building up a rapport with the person.

Giving your name and your purpose helps put the person at ease. It also helps you to assess short-term memory. You can ask the person subsequently 'Can you remember my name?' If they cannot, it may indicate cognitive impairment, but more usually suggests that the person wasn't listening too carefully. It may be useful to write your name down for the person, with your contact address or phone number. This helps build up trust between you and the person.

Ask the person 'What is your name?' Be on the lookout for hearing impairment at this stage. The reply should give an idea about how the person wishes to be addressed. A first name, if given in response, should not be assumed to be the preferred form of address. For example, ask the patient, 'Would you like me to call you Mary?' By doing this you avoid calling a spinster Mrs, rather than Miss, and you also avoid being over formal with those people who would rather be known by their first names.

POSITIONING, VISION AND HEARING

If you or your patient are uncomfortable you will not get very far. Make sure that the patient is in an appropriate position for what you plan to do. If you are going to simply talk to the patient, make sure they are sitting up, and preferably in a chair. If you are going to examine the legs, make sure the patient is in bed or on a couch. Get yourself a chair, and sit down so that you are not towering over the patient in an authoritarian way. It only takes a moment, and saves time later.

Remember that if you or the patient wants to go to the lavatory, the interview will be a tense business. Ask patients if they are comfortable, check that they do not want to go to the lavatory. You may be the first person who has come near them and stopped long enough to ask since they came into hospital.

Ask the patient if they usually wear glasses and ensure that the patient puts them on. If speech sounds slurred and the patient does not appear to have false teeth in place, ask where they are, and suggest they be put in. Ask about a hearing aid and make sure it is switched on. It is important in a hospital or nursing home to note the presence of such aids. Frequently they are 'lost' and a note stating that they were left at home is invaluable in finding them. Also any regularly used aids should be obtained and used while the patient is in hospital.

Deafness is such a common problem that any situation where elderly people are seen regularly should have a communication aid for deaf people. The simplest form of ear trumpet is often as effective as much more sophisticated electronic aids. Doctors should carry a small plastic trumpet in their 'black bags', and every ward in a hospital should have a supply. Shouting in the ear of a deaf patient is exhausting for everyone. Avoid doing it.

THE ENVIRONMENT

Talking at the bedside in a busy hospital ward is accepted practice in the UK. Provided the conversation is about general matters, and you are not too bothered whether the patient tells you the truth or not, go ahead and continue with the traditional approach. If you wish to talk about sensitive matters, or give the patient an opportunity to raise serious issues do not try to do it behind the curtains in a shared room. This is not privacy, and it is only an institutionalized doctor who could possibly believe it is. It takes time to take a patient to the ward interview room, or to a quiet treatment room. But it is worth the time if you want to do the job properly. Your patients will notice the difference. A busy, noisy ward environment is exactly the wrong place to be talking about incontinence, testing for cognitive impairment, and exploring depressive symptoms and your patient's doubts and fears.

Furthermore, your pockets are never big enough to include the vision test board (Snellen chart), the auroscope and ophthalmoscope, the blood pressure machine, the rectal examination tray, the neurological examination kit, the tape measure, the goniometer, and so on. These should all be kept in one place, preferably a ward examination room.

If you do have to work in the main ward area, behind the curtains, do not forget that everyone else can hear what is going on. Furthermore, if you are called away, do not forget to pull back the curtains so that your patient is not left in limbo.

GETTING THE STORY

Let the patient tell the story as they wish, but help them with time sequence. It is useful to ask the patient 'What happened to you today, why have you come into hospital?' This encourages the patient to focus on recent events. Inevitably, some patients will start 'It all really started when I was gassed in the First World War'. Politeness dictates that you should listen to a little of the story. What the patient is saying to you is 'I am a person who has been around, I've fought for my country, I am somebody'. You may use the story to collect information that you were planning to ask about later. For example, you might go on to ask about occupational history, about major life events besides the war, about past medical history. Although medical students are taught to start with the history of the presenting complaint, our patients are not taught this!

It is not worth spending time collecting information directly from the patient that can be more easily obtained from the case records, or family doctor's letter. Check important facts, but do not press the patient for dates of operations or consultants' names. It is worth asking patients about their medication. Do they know the names of drugs, their purposes, and when they are meant to take them?

Interruptions

Try to avoid interrupting a patient's story if possible. Some patients give a rapid account of things, others are much slower. Try to adjust your pace to that of the patient. Elderly patients have been around for a lot longer than younger patients, and have more to tell you. However, it is often necessary to interrupt and redirect the conversation. It is not impolite to do this, and you need to develop your own technique to avoid embarrassing the patient, or losing rapport. A comment to demonstrate you have been listening to what has just been said, followed by 'Can we just get back to the pain you were telling me about. Exactly where was it?', should help you get back on track.

Time

Doctors and nurses are busy people, they even walk quicker than most normal people! But do not fall into the trap of behaving like a 'busy person'. Your job is to talk to patients, and part of the skill is to make the patient feel that they have your undivided attention. If you can, leave your bleep with the ward receptionist or with a colleague who can call you if the message is really urgent. Make sure you are not trying to do a 30-minute task if you have to be somewhere else in 10 minutes. Rather than do a rushed job, initially do a much more limited history or examination and come back later. If you are called away in the middle of the interview, apologize and explain what is happening. Do not just run out of the room.

Embarrassing questions

Asking about incontinence, about sex life, about depressive symptoms can be embarrassing for both patient and doctor. It is even more difficult if you are not sensitive about how you ask the questions. Avoid asking direct questions like 'Are you ever incontinent?' Some patients may not understand the term 'incontinence', others may deny the symptom. A gentler and more effective question is 'Do you ever have trouble holding your water?' It may be helpful to start a sensitive question like this: 'Some women find that sexual intercourse becomes quite painful after the menopause. Have you ever found that?'

It is sensible to keep sensitive questions until you have built up a rapport with a patient. Come back later. Start by showing that you respect the patient as a person. Admire a bedside photograph or Get Well card, or the patient's appearance. After the interview thank the patient for their clarity and helpfulness in giving a good history.

Language problems

We live in a multicultural society but we tend to expect our patients to speak English (see Chapter 33). It is impossible to be fluent in every language spoken in a big city like Manchester or London. However, it is quite easy to remember how to say 'hello' in several languages, which will almost certainly make your patient and their family feel that you are sympathetic at the very least. *Salam halikum* is the general greeting for any Islamic patient, literally 'peace on you'.

Patients from ethnic minorities are used to communication problems and usually bring a relative or friend with them to translate. This can lead to difficulties if the interpreter is inexperienced and you have little experience of consulting through another person. In general, keep the questions simple and do not allow a long rambling conversation to go on between the interpreter and the patient. You have to keep control of the consultation.

Children interpreting for their parents or grandparents will be emotionally involved in what is happening and you should not attempt to cover all the ground. The patient may not wish to admit what is really happening in front of the children. It is always best to check with the patient or general practitioner whether an interpreter will be needed and to make arrangements beforehand. Some districts have a 'language line' which is a telephone interpreting system. If all else fails, re-book a new appointment with a trained interpreter.

THE CONFUSED PATIENT

'Patient confused, no history available' speaks volumes about the training and attitudes of the medical profession. Confused patients deserve better. They are suffering from acute or chronic brain failure yet doctors seem inadequately trained to face up to the challenge of making a diagnosis and initiating management. Failure of almost any other organ system in the human body causes doctors to get excited and strive to find the underlying cause. Not so brain failure.

Many patients with major cognitive impairments (e.g. short-term memory loss, problems of recognition, language problems) are passed as normal by inexperienced (and sometimes experienced) professionals. In part this is because a patient needs a very small repertoire of social skills to maintain a façade of normality in the typical hospital ward, and even in front of their GP.

It is crucial to establish early on whether the patient is orientated in place, time and person. You also must decide whether the patient is alert or not. Mild degrees of clouding of consciousness are difficult to detect. The patient may appear to be 'not quite all there'.

Most geriatricians now use a standard test of mental function (Fig. 18.2). Beware of announcing to the patient, and usually the rest of the ward, that you are about to ask him or her some 'silly questions'. By implication either you or the patient is silly to want to use 'silly' questions! Rather explain that you want to test your patient's memory, and ask them whether they mind you doing this. With experience it is possible to check most of the items in a mental test score by working them into your introductory talk with the patient. This is preferable to simply going through them like a shopping list. Remember that subtle impairment may not be detectable with a simple mental test score. You can try asking patients about current affairs, about their families, or carry out a more detailed assessment such as the Mini-Mental State Examination.

> **ABBREVIATED MENTAL TEST (AMT)**
>
> - Age
> - Time (to nearest hour)
> - Address for recall
> - Year
> - Where do you live (town or road)?
> - Recognition of two persons
> - Date of birth (day and month)
> - Year of start of First World War
> - Name of present monarch
> - Count backwards 20 to 1
> - Don't forget to ask for the address!

Figure 18.2 Abbreviated mental test (AMT)

Always remember that deafness and speech impairments, such as nominal dysphasia, can make patients appear very cognitively impaired, and that depressed patients do not do well on mental test scores.

Confused patients can often reliably tell you about symptoms they are experiencing at the time. For example, do ask about pain and breathlessness.

ACTIVITIES OF DAILY LIVING (ADL)

Elderly people typically suffer with multiple pathology, some of which may be related to the reason for admission to hospital, or for consultation, some of which may not. A patient may give a symptom of chest pain suggesting a heart attack, prompting a detailed enquiry about cardiovascular and respiratory symptoms.

In younger patients, a brief 'systems enquiry' concerning gastrointestinal, neurological and locomotor systems is all that is necessary to rule out any other significant problems.

In older patients this approach does not work. A systems enquiry in an older patient can take almost forever, producing spurious symptoms. This is because elderly people often have so many symptoms, many of which are not relevant to the problem in hand. Some sort of screening is needed, and enquiry about activities of daily living (ADL) provides a useful screen (Fig. 18.3).

In general, patients who can dress, get about outdoors, are continent, can do their own housework and cooking, manage their own pension, do not require much more enquiry other than their presenting problem. Such patients are the exception in usual practice with very old people.

If a daily living task cannot be carried out, then it is necessary to make a detailed enquiry focused on the reasons for this.

It is useful to obtain a 'pre-morbid' ADL, enabling you to describe what the patient was usually able to do before they became ill. This provides a rough goal for the outcome of treatment. A patient who was unable to get in and out of the bath, who could not dress, and who was incontinent prior to suffering a stroke or heart attack is not likely to get back to a trouble-free life. With younger patients we make the assumption that they were disability-free before the onset of an acute illness. With older people, this assumption is seldom worth making.

A DRUG HISTORY (Fig. 18.4)

Old people are the pharmaceutical industry's greatest friend. They take more medication than any other age-group. Many patients do not take all their prescribed medication. Check dates on tablet bottles and count the number of pills remaining as a rough guide to compliance. Everyone, young and old, hoards medicines against some future catastrophe. There are few medicine cabinets in the country that do not contain some out-of-date hypnotics, skin ointments and analgesics. Remember that sharing of medication is commonplace

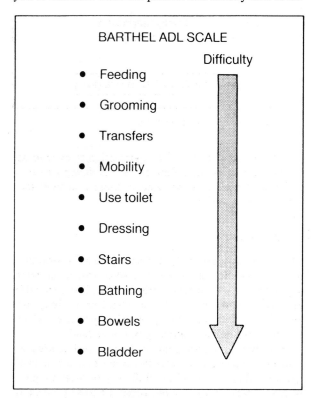

BARTHEL ADL SCALE

Difficulty

- Feeding
- Grooming
- Transfers
- Mobility
- Use toilet
- Dressing
- Stairs
- Bathing
- Bowels
- Bladder

A TREATMENT HISTORY

- Current medication
- Previous hospital and family doctor medication
- Treatment from 'alternative' practitioners
- Self-medication
- Past bad experiences with medicines
- Other non-drug treatments
- Medicines kept in the home

Figure 18.3 Barthel ADL (activities of daily living) scale

Figure 18.4 A treatment history

as part of the self-help culture of elderly people — people swap stories about symptoms and try each other's drugs. Traditional remedies may also be used, and some people are naturally reluctant to divulge their secret remedies.

CORROBORATION OF THE EVIDENCE

None of us is a perfect witness of events, even if they concern us intimately. In medicine it is necessary to be critical of the history and check key points. Most students are familiar with that sinking feeling when the consultant, having heard the student's history-taking, asks two or three questions of the patient that appear to totally contradict the main thrust of the history. Patients change their story not because they are contrary, but because they become more astute to the importance of certain symptoms, they remember time relationships better, and sometimes it really is very difficult to be precise about a symptom.

The simplest form of corroboration is to go over the key symptoms with the patient after a few hours. It is essential to get whatever help you can from collateral sources of information. Do get hold of the old case notes from the other hospital, because buried in them may be important information. Ring up the family doctor for clarification of points not covered in a referral letter. Most important of all, talk to a close relative or friend if at all possible. The telephone is a vital piece of equipment for history-taking with elderly patients. If you have not had to use it, ask yourself why not.

EXAMINATION (Fig. 18.5)

It is impossible to take a history and examine an elderly patient fully in under an hour. It is also unwise to try to spend an uninterrupted hour doing this. You will be exhausted and so will your patient. Your examination findings may well be inaccurate because of tiredness. So do not even try to do it all in one go. Take your history and then go away and write it down. You will inevitably have forgotten to ask some vital piece of information, and you will almost always need to check important facts with case notes, the family doctor or a relative.

Come back to do your examination when you have thought through what it is you need to examine. Does the history suggest a neurological problem? Does the

EXAMINATION OF A PATIENT	
System	*Don't forget!*
General	Appearance, mood, skin, Parkinson's, myxoedema, anaemia, breasts, temperature, nutrition
CNS	Higher cortical tests, apraxia, agnosia, speech, hemiparesis, wasting, vision, hearing
CVS / respiratory	Respiration rate, postural BP, scars
Abdominal	Bladder, PR, urine
Locomotor	Gait, transfers, feet, hips, knees
Aids / appliances	Stick, hearing aid, spectacles, teeth

You can't do it all in one go!

Figure 18.5 Examination of a patient

patient look Parkinsonian? Are you going to have to do a pelvic examination? Often it is worth doing a neurological examination as a separate exercise to achieve satisfactory cooperation.

Be gentle!

Elderly skin bruises easily, and a rough hand does nothing to promote confidence that what will come later (e.g. taking blood, rectal examination) will be done with care. Always explain what you intend to do first, and help the patient into the appropriate position. Make sure your instructions are easy to understand.

Elderly people once possessed bodies as beautiful as your own, and they are only too aware of the effects of age on collagen, and of the difficulty of looking good with a wayward body. Do not aggravate this by a look of distaste as you examine a corpulent belly, or slide your stethoscope and fingers into severe intertrigo under a pendulous breast. You are not immune to the ageing process.

Always thank a patient for their cooperation and performance. Do not do the examination in total silence — this can only mean you have discovered something terrible. Explain what you are doing as you go, and comment reassuringly on what you find.

Clothing

It sometimes seems that the principle of dressing elderly hospital patients in their own clothes is done simply to stop doctors getting on with examining patients! It takes time to undress patients, but it is useful to use that time to observe your patient's abilities. Ask patients to remove clothes themselves. Consider whether the patient can reach her feet, can she manage her buttons, can she unhook her bra strap? Is her balance good, can she get on to the examination couch herself? These points may be of use in making the diagnosis, and any difficulty with undressing should be assessed by the occupational therapist.

Having got the patient undressed, be sure to keep him or her comfortable. Make use of a blanket to protect the patient's dignity, and never leave a patient undressed while you get on with seeing another patient — it always takes longer than expected.

If you are planning to do a vaginal or rectal examination ask a nurse to help you.

'EXTRAS' FOR THE ELDERLY PATIENT

Elderly patients require the same examination as younger patients but there some extras that are often forgotten. Check visual acuity and hearing, take off the shoes and examine the feet, and do not forget the patient's teeth — false or real. Check pressure areas (heels, hips, sacrum, shoulders, elbows) for signs of skin breakdown. A lying and standing (sitting will do) blood pressure is mandatory for all patients. Counting the respiratory rate is a more useful examination than listening to the chest. Most elderly people have noisy lung bases, but if the respiratory rate is not raised it is unlikely that there is an acute problem. Rectal examinations are a required part of a full examination, yet are often omitted in all age-groups.

A common deficiency in neurological examination is to omit any consideration of higher cortical function — the bits that make us human. The examination tends to focus on cranial nerves and spinal reflex arcs rather than testing language, perception and memory. Pencil and paper tests can be invaluable in providing a global test of competence. A favourite test is to present the patient with a circle (about 10–15 cm diameter) and ask them to fill in the numbers to make a clock face. This test will be abnormal in patients who have visual impairments, who have difficulty carrying out purposeful actions (apraxia), who have perceptual problems or who are cognitively impaired (Fig. 18.6).

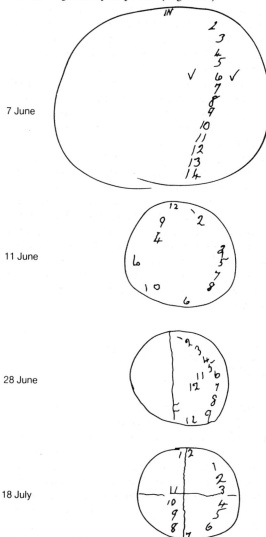

Figure 18.6 Clock face drawings: this patient showed some obvious improvement over the period

It is essential to examine every patient's walking — or gait pattern. Subtle evidence of hemiparesis may show up, as may poor balance, or the clutching 'furniture- cruising' gait of long-standing mobility problems. This also provides an objective check of at least one activity of daily living. Occasionally patients report that they are capable of carrying out activities when in reality they cannot.

Aids and appliances

Many patients have spectacles, hearing aids, dentures, walking sticks, wheelchairs, and many other aids. It is sensible to give them an examination too. A hearing aid that is not working is no use, so arrange to get it fixed. A walking stick with a worn ferrule may be dangerous on wet pavements — change it. A wheelchair with flat tyres or with worn brake pads is both dangerous and an effort to use — get it overhauled. Elderly people's footwear is often ill-fitting and painful — get the therapist and surgical supplies staff to see what they can do.

With elderly patients, more than any other group of patients, it is attention to small, seemingly unimportant details that makes the difference between success and failure. Because the details are not viewed as sufficiently important they are neglected, and not surprisingly, elderly patients fail to get better and get home. The satisfaction for health professionals in dealing with the details comes from the gratitude shown by patients who have had chiropody for painful feet of years' duration, or who can now hear after removal of impacted wax, or who simply appreciate the fact that someone has listened.

EXPLANATION AND REASSURANCE

At the end of your history and examination you should always explain what will happen next and when. Give a summary of what you think is the matter, and write down what you have told the patient. Check that the patient understands, by asking them to repeat the key points. Always ask patients if there is anything that has not been covered that they think you should know. Be sure to allow time for patients to ask you to clarify information.

Whether you have good or bad news for the patient at the end of the examination, be sure to reassure that everything will be dealt with properly, that the patient will be involved in deciding on how treatment will be organized, and leave the patient in no doubt that, no matter how serious the disease, you intend to do something helpful.

FOLLOW-UP

You are likely to want to see the patient again. But ask yourself, why are you bringing the patient back? If it is simply to review an X-ray or a laboratory test, why not do that on your own and phone or write to the patient and general practitioner? Too often, patients are brought back for no very good reason and this is often perpetuated by generation after generation of junior doctors.

Check how the patient got to the health centre or the hospital. Were there problems with transport? Did the neighbour or a relative have to go in to get the patient ready in time? Are they out of pocket from paying taxi fares? Did the appointment clash with a regular engagement?

Ask yourself whether the facilities you use are user-friendly for older people. Is it easy to find the clinic? Are lavatories signposted clearly? Are appointment times kept? What happens after the patient leaves you — is it an even longer wait for venepuncture and X-rays? Are refreshments available?

These factors will determine whether the patient will be willing and able to come back.

Key points

- Information obtained from the history is crucial in subsequent diagnosis and management. Even in a confused or dysphasic patient a history must be obtained by enquiry from relatives, friends, family doctors, nurses, wardens, and even the ambulance crew.
- Both you and the patient must be comfortable. A warm quiet room containing all the relevant equipment needed is essential.
- History and examination takes a long time with a person who has lived a long time and has suffered many illnesses. Do not waste time establishing information that can be better obtained from old case records. Split the interview up to give both you and the patient a break.
- Use of a routine mental test examination, enquiry about performance of activities of daily living, and a careful drug history are essential.

- Elderly people take time to get undressed: observing any problems with undressing is an important part of the examination.
- Thank your patients for their help and cooperation, and reassure them as you carry out the examination. Explanations of what is the matter and what might be done are essential. Allow time for questions.
- Do not forget: visual acuity and hearing; feet and shoes; pressure areas; postural blood pressure; respiratory rate; higher cortical impairments (e.g. apraxias, agnosias); aids and appliances.

FURTHER READING

Applegate WB, Blass JP, Williams TF. Instruments for the functional assessment of older patients. *N Engl J Med* 1990; **322**(17): 1207–1214.

Bendall MJ. The examination of the elderly patient. In: Toghill P (ed.), *Examining Patients. An Introduction to Clinical Medicine*. Edward Arnold, London, 1990.

Fields SD. History-taking in the elderly: obtaining useful information. *Geriatrics* 1991; **46**(8): 26–28, 34–35.

19 IMMOBILITY

- The cause
- The pattern of immobility
- Is the patient really immobile?
- What next?
- Mobilization

The immobile elderly patient is one of the classic and most common presentations. However, every case requires careful history-taking to discover the underlying problems.

THE CAUSE

Ask the patient what has happened. Although obvious, this is frequently omitted, and a simple enquiry may lead to a direct lead (e.g. pain in the hip) or an indirect lead (e.g. recurrent falls leading to fear of walking), or may suggest important contributing factors (e.g. dementia or depression).

Separate cause from effect. It is all too easy to discover a diagnosis in an elderly patient and assume that this disease process is the cause of the patient's immobility. For example, a toxic confusional state may cause immobility, but immobility may be the cause of orthostatic pneumonia and dehydration.

Frequently it is not clear which way round events have occurred. The patient has several problems of which immobility is one. The management of the patient is not greatly influenced by sorting out the causal sequence, but the prognosis for recovery is largely determined by the underlying cause of the patient's immobility.

The last straw. Your patient may have been struggling along with several disabilities until a final event tipped the balance and pushed the patient into immobility. Often the last straw is a comparatively trivial problem (an inflamed bunion, or upper respiratory tract infection), or may be a 'social problem' such as a carer being taken ill, or a familiar home help going on holiday.

If the last straw that led to admission to hospital does seem trivial to you, remember that this is simply an indication of the vulnerability of your patient. A trivial final cause of immobility does not make the fact of immobility any the less urgent a medical problem.

THE PATTERN OF IMMOBILITY

The crucial part of the history of immobility is to get an indication of the time frame. The graphs in Fig. 19.1 show several different possibilities. By the time you

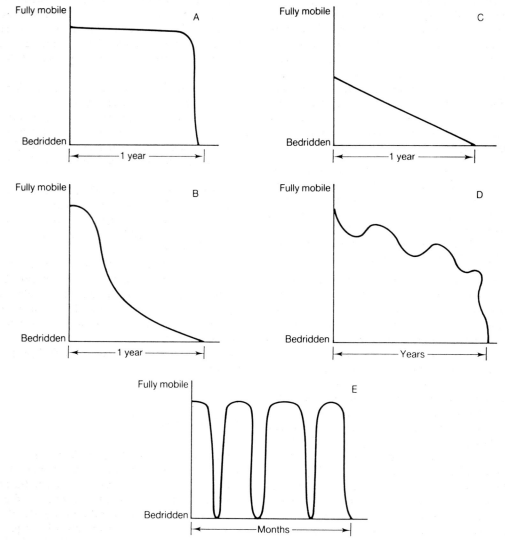

Figure 19.1 Five possible patterns of immobility

have finished taking the history you should be able to fit your patient into one of these types of mobility–time graphs.

Patient A should be easy to sort out. Whatever caused the plunge into immobility occurred suddenly and recently. Easy diagnoses to miss are stroke, impacted subcapital hip fracture (often previously X-rayed in the Accident and Emergency department), toxic confusional state, and other acute medical diagnoses. Investigations will depend on your examination findings, but if these do not point to a clear diagnosis make

sure you do a chest X-ray, ECG, cardiac enzymes, blood and urine cultures.

Patient B has a progressive disease process leading to steady deterioration in mobility. The disease may well have been diagnosed several years previously, so obtain the old medical records and go through the primary health care record in some detail. Old records may help chart the rate of decline, confirming its pattern. Parkinson's disease, myxoedema and osteoarthritis may show this sort of pattern.

Patient C is very difficult. Whatever caused the immobility happened a long time ago, and the picture is now clouded by complications of immobility. This patient will often have several diagnoses, none of which is the cause of the immobility. For example, the patient may have pneumonia, dehydration, pressure sores, muscle wasting, contracted joints and a confusional state. The main tasks here are to decide on priorities for treatment (dehydration is usually top of the list for treatment), systematically ensuring that each problem is managed. As the patient's problems are solved, so it may become clearer what caused the original immobility.

Patient D has a stepwise decline, caused by a disease that has periods of exacerbation and of remission. Multiple sclerosis is the classic example, and can occur for the first time in old age. Chronic obstructive airways disease may produce this picture, as can recurrent heart attacks. Probably the commonest causes are recurrent minor strokes and rheumatoid arthritis.

Patient E is interesting because of the rapid swings from full mobility to total immobility over a matter of days. Recurrent medical problems are a likely cause: heart failure, urinary tract infection, transient ischaemic attacks. Falls from whatever cause may lead to this sort of picture, with short periods of loss of confidence and immobility. If the periods of immobility are short, less than a day, it is worth considering Parkinsonian 'on–off' syndrome. Recurrent episodes of immobility often lead to recurrent hospital admissions. It is always worth making the effort of going through the notes, however thick they may be. It is all too tempting to label such patients as suffering from a behavioural or psychiatric problem, particularly when they get better without any apparent intervention. In such cases never overlook the possibility of alcohol abuse, other drug use (including prescribed medications), epilepsy, carbon monoxide poisoning from blocked flue pipes, and self-neglect due to depression or an early dementia syndrome.

IS THE PATIENT REALLY IMMOBILE?

Having obtained an idea about the pattern of decline and any symptoms, together with a clinical examination, it is necessary to decide just how immobile your patient is. Within the bounds of common sense, you should get the patient standing and attempting a few steps.

This exercise may reveal that the patient can walk, but is immobile because he or she is unable to get out of a bed or chair unaided. Alternatively, a confused patient may not have mentioned unbearable pain on standing and walking, which has prevented them from attempting to move.

A chair-shaped patient indicates a duration of immobility longer than a few days.

If the patient has no concept of walking, suspect apraxia (inability to carry out a purposeful sequence of activity despite normal power and sensation) due to a stroke, dementia syndrome, or a confusional state.

Tentative steps, with clutching of helpers, may indicate loss of confidence following a fall.

If there is dramatic staggering to the nearest bed, chair or nurse followed by an Oscar-winning collapse, a behavioural cause is likely.

Sometimes a diagnostic gait pattern is found. Examples are: broad-based gait of ataxia (poor balance); feet stuck to the floor — Parkinsonian syndrome; dragging of one leg — a stroke; waddling — weak proximal muscles (e.g. osteomalacia); or a limp — joint disease (but also check feet).

Make sure the patient can see. Blind people do not always tell the doctor!

WHAT NEXT?

There is seldom a shortage of diagnoses in an immobile patient, usually there are too many. A sensible strategy is to draw up a problem list, indicating possible causal relationships. The pattern and duration of immobility will give some indication of the chances of recovery. Each medical diagnosis will require treatment, although it is wise to set priorities and not attempt to treat everything at once. Rehydration and further use of the telephone are usually the first steps of management. A good problem list will ensure that you do not forget management of other less pressing problems.

Immobility in elderly patients is almost always a multifactorial problem, so beware of coming down on a single diagnosis as the cause of immobility. 'Immobility due to Parkinson's disease' is more likely to be 'Immobility in a Parkinsonian patient because over-caring daughter tucked her up in bed when she had a cold. Unable to remobilize, now she has pneumonia.'

MOBILIZATION

The patient remains at risk of the complications of immobility even in hospital, so it is vital that a planned programme of mobilization occurs as soon as possible. It is important not to confuse mobilization with moving the patient from bed to chair. Very few elderly patients benefit from being nursed in a chair for long periods.

Some patients may find mobilization quite exhausting. It is always worth re-examining patients who are not progressing well. Often their poor exercise tolerance is due to undiagnosed heart failure, depression, muscle weakness, arthritis or pain. Appropriate treatment and advice usually allows continued, but slower mobilization. Patients with dementia syndromes can be particularly difficult to mobilize, often appearing completely unwilling to do anything, and with virtually no ability to learn how to get back on their feet. In these cases it is important not to give up too soon, and a supportive team approach is vital. The physiotherapists cannot hope to mobilize such patients alone.

A few patients should not be mobilized rapidly: those with unstabilized fractures, vertebral collapse, bony secondaries, acutely inflamed joints or joint effusions. In these cases, the underlying disease process should be controlled first, and then mobilization started. For the majority, a progressive increase in activity from lying to sitting on the edge of the bed, regaining postural reflexes, to taking a few steps with two helpers, to walking with a frame, to independent walking should be attempted. It is not necessary to have a full diagnostic work-up before starting mobilization.

Key points

- Immobility is a classic presentation of disease, and may be caused by a wide range of different disease.

The aetiology is usually multifactorial, but often a single factor becomes 'the last straw'.

- The pattern of decline in mobility is fundamental to making a diagnosis and prognosis. Patterns are: sudden decline, progressive steady decline, sudden decline in distant past, stepwise decline, fluctuations.
- An essential part of the examination of all patients is to watch them stand up and walk, with assistance if necessary.
- Mobilization should begin as soon as any acute medical problem has been controlled, but should not wait until the whole team has completed their work-ups.

FURTHER READING

Andrews K. *Rehabilitation of the Older Adult.* Edward Arnold, London, 1987.

Bendall MJ, Bassey EF, Pearson MB. Factors affecting the walking speed of elderly people. *Age & Ageing* 1989; **18**: 327–332.

Creditor MC. Hazards of hospitalization of the elderly. *Ann Intern Med* 1993; **118**(3): 219–223.

Guralnik JM, Simonsick EM. Physical disability in older Americans. *J Gerontol* 1993; **48**: 3–10.

Heinemann AW, Linacre JM, Wright BD, Hamilton BB, Granger C. Prediction of rehabilitation outcomes with disability measures. *Arch Phys Med Rehab* 1994; **75**(2): 133–143.

Imms RJ, Edholm OG. Studies of gait and mobility in the elderly. *Age & Ageing* 1981; **10**: 147–156.

Redford JB. Seating and wheeled mobility in the disabled elderly population. *Arch Phys Med Rehab* 1993; **74**(8): 877–885.

Shephard RJ. *Physical Activity and Aging*, 2nd edn. Croom Helm, London, 1987.

20 FALLS

- Causes
- Key questions to ask
- Psychological consequences of falls

Falls are common in old age, and commoner amongst women than men. The reported prevalence of falls over a period of a year is approximately 30 per cent, although prospective studies have given lower rates, suggesting that elderly people tend to overestimate their experience of falls when asked to recall past events.

As people age, various physiological changes take place that increase their risk of falling (Table 20.1). So-called accidental falls are often caused by a failure to respond quickly enough to changes in the body's centre of gravity. Poorer proprioception is a factor, coupled with the need to use vision much more than at younger ages to correct and maintain balance.

Table 20.1 Physiological ageing changes

Reduced muscle strength
Slower psycho-motor responses
Increased body sway
Poorer proprioception
Slower visual accommodation reflexes

Clearly it is sensible practice to make the home environment as safe as possible by removing loose mats and stair carpets, ensuring that lights are left on in dark hallways, fixing stair rails that go down beyond the last step, replacing wall sockets to waist height to avoid bending down, and re-siting kitchen cabinets and shelves at a height where things can be reached easily. However, many elderly people may view such alterations with little enthusiasm, so it is as well to consider such changes as part of a peri-retirement plan when behaviour may be easier to change.

CAUSES

Falls range from minor, trivial trips with no lasting consequences to major, life-threatening events. The underlying pathologies that cause falls are wide, as are the consequences of a fall. The aim of history-taking and examination of a person seen because of falls is to attempt to diagnose the underlying pathological processes (Table 20.2). The physiological changes of ageing may well be superimposed on disease processes, making it a difficult task to sort out the underlying cause.

Premonitory falls occur in the run-up to a serious illness, and it is common for an elderly patient to have presented with a fall to an Accident and Emergency department the day before admission with pneumonia. Often careful assessment at the time of a premonitory fall will reveal signs of underlying acute illness. Casual assessment will not!

Table 20.2 The causes of falls

Premonitory falls
  Forerunner of acute, usually infectious, illness

Prescribed medications
  Multiple drugs
  Psychotrophic drugs
  Diuretics
  Antihypertensives
  L-Dopa

Neurological disease
  Stroke
  Transient ischaemic attack
  Parkinson's disease
  Cerebellar disease
  Spinal cord degeneration
  Epilepsy

Circulatory system diseases
  Silent myocardial infarction
  Vasovagal attack (faints, micturition syncope)
  Dysrhythmias
  Postural hypotension
  Vertebrobasilar syndrome
  Carotid sinus sensitivity

Musculo-skeletal disease
  Generalized muscle weakness
  Wasting secondary to arthritis
  Unstable knee joint
  Proximal myopathy

Miscellaneous
  Drop attacks
  Hypoglycaemia
  Electrolyte imbalance
  Pain (e.g. feet)
  Abuse
  Labyrinthitis
  Cervical spondylosis
  Alcohol
  Environmental hazards
  Poor vision

The more medications a patient takes the greater the risk of falling. This may be because of the drugs themselves, but is more likely a marker of serious underlying disease. However, drugs that cause low blood pressure, particularly on standing up (postural hypotension) may cause falls. The most notorious are diuretics and anti-depressants.

Neurological diseases are commonly associated with falls, and may be quite subtle and difficult to detect. Mild strokes are frequently not detected by a superficial examination. Parkinson's disease may not be associated with a tremor and can often be mistaken for 'ageing'. Cerebellar disease is quite rare, but since the cerebellum is responsible for coordination and balance, often leads to a very unsteady, drunken gait. Causes of cerebellar disease are strokes, myxoedema, alcoholism,

and degenerations associated with cancers (especially of bronchus and breast).

The spinal cord carries both motor nerve fibres (pyramidal tracts) and position sensory fibres (posterior columns) to the brain. Vitamin B_{12} deficiency (pernicious anaemia) and neurosyphilis (tabes dorsalis) can both affect the spinal cord, and lead to a degeneration of both types of nerve fibre. Epilepsy is usually due to a previous stroke in elderly people, although brain tumours can also cause epilepsy. An epileptic attack will lead to a fall, and without a witness to the attack, can be difficult to diagnose.

Circulatory system diseases are common. 'Silent' myocardial infarction (i.e. without characteristic chest pain) may present with a fall because of reduced cardiac output and low blood pressure, and associated heart failure. Vasovagal attacks (faints) can also occur in elderly people and may be precipitated by straining — for example on micturition. Dysrhythmias, often due to ischaemic heart disease, may lead to an abnormally slow heart rate or a very rapid heart rate. In both cases, cardiac output is reduced and a fall may result. Postural hypotension of up to 40 mmHg between lying and standing systolic blood pressure occurs in up to 5 per cent of elderly people, for no apparent reason. Such patients may feel extremely light-headed and dizzy on standing and are therefore at risk of falling. In many cases an underlying cause is found: drugs, myocardial infarction, dehydration, acute blood loss from a bleeding peptic ulcer. Vertebrobasilar syndrome is probably overdiagnosed, and is thought to be due to interruption of the blood supply to the brainstem on upward or sideways movement of the head associated with cervical spondylosis. In true cases, associated symptoms of tinnitus, double vision and vertigo are found.

Musculo-skeletal diseases are usually obvious, and may be due to general effects of widespread cancer, or local effects of arthritis. Osteoarthritis of the knee joints may lead to instability of the joint and the sensation of the joint 'giving' and may precipitate a fall. Less often seen is a proximal myopathy of the limb girdle muscles (shoulders or pelvis) which leads to difficulties getting out of a chair and climbing stairs. Osteomalacia sometimes causes this problem and improves with treatment with vitamin D and calcium.

Miscellaneous causes of falls are many, but drop attacks deserve special mention. The patient is usually walking outdoors, and in previously good health. Without any warning, the legs give way and the patient is unable to get up. The legs feel useless, but after a variable time (up to several hours) the use comes back into the legs and the patient is able to walk again. The underlying cause of drop attacks remains unknown.

Occasionally it is necessary to pose the question 'did the patient fall or was she pushed?' Elder abuse is increasingly recognized as a cause of trauma in frail elderly people.

The inner ear contains sensitive mechanisms for maintenance of balance, and acute viral labyrinthitis will lead to severe vertigo and nausea. The presentation is usually so acute and the symptoms severe, that diagnosis is not difficult. Lesser degrees of chronic dizziness are very common in elderly people and are frequently attributed to cervical spondylosis. However, X-ray changes in the cervical spine are so common that it is difficult to be certain that this is really the cause of the symptoms, and is seldom the cause of recurrent falls.

Too much alcohol is a common cause of falling over at any age. It has to be remembered that some elderly people are likely to overindulge in drinking and, together with their poorer physiological mechanisms for maintaining balance, are more likely to fall over after a relatively modest amount of alcohol.

KEY QUESTIONS TO ASK

It should be obvious that even a single fall should lead to a detailed history and examination and any witnesses should be questioned too; often this is not done, and opportunities for early diagnosis and treatment are missed. The family doctor and Accident and Emergency department staff are likely to be the first doctors to assess such patients, and need to give time, sympathy and a systematic approach. Often, referral to the Department of Health Care for Elderly People/Medicine of Old Age will be needed for diagnosis and treatment.

Is the patient in good health?

A fall in a patient who is suffering with a chronic disability should lead to a different line of enquiry. Many falls occur in the course of daily living (for example, transferring from bed to chair, or in the bathroom) in patients with previous strokes, Parkinson's disease and arthritis. It is essential to make a careful enquiry about medication, and any recent changes.

In a patient who is previously well, a search must be made for new acute illness, and if none is present, then the fall may be 'accidental' and due to ageing physiol-ogy, or due to environmental factors (poor lighting, loose mats).

Has the patient had previous falls?

Unless a fall leads to a severe consequence, such as a fracture, patients often do not seek any medical attention. It is often only after recurrent or bad falls that help is sought. Recall of the pattern of previous falls can be helpful, in particular their frequency, relationship with posture, time of day, any residual symptoms following the fall, and any avoiding steps taken by the patient.

What was the patient doing at the time?

Falls that occur on changing posture, particularly lying to standing, suggest postural hypotension, verte-brobasilar insufficiency or accidents. Coexisting diseases may lead to falls on transfers (see above).

Did the patient trip?

A trip may occur simply as the result of poor postural reflexes associated with ageing, but may be aggravated by poor vision. Sometimes bifocal glasses can give a distorted view leading to an accidental fall. Outdoor falls may be due to uneven pavements, or being pushed by other people. Frequently, patients admit that they were trying to do two things at once; for example, boiling some soup when the door bell rang, and in the moment of confusion over which task to attend to, a fall occurred.

Did the patient get any warning?

The absence of any warning implies a sudden event, usually neurological or circulatory diseases. However, prior to an epileptic fit patients may feel peculiar, and may feel dizzy with the onset of any cause of a reduced cardiac output.

Is the patient able to walk normally?

Perhaps the single most useful investigation of elderly fallers is to watch them walking, as the signs of diseases that frequently cause falls may be ruled out: Parkinson's disease, stroke, arthritis, muscle weakness, neuropathy, cerebellar disease.

If the patient has a normal gait, it is necessary to rule out the transient causes of instability: epilepsy, dys-rhythmias, postural hypotension, effects of drugs and alcohol, myocardial infarction, hypoglycaemia, transient ischaemic attacks.

PSYCHOLOGICAL CONSEQUENCES OF FALLS

A fall is a tremendous psychological blow to many elderly people. It reminds them of their increasing frailty, and may lead to dramatic loss of confidence, particularly walking outdoors. This in turn may lead to becoming housebound, and a reduction in social contacts, and depression. Many patients require protracted rehabilitation, with practice in their own homes and nearby shops to restore confidence. A medically trivial fall may have far-reaching effects on the individual.

Key points

- Falls are extremely common, with up to a third of people having a fall in the course of a year.
- Physiological ageing changes make older people more vulnerable to falling, but a search must be made for underlying diseases.
- Important points in the history are: is the patient in good health; has the patient had previous falls; what was the patient doing at the time; did the patient trip; was there any warning?

- The single most useful part of the examination is to watch the patient walking. A postural blood pressure is essential.

FURTHER READING

Blake AJ, Morgan K, Bendall MJ *et al*. Falls in elderly people at home: prevalence and associated factors *Age & Ageing* 1988; **17**: 365–372.

Costa AJ. Preventing falls in your elderly patients. *Postgrad Med* 1991; **89**(1): 139–140, 142.

Campbell AJ, Spears GFS, Brown JS, Busby WJ, Borrie MJ. Circumstances and consequences of falls experienced by a community population 70 years and over during a prospective study. *Age & Ageing* 1990; **19**: 136–141.

Guickel J. Falls among elderly people living at home: medical and social factors in a national sample. *J Med Sci* 1992; **28**: 446–453.

Marks W. Physical restraints in the practice of medicine. Current concepts. *Arch Intern Med* 1992; **152**(11): 2203–2206.

Meunier PJ. Prevention of hip fractures. *Am J Med* 1993; **95**(5A): 75S–78S.

Morris J. Falls in older people. *J Roy Soc Med* 1994; **87**: 435-436.

Tinetti ME. Falls. In Cassel CK, Riesenberg DR, Sorensen LB, Walsh JR (eds), *Geriatric Medicine*, 2nd edn, Springer-Verlag, London, 1990.

21 CONFUSION

- Acute confusion
- Chronic confusion
- Alzheimer's disease
- Multi-infarct dementia
- Laboratory investigations

A confusional state is best described as being either acute or chronic.

ACUTE CONFUSION

Acute confusion (delirium) is one of the most common forms of organic brain syndrome with both physical and mental abnormalities needing urgent assessment. The clinical features are listed in Table 21.1. It is relatively uncommon in young people as their confusion threshold is high, although conditions such as malaria and severe pneumonia may cause confusion. The threshold for confusion is much lower in older people and it may be the presenting feature of such conditions as myocardial infarction, pneumonia or urinary tract infection. Failure to recognize it and hence to diagnose and treat the underlying condition can have fatal consequences for the patient. This is most likely to occur in patients already suffering from a chronic confusional state whose acute exacerbation is misinterpreted as simply a worsening of the 'dementia'. Failure to assess a person's level of cognitive functioning on admission and to monitor it periodically during hospitalization

can also result in a missed diagnosis of acute confusional state. 'Acute' can mean an onset ranging from a few minutes through hours and days up to three months.

Table 21.1 Clinical features of acute confusion (delirium)

Clouding of consciousness
Disorientation in time and place
Onset usually over hours and days (fluctuating course)
Poor short-term memory
Hallucinations or misinterpretations
Altered activity levels (agitated, restless and wandering or drowsy and lethargic)
Evidence of the disease process causing the confusion with physical signs — tachycardia, sweating, etc.
Speech abnormalities (mumbling, rambling)

There are various major groups of causes of acute confusion (Table 21.2), though it is common to find multiple causes.

Prodromal features such as restlessness, hypersensitivity to visual and auditory stimuli, nocturnal insomnia and daytime sleepiness may all be found.

The factors shown in Table 21.3 are thought to predispose to acute confusion.

Table 21.2 Major causes of acute confusion

Neurological conditions
  Head injury
  Stroke (especially small cortical lesions without focal neuro-
  logical signs)
  Epilepsy

Systemic conditions
  Infections
  Hypoxia/hypercarbia
  Uraemia
  Hypo/hyperglycaemia
  Hypo/hyperthermia
  Heart failure
  Myocardial infarction
  Pulmonary emboli
  Acid–base disturbance
  After a 'fall'

Drugs
  Side-effect of prescribed medication (anticholinergics,
  hypnotics/sedatives/tranquillizers, antidepressants,
  analgesics, L-dopa preparations)
  Overdose or withdrawal (alcohol, hypnotics)

Environmental changes
  A move to new surroundings, e.g. admission to an institution (translocation effect)
  'Sundowner' syndrome (increased agitation/confusion in
  people with chronic confusion in the evening)

Table 21.3 Factors that predispose to acute confusion

  Ageing process (decreased threshold)
  Impairment of vision and hearing
  Presence of chronic physical and chronic brain diseases
  Age-related changes in drug effects

Early diagnosis is important because most patients can recover with appropriate treatment. However, advanced age and longer duration of illness worsen the prognosis and mortality rates range up to 30 per cent. The differential diagnoses include acute or chronic confusion, chronic state (e.g. the dementias) and acute functional psychosis (pseudodelirium).

An assessment of mental state is not complete without a mental test score. This appraisal of memory (short- and long-term), orientation and numeracy skills can be performed using a simple 10-point plan (Table 21.4) or more elaborate forms such as the Mini-Mental State Examination. Highly complex tests (some using user-friendly computers) are available and advice can be obtained from a clinical psychologist for both acute and chronic confusional states.

The mental test score is most valuable when used on the same patient over a period of time. A low initial score becomes more relevant if an underlying diagnosis of dementia is suspected and it does not improve after treatment of any acute problems. A score that rapidly improves over a few days obviously helps rule out a chronic 'dementing' illness.

Table 21.4 The mental test score

  1. Name
  2. Date of birth
  3. Age
  4. Date and time of day
  5. Address
  6. Name of Prime Minister
  7. Date of First World War
  8. Place
  9. Remember an address 5 minutes later
  10. Count back from 20 to 1

CHRONIC CONFUSION (DEMENTIA)

Chronic confusional states must have been present for at least three months to be labelled as such. There is usually loss of function in multiple areas (e.g. intellectual function, memory, language). There are, however, *reversible* causes, so diagnosis and treatment may produce improvement. Chronic confusional states become increasingly common in old age (10 per cent > 65, 20 per cent > 80) but are obviously not a component of normal ageing. Regardless of age a search for the cause is warranted in most cases (Table 21.5).

Table 21.5 Causes of chronic confusion

Reversible causes (about 20% of cases)
  Drugs (e.g. long-acting tranquillizers)
  Endocrine disorders (e.g. hypothyroidism)
  Systemic illness
  Vitamin deficiencies (e.g. B_{12}, thiamine)
  Undernutrition
  Intracranial masses (benign and resectable) (e.g. menin-
  gioma)
  CNS infections (e.g. syphilis)
  Normal pressure hydrocephalus (see Fig. 21.1)
  Depression
  Alcohol

Irreversible causes
  Alzheimer's disease
  Pick's disease
  Multi-infarct dementia
  CNS malignancy
  Creutzfeldt–Jakob disease
  Huntingdon's disease
  Parkinson's disease
  Post-infective brain damage
  AIDS 'dementia'
  Post-traumatic/anoxic brain damage

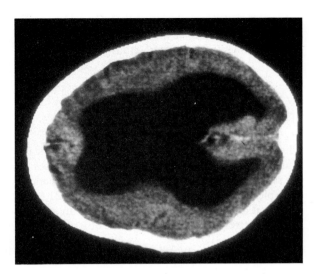

Figure 21.1 A rare cause of confusion: normal pressure hydrocephalus shown on a CT scan

The differential diagnoses include acute confusional states, benign (senile) forgetfulness, amnesic syndromes and depression (pseudodementia).

Acute confusional states (or acute on chronic) should be picked up by the presence of specific features (clouding of consciousness, evidence of the disease process with physical signs, etc.). Benign (senile) forgetfulness involves a minor degree of forgetfulness, especially for recent memory (sufferers are forever losing keys, spectacles, etc.). It was portrayed to perfection by Margaret Rutherford in the film *The VIPs*. It is not progressive. The amnesic syndromes include alcohol abuse (Korsakoff's syndrome secondary to thiamine deficiency), trauma (including the repeated head trauma of boxers — dementia pugilistica), hypoxia and stroke. Transient global amnesia is a condition of short-lived amnesia (usually hours) secondary to either migraine or cerebral microemboli. Depression can be difficult to distinguish from a primary chronic confusional state and in some cases a psychiatric opinion should be sought. A diagnosis of depression may be helped by the findings of a more rapid onset and progression of symptoms and a depressed mood. Attention and concentration as well as learning abilities are often intact.

The multiple cognitive 'losses' are of sufficient severity to interfere with social and occupational functioning. The deficits being multifaceted involve memory, judgement, abstract thought and a variety of higher cortical functions. Changes in personality and behaviour also occur and these may cause the greatest distress to carers.

Memory impairment is the most prominent symptom, especially recent memory. In mild cases there is forgetfulness in daily life and the need for repetition to facilitate remembering. In severe cases long-term memory is also affected. Impairment of abstract thinking can be assessed by testing the ability to interpret proverbs. Language (a higher cortical function) is often impaired; it may become vague, stereotyped, imprecise or aphasic. Dyspraxia (the inability to perform common tasks such as dressing or walking) also occurs. Judgement becomes impaired and personality changes including the accentuation of pre-existing traits (e.g. aggression, paranoia) are common. Some people retain a degree of insight and not unnaturally become depressed; others suffer from anxiety. In advanced cases they may have delusions or hallucinations.

The above description applies mainly to the largest group of non-reversible causes of chronic confusion — the dementing syndromes.

The two most common causes of dementia are Alzheimer's disease and multi-infarct dementia. Alzheimer's disease is seen more frequently in clinical practice but a positive diagnosis of either of the two conditions requires careful assessment. Post mortem histological studies of brain tissue, however, show a great deal of overlap between the two conditions.

ALZHEIMER'S DISEASE

Alzheimer's disease was named by Alois Alzheimer in 1907. He described senile plaques and neurofibrillar tangles in the brain sections of a 57-year-old woman who died of 'dementia'. His name became attached to this pre-senile form although it is very rare. The similar condition in the elderly was termed senile dementia of the Alzheimer type (SDAT). Now all cases are termed Alzheimer's disease (AD).

AD is a clinical diagnosis made by excluding other disorders. A definitive diagnosis can only be made by biopsy (not usually feasible) or at autopsy. The characteristic histopathological changes are neurofibrillar tangles, neuritic plaques and amyloid angiopathy, especially in the hippocampus and cortex. Other findings include diffuse cortical atrophy, diminished brain weight, gliosis and granulovacular degeneration. These findings are not pathognomic for they occur in other disease processes and in *normal ageing*, the difference being quantitative and in the location of the changes.

Investigations are usually normal, although a CT brain scan may show some non-specific cortical atrophy.

The discovery of cholinergic deficiency in AD was a major advance in pathogenic research. The replacement of neurochemical transmitters is a fundamental research area and may produce new treatments in the future.

Finding a 'cause' for Alzheimer's disease revolves around three other research topics: the role of aluminium; a viral aetiology; and the role of genetics. Aluminium is the world's most abundant metal, being present in all food chains and the water supply. It forms the core of the neuritic plaque found in the disease. In parts of the world where the element is present in high levels there appears to be a higher incidence of neurological disorders (in some places clinical combinations of AD, Parkinson's disease and multiple sclerosis). Aluminium is certainly neurotoxic as evidenced by the damage caused to renal dialysis patients when dialysis fluid was originally found to contain high aluminium levels.

There is currently no evidence to favour a viral/slow virus aetiology for AD, although it is well recognized that transmissible agents (probably smaller than viruses), are responsible for at least two dementia syndromes — kuru in Papua New Guinea, and Creutzfeldt–Jakob disease.

Down's syndrome may help provide a genetic 'marker' for the disease. Down's patients develop histopathological changes similar to AD at an early age. The genetic defect is known in Down's syndrome, so presumably the 'code' for the brain damage is present in this segment and when accurately located could be isolated, possibly providing a marker to susceptibility. It is now known that the precursor protein for amyloid is coded for by a gene on the long arm of chromosome 21 and another gene in this location governs the familial form of AD that affects younger people.

MULTI-INFARCT DEMENTIA

Multi-infarct dementia results when patients have sustained recurrent cortical or subcortical strokes. Most of the strokes are too small to cause permanent damage or even residual focal neurological deficits. The clinical criteria for vascular dementia include the presence of a dementia with a stepwise deteriorating course, a patchy or uneven distribution of cognitive deficits and focal neurological signs. Other characteristic features include the presence of hypertension, signs of atherosclerotic disease elsewhere, emotional lability, pseudobulbar palsy, dysarthria and transient depression. The Hachinski score gives 'marks' for each of the above and a score over 4 is consistent with multi-infarct dementia.

LABORATORY INVESTIGATIONS

The use of investigations in chronic confusional states is aimed at identifying potentially reversible causes. At the same time one must not subject vulnerable patients to unpleasant tests or waste resources. Table 21.6 lists investigations that should be considered in patients with a relatively short history who are otherwise well.

Table 21.6 Investigations for chronic confusion

Necessary
  Blood count and film
  ESR
  Kidney and liver function
  Glucose
  Calcium and phosphate
  Thyroid function
  Vitamin B_{12} and red cell folate
  Syphilis serology
  Chest X-ray
  ECG
  CT brain scan

In selected cases
  EEG
  HIV screen
  Lumbar puncture
  Blood cultures
  Blood gases
  Toxicity screen

Key points

- A confusional state is best described as being acute or chronic.
- Acute confusion (delirium) has both physical and mental abnormalities needing urgent assessment.
- Clouding of consciousness is an important feature of acute confusion (others include disorientation, poor short-term memory, hallucinations and evidence of a disease process).
- Acute confusion may be the presenting feature of almost any medical condition in an elderly person.
- Common causes of acute confusion include stroke, infections and medication.
- Assessment of the mental state is essential in all cases of confusion.

- The mental test score is most valuable when used on the same patient over a period of time.
- Twenty per cent of cases of chronic confusion have a potentially reversible cause.
- Reversible causes of chronic confusion include drugs, endocrine abnormalities and depression.
- Alzheimer's disease and multi-infarct dementia are two of the most common dementia syndromes.
- Research in Alzheimer's disease involves cholinergic pathways and replacement as well as the role of aluminium, viruses and genetic markers.
- In most cases patients with chronic confusional states require investigation.

FURTHER READING

Arie T. Confusion in old age. *Age & Ageing* 1978; **7** (suppl.): 72–76.

Bennett GCJ. *Alzheimer's Disease and Other Confusional States*, 2nd edn. Macdonald Optima, London, 1994.

Hachinski VC. Multi-infarct dementia — a cause of mental deterioration in the elderly. *Lancet* 1974; **ii:** 207–209.

Small GW, Jarvik LF. The dementia syndrome. *Lancet* 1982; **ii:**1443–1446.

22 MANAGEMENT OF CONFUSIONAL STATES

- Supportive care
- Medication
- Management of chronic confusion
- Multidisciplinary help

Specific management of acute confusional states is directed at the underlying pathology and may involve treating acute illnesses such as infections or myocardial infarction, using appropriate drugs and other help (e.g. nursing care, physiotherapy).

SUPPORTIVE CARE

Initially the patient may need intensive nursing care best carried out in a well-lit single room with the minimum of disturbance. It is best to avoid frequent changes of staff, loud noises, and other disruptions. Cot-sides should not be used. If the person is severely agitated, and whilst waiting for medication to work, the mattress can be placed on the floor (after explaining to carers) thus avoiding serious injury. Severely ill patients may need intravenous therapy. Less ill but still restless patients may prefer to sit in a chair.

Once a diagnosis has been made and a plan of treatment organized it is best if at all possible to let the specific medication work and the confusional state settle. This may require a dedicated nurse to encourage fluids, reassure, monitor vital signs and help prevent restlessness. However, some patients are very agitated and occasionally violent or are a danger to themselves by being so unsteady that some calming medication is necessary.

MEDICATION

All types of psychotropic medications have side-effects which are usually more pronounced in elderly people. The smallest effective dose should be used; the aim is *not* to render a difficult patient unconscious only to wake up for someone else to deal with. The clinician should use and get to know a small group of drugs for use in confused, agitated or aggressive patients. In this way a confident yet therapeutic approach is used, always remembering that medication is only part of the treatment process.

Haloperidol

This is a neuroleptic butyrophenone used especially in paranoid psychoses, severe agitation and aggressive disorders. It has a flexibility of dosage and administration, though as with most drugs a lower dose should be used initially, e.g. 0.5–1.0 mg, and increased in frequency under supervision. Its main adverse effects include extrapyramidal symptoms (avoid in patients with Parkinson's disease) and postural hypotension.

Thioridazine

This is a phenothiazine antipsychotic agent. It is not only used in psychotic states but in agitation and restlessness in elderly people. It is well tolerated but postural hypotension and anticholinergic side-effects can occur. It appears to cause less tardive dyskinesia. It is available in suspension syrup and tablet form with initial dosages in the 10–25 mg range.

Other drugs

Chlorpromazine should be avoided, it is long lasting and has a higher profile of potential side-effects in elderly people. Benzodiazepines should not be used for sedative purposes in confusional states; rebound hyperagitation can occur. The drugs should only be given for a short period and withdrawn as soon as the organic cause of the confusion state responds to treatment.

MANAGEMENT OF CHRONIC CONFUSION

Elderly people with chronic confusional states at home or in some form of institution usually present a comparatively stable but declining picture. This steady state can include types of behaviour that are particularly difficult to manage, including wandering, verbal or physical violence (sometimes both), sexual disinhibition or a perplexed agitated restlessness. The stress, anxiety and concern of relatives and carers cannot be overestimated.

Occasionally there is a sudden change in mental state with a clinical picture more of delirium superimposed upon the chronic episode. This is usually due to an acute event, e.g. infection process, reaction to medication or a new organic process. These new medical complications need to be identified quickly and treated. Psychotropic medication may be necessary in addition to disease-specific drugs. The same general measures apply: calm atmosphere, a well-lit room avoiding shadows, no loud noises and consistency of care as far as it is feasible.

In addition to a new organic cause, other significant events, e.g. a fall, a move or a bereavement, can trigger an acute or chronic episode.

MULTIDISCIPLINARY HELP

Help should be multidisciplinary, whatever the elderly person's setting. Key people include those listed in Table 22.1.

Table 22.1 Key people involved in the management of chronic confusion

General practitioner
Community nurse
Community psychiatric nurse
Psychiatrist (old age)
Community crisis intervention team (or equivalent)
Day hospital staff (including outreach duties)
Physician (Health Care of Elderly)
Continence adviser
Pharmacist
Clinical psychologist
Voluntary sector (including Alzheimer's Disease Society)
Social services
    Respite schemes
    Sitting services
    Assessment (OT/physio)
    Day care

The formidable task is to provide effective help in a coherent way, help that meets both the patient's and the carers' needs and wishes. A key task is to have effective assessment without either overlap or gaps in the service provision. The process of seeking and then receiving help can seem a bureaucratic nightmare.

Early assessment and, where necessary, intervention should be made to help with problems such as wandering, aggressiveness, incontinence or sexual problems with appropriate referral. Wandering is hard to control and restrictions or restraints usually make matters worse. The balance of risk-taking on someone else's behalf is a difficult one. Wandering may indicate an inability to find the toilet etc. and simple behavioural therapies can be effective. Much can be achieved to help incontinence (see Chapter 23). Sexual disinhibition may need the intervention of psychiatrist, psychologist and pharmacist to help control, distract and manage. Aggressive behaviour can have many causes (medication, attempts at restraint, etc.) and if simple measures fail (allowing greater freedom of wandering, altering medicine after checking with pharmacist) an expert witness opinion via psychiatrist or psychologist should be sought.

As far as possible this should occur in the client's own home though short-stay assessment or respite may be more appropriate in some cases.

Ideally there should be regular reassessments of

function and medical checks and this should prove administratively easier with the over-75 GP health checks. Family and carers (including rest and nursing home staff) should be regularly updated on the non-confidential aspects of the client. It is important that they have medication explained and that they are supported in the caring role. This includes an acknowledgement of the difficult task they are doing (usually extremely well) as well as education on the disease process, role of the key other members of the team and an explanation of why certain things are happening. The other members of the team should also explain their input, i.e. how they hope to achieve continence, stop aggressiveness, etc. Counselling aspects are particularly important with a view to identifying and resolving family conflict, handling anger and guilt, helping with decisions over respite or institutional care, legal and, indeed, ethical issues.

Links should be made early with social services and voluntary organizations including the Alzheimer's Disease Society, Demential Relief Trust and Carers National Association. These organizations can provide invaluable practical and emotional help and support. Locally, each district provides different and sometimes unique services (night sitters, legal and financial counselling, relative support groups).

Discharging confused elderly people from hospital back into the community requires a great deal of communication with the (usually) wide range of people involved. It must be well planned and organized (see Chapter 46).

Key points

- Treatment is specifically directed at the underlying pathology. Supportive measures include a well-lit room and the minimum disruption.
- All psychotropic medications have side-effects in older people, especially postural hypotension.
- Get to know and use a few drugs to establish confident prescribing.
- The new medical complications in acute or chronic confusion need to be quickly identified and treated.
- Key members of the multidisciplinary team will need to be involved to help with specific symptoms, e.g. incontinence, wandering, sexual disinhibition, aggressiveness.
- Support the carers (both at home and in institutions).

23 INCONTINENCE

- Acceptable places
- Getting there
- History and examination
- Urinary incontinence
- Faecal incontinence

As babies our bladders and bowels function involuntarily and automatically. In early childhood we are trained to identify acceptable places and control excretion by the discipline of praise (keeping dry and not wetting the bed). Once control has been achieved any failure causes embarrassment which continues to occur at any age. To avoid this, only 'acceptable' voiding is allowed so a given individual must be able to identify an acceptable place and get there safely. Advancing age and increasing disability can lower the threshold for control but incontinence is not an inevitable outcome of ageing.

Incontinence is an involuntary loss of urine or faeces in an inappropriate place. This implies that there were no physical or psychological barriers preventing access to an acceptable place but despite this the person excreted inappropriately. This necessitates a thorough investigation as many causes of involuntary loss of control are amenable to medical and surgical management.

ACCEPTABLE PLACES

These are dependent upon a host of factors such as age, sex, social class, society, nationality and present circumstances. The driver of a hansom cab is allowed by law to urinate against the rear offside wheel of his cab. This law has never been repealed, but putting it to the test would probably result in an arrest for obscene behaviour in a public place. Peasant farmers squat down in fields around the world, but Oxford Street (which was once a field) is certainly not now acceptable; society here has decreed the use of private lavatories or public conveniences. Most people have no problem in identifying acceptable places. Difficulties arise, however, when one is unaware of the location. This can happen to anyone in a strange town or building and is a plight experienced by people with dementia; they know they should get to an acceptable place but they cannot find it. If directed, continence results; if not, the nearest suitable alternative (bin or sink) is used rather than be wet. There is no difference in behaviour between the demented patient and someone unable to find a toilet who urinates in the bushes or up against a wall.

In hospitals the lack of suitable toilets is a common cause of loss of continence. Patients may be aware of the need to go, of where to go and of acceptable alternatives (commodes) but are unable to get to them in time. Some patients are placed on incontinence pads in bed, psychologically inviting loss of control. The necessity to get up at night to urinate increases with advancing age. High beds, night sedatives, cot-sides and shortage of help combine to prevent patients from getting to the toilet. It is essential that commodes and toilets be near the beds and chairs of elderly patients.

GETTING THERE

Psychological barriers

The indignity of being inadequately clothed (split-back nightdresses, pyjama bottoms that fall down) means that many people are incontinent rather than shame themselves crossing a semi-public ward area 'naked'.

Loss of mobility

This is the commonest cause of difficulty both in the community and in institutions. Most public conveniences were designed for the physically able. There are few with access and facilities for the disabled. People taking diuretics or those with bladder or bowel control difficulties often have to plan routes on the basis of available toilet facilities; more commonly they become house bound. There is no need for architects and town planners to experience being old, a test dose of a fast-acting diuretic taken in the middle of a shopping precinct should concentrate the mind!

Location of toilet

An outside toilet requires that to be continent one must get outside (whatever the weather) or use another receptacle. Toilets upstairs depend on good physical mobility. Thus many elderly people who are ill at home have been 'incontinent' before they enter hospital, their illness preventing them from reaching the toilet. The loss of control is due to illness and associated immobility, not their age. A bedside commode may have enabled them to remain continent. How they are treated in hospital will influence whether incontinence becomes an established pattern or not.

Ward toilets

The majority of hospital wards have too few toilets, often providing only two for 20–30 people. If we really expected people to be continent we would provide (as in hotels) a lavatory for each patient next to the bed. Most patients have to walk long distances then wait.

Toilet doors are often heavy and the space may not permit a wheel chair or walking frame. Unless specifically designed, the seat will be too low, with no hand rails and toilet paper on a roll. Try going to the toilet using only one hand, balancing on one leg and get a few pieces of paper off the roll at a time (this is often a situation stroke patients find themselves in).

Bad design

Many hospitals are still equipped with old-fashioned high beds so that nearly all elderly patients need assistance to get in and out. If someone does try to get out unaided they either fall or sides are put up. If the bed is adjustable and set correctly most patients can get out unaided and cot-sides are certainly unnecessary.

Use of bed pans

The gymnastic prowess necessary to straddle a bed pan and maintain balance and position on it is difficult and exhausting for most elderly patients. The sheer act becomes one of dread and putting off its use can lead to retention and constipation with later faecal incontinence due to overflow (spurious diarrhoea). A bedside commode is easier to use.

Chairs

The correct chair is one that a person can get out of easily. Properly dressed (with underclothes), sitting in a chair of the correct height with a walking frame nearby, the majority of elderly patients can get to the toilet independently. They cannot do this if the chair is too high or too low, if they are trapped by a fixed table or if they feel inadequately dressed or cannot reach their walking frame.

HISTORY AND EXAMINATION

A full clinical history with careful attention to the history of bladder and bowel function prior to the present illness (from both patient and relatives) will help to differentiate between loss of ability to control excretion and failure to identify or get to an acceptable place. Clinical examination, including a rectal and a vaginal examination, and culture of a mid-stream specimen of urine are all essential (and will often give a good indication as to the cause of the problem).

An incontinence chart kept for a few days only (it is a very nurse-intensive process) may give a recognizable pattern of urine and/or faecal incontinence, e.g. morning incontinence associated with fast-acting diuretics. The specialist help of a continence adviser may be needed at times.

URINARY INCONTINENCE

The common causes of urinary incontinence are listed in Table 23.1 and the mechanisms in Table 23.2.

Table 23.1 Common causes of urinary incontinence

Urinary tract infection
Stress incontinence
Detrusor instability (unstable bladder)
Retention with overflow
Prostatism
Uninhibited neurogenic bladder
Reflect neurogenic bladder
Atonic neurogenic bladder
Others
   Uterine prolapse
   Cystocele
   Atrophic vaginitis

Table 23.2 Mechanisms of urinary incontinence

Involuntary detrusor contractions
Loss of normal elasticity of bladder wall
Incompetence of bladder neck and distal sphincter
   mechanisms
Loss of higher CNS control of micturition function
Abnormalities of bladder sensation

Infection

Urinary tract infections are common (Table 23.3) and potentially very serious. The incidence is 20 per cent in people over 65 years, compared with an incidence of 3.2 per cent in those aged 45–65.

Table 23.3 Causes of neurogenic bladder

Uninhibited neurogenic bladder
   Cerebrovascular disease (multi-infarct dementia or stroke)
   Frontal lobe tumour (precipitant micturition)
   Parkinson's disease
   Normal pressure hydrocephalus

Reflex neurogenic bladder
   Spinal cord disease (disc prolapse, spinal cord tumour, etc.)

Atonic neurogenic bladder
   Diabetes mellitus
   Tabes dorsalis

Less efficient bladder emptying (especially if there is any degree of bladder neck obstruction) may predispose to an increased frequency of infection. Women wiping bowel organisms forwards to the urethal area can also precipitate infection. Other pathologies in the urinary tract presenting with infection (e.g. bladder tumours, stones) should be considered. The classic history of frequency and dysuria is often absent. A urinary tract infection may present as an acute confusional state or a series of falls and because it is so common should always be ruled in or out by appropriate testing, including Dipstix tests done on the ward.

Stress incontinence

In this condition there is bladder neck incompetence, the distal urethral mechanism is unable to cope with the intra-abdominal pressure rise that occurs on coughing and laughing. It is extremely common in women and has been related to the 'damage' that occurs to the pelvic musculature during childbirth. In addition the post-menopausal changes (due to the lack of oestrogen) give rise to atrophic change affecting the muscular sphincter mechanisms.

Detrusor instability

This accounts for about two-thirds of cases and is also called 'unstable bladder' incontinence. In this condition the uninhibited detrusor contractions result in the bladder neck mechanism failing, leading to the distal urethral mechanism also failing and incontinence resulting.

The incontinence episodes may be reported by the relatives as 'wilful', typically the person had been on the toilet for ten minutes, went into the living room and then incontinence occurred. After diagnosis the cause (involuntary contractions triggered by many things, movement, coughing, volume of urine, etc.) must be carefully explained. The diagnosis, however, is best made after urodynamic studies, though the confused and/or severely immobile patient should not be subjected to these investigations without appropriate consultation.

Overflow incontinence

The commonest cause in both sexes is a loaded rectum. In men, prostate enlargement is also a common factor. A constant dribble of urine is a typical symptom and it is then mandatory to examine the abdomen for a distended bladder and do a rectal examination. Women go into retention less easily than men and, in addition to constipation, a pelvic mass should be excluded. Drugs can cause retention (anticholinergics) as well as urethral strictures (often post-catheter or surgical trauma).

Prostatism

This common condition of elderly men presents with a history of delay in the start of micturition and a poor stream with terminal dribbling. Sufferers may be incontinent due to urgency (75 per cent of patients also have some evidence of detrusor instability), overflow (if they have gone into retention) and post-micturition dribble (PMD). This is an exaggerated form of a condition that affects most men of all ages (the leakage of small amounts of urine after micturition has ceased). When prostatism is not a problem PMD can be avoided. At the end of micturition the scrotal sac should be lifted gently and the base of the urethra gently pushed upon, to allow a few extra millilitres of urine to be passed.

Neurogenic bladder

Damage to the innervation of the bladder and cortical damage can lead to a neurogenic bladder (see Table 23.3). There is usually a lack of awareness and voiding occurs automatically once a certain volume has been reached. Some patients, however, learn to control voiding by increasing intra-abdominal pressure.

Investigations

Not every patient requires a full work-up, including invasive bladder studies. Usually the diagnosis is clear once a basic history and examination, coupled with a continence chart, have been completed (Table 23.4). If the problem appears complex (e.g. elements of stress and urge incontinence), then referral to a urodynamic clinic is often worthwhile.

Treatment

Antibiotics should be used to treat a urinary tract infection (>1000 wbc and > 1.0 million colony count). If associated with a catheter this should be removed, albeit temporarily. If there are accompanying systemic symptoms and signs (e.g. confusion, hypotension and rigors) then parenteral antibiotics should be used. Precipitating causes of urinary incontinence (e.g. drugs) should be altered where possible. Outflow tract obstruction can be managed conservatively in some

Table 23.4 Investigative process

History
    Medication (diuretics, laxatives, tranquillizers)
    Medical and surgical history

Examination
    Mental state
    Mobility
    Neurological examination
    Rectal examination
    Vaginal examination
    Abdominal examination

Investigations
    Continence chart
    Mid-stream urine
    Blood sugar
    Urea and electrolytes

Possibly:
    Plain abdominal X-ray
    U/S
    Kidneys, ureters and bladder
    Intravenous urogram
    TPHA/UDRL (syphilis serology)
    Cystometry
    Urodynamics

selected cases (severe frailty, personal choice) by the use of a long-term catheter. Most other cases benefit from referral to a specialist urologist. Gynaecological advice should be sought in patients with a uterine prolapse, cystocele and atrophic vaginitis (the latter is usually helped markedly by the application of oestrogen cream).

The ward environment (clearly marked toilets) and mobility exercises assist patients greatly. Confused patients may be helped by reality orientation techniques. Praise and the short-term use of a two-hourly toileting regime should begin the process of assessment. Hourly toileting is difficult and the charts fail to be filled in after a few days. The chart should provide a 'pattern' and help with diagnosis and management, and not become an end in itself.

There is very little evidence that anticholinergic drugs confer significant benefit to most elderly people with unstable bladders. The use of anticholinergics is not without risk of side-effects and, as their benefits are usually minimal, careful consideration should be given to their use (especially their continued use) if improvement does not occur.

Catheters have their uses, intermittently for some, permanently for a carefully selected group of patients where there is also user acceptance and satisfaction. Acutely ill people often need catheterizing, though it should be removed at the earliest opportunity in the rehabilitation process. Catheters should never be used for ease of nursing/caring but only if the patient also benefits. The vast range of different catheters and all advice on continence aids, their use, selection, comfort and suitability are part of the expertise of continence advisers and their help should be sought.

Pads have reduced the laundry problems of people with persistent incontinence and are now widely used. Most are only able to cope with a dribble of urine rather than an intense void of half a litre, however. Better, more absorbent pads cost more, and most health authorities are finding that bills for pads are escalating, so the range of pads available may be limited. It is usual for most people with persistent incontinence to use pads in preference to regular trips to the toilet. Pads tend to give a feeling of security, particularly on long journeys. Pads have certainly reduced the use of indwelling catheters in institutions and probably reduced the risks of septicaemia and death due to catheter-related infections.

FAECAL INCONTINENCE

Faecal incontinence is far less common than urinary incontinence but much less well tolerated and a cause of great distress by its nature to both patient and carer. There are three main groups of causes (Table 23.5).

Table 23.5 Causes of faecal incontinence

Bowel disease
  Carcinoma of colon/rectum
  Diverticular disease
  Ischaemic bowel
  Ulcerative colitis/proctocolitis
  Diabetic neuropathy
  Laxative abuse

Faecal overloading/impaction

Neurogenic bowel
  Dementing syndromes
  Normal pressure hydrocephalus
  Spinal cord disease

The overwhelming number of cases are due to faecal overloading/impaction either resulting in solid stool being passed involuntarily or as diarrhoea (spurious) due to the impaction extending back up the colon and liquid stool seeping past. Disimpaction may initially need manual removal followed by enemas. Stimulant (e.g. senna) should never be given until the lower bowel and rectum has been cleared as their use can cause colic and precipitate subacute and acute obstruction.

INVESTIGATION AND MANAGEMENT

In all cases a rectal examination must be carried out and a sigmoidoscopy considered. If the rectum is empty a plain abdominal X-ray will confirm a diagnosis of high faecal overloading. A rectal examination will confirm impaction and help exclude a rectal carcinoma which can impair rectal tone. Also, conditions which inhibit defaecation through fear of pain during a bowel movement (e.g. haemorrhoids or fissure) will be revealed.

Diarrhoea may need investigating further, including stool specimens and rectal biopsy. Other bowel disease may need investigating via barium enema or colonoscopy. Diarrhoea (from whatever cause) can cause incontinence in any age group. Neurogenic bowel (with similar aetiology to the bladder conditions) is usually diagnosed from the history. Manometry studies are available in some research centres. People suffering from dementia syndromes may have voluntary incontinence if they cannot find the toilet. At the end stage of the disease they may lose higher control of the bowels and bladder.

Excessive consumption of laxatives can cause faecal incontinence. This abuse may be suspected by the biochemical findings of hypokalaemia, melanosis coli (black mucosal discoloration) on sigmoidoscopy and the fact that the laxatives are kept hidden.

An active and energetic approach will enable many patients to regain continence. For the person who does not, a sympathetic and enlightened approach is essential. In a well-managed environment overt evidence of urinary or faecal incontinence should be unacceptable.

Key points

- Incontinence is an involuntary loss of urine or faeces in an inappropriate place.
- To be continent an elderly person must be mobile, to be able to find the toilet, be appropriately clothed for the journey and use a suitably designed toilet.
- History and examination includes rectal, vaginal and urine microscopy and culture.
- Causes of incontinence of urine include infection, stress incontinence, detrusor instability, overflow, prostatism, neurogenic bladder, uterine prolapse, cystocele and atrophic vaginitis.

- Limited benefit is derived from drug usage in urinary incontinence.
- Urinary catheters may be used intermittently or permanently.
- Causes of faecal incontinence include bowel disease (carcinoma of rectum, diverticular disease, laxative abuse), faecal overloading and impaction and neurogenic bowel.
- The overwhelming number of cases of faecal incontinence are due to faecal overloading/ impaction.
- Stimulant laxatives should never be given until the lower bowel has been cleared. Investigation and management of faecal incontinence include history, examination, rectal examination, sigmoidoscopy and laxative review.

FURTHER READING

Brocklehurst JC. Treatment of constipation and faecal incontinence in old people. *Practitioner* 1964; **193**: 779–782.

Brocklehurst JC (ed.). *Urology in the Elderly*. Churchill Livingstone, Edinburgh, 1984.

Castledon CM, Duffin HM. Guidelines for controlling urinary incontinence without drugs or catheters. *Age & Ageing* 1981; **10**: 186–190.

Mandelstrom D. *Incontinence*. Disabled Living Foundation, London, 1977.

Percy JP, Neill ME, Kandiah TK, Swash M. A neurogenic factor in faecal incontinence in the elderly. *Age & Ageing* 1982; **11**: 175–179.

24 CHRONIC WOUNDS: PRESSURE SORES AND LEG ULCERS

- Prevalence of pressure sores
- History and aetiology of pressure sores
- Pathology and healing of pressure sores
- Prevention and treatment of pressure sores
- Prevalence of leg ulcers
- Aetiology and pathology of leg ulcers
- Management of leg ulcers
- Diabetes mellitus

Necrosis of skin, adipose tissue and muscle caused by pressure occurs rapidly in acutely and chronically ill elderly people. Necrosis of any other tissue (e.g. myocardial infarction) causes considerable medical attention whereas death of skin and muscle overlying hips and buttocks — often caused by and causing whole body complications — attracts very little notice. This state of affairs is changing for many reasons, increasing awareness of medical responsibility, medical audit, scientific research, cost management and the new spectre of litigation being a few. Some groups of people appear especially at risk (Table 24.1).

Table 24.1 Groups of people at risk of pressure sores

Acutely and chronically ill elderly
Neurological disease (stroke, Alzheimer's disease, Parkinson's disease, multiple sclerosis)
Spinal cord injury
Peri- and post-orthopaedic surgery
Postoperatively (general surgery)
The very ill (ITU all ages)
The dying

PREVALENCE OF PRESSURE SORES

Large-scale studies in the 1970s indicated a prevalence rate of about 9 per cent of all UK hospital patients with some form of pressure sore. This contrasted with about 5 per cent in Scandinavian research. However, more recent data indicate that the UK range is wide (2.7–66.0 per cent), the highest figures being in elderly people with fractured femurs. The lowest figures come from units where dedicated individuals apply education and resources to considerable patient benefit. The total cost to the Health Service in purely financial terms is enormous, each health district spending close to £1 million per year on treating this one condition. Prevalence data are becoming more easily available, with many purchasers insisting upon pressure sore prevalence data as part of the quality standards information. Clinical audit is another area where pressure sores are an important topic. Incidence, however, is an area that requires further development. Increasingly clinicians and teams need to know how many new cases develop to organize more effective intervention strategies.

HISTORY AND AETIOLOGY OF PRESSURE SORES

Pressure sores are not a new phenomenon. The earliest reference concerns an Egyptian twelfth-dynasty Priestess of Amen. When unwrapped following her arrival at the British Museum she was noted to have a sacral pressure sore (which had presumably occurred whilst she was ill and dying thousands of years ago). Her claim to immortal fame continues in that her pressure sore was covered with a piece of gazelle skin, making her the first known recipient of a skin graft. There are Biblical references to pressure sores (Isaiah) and subsequently all the great names in medicine (Quesnay, Fabricius, Brown-Sequard, Charcot) all wrote learnedly on the subject. Many of their themes carry through to current thoughts on aetiology (Table 24.2).

Table 24.2 Causes of pressure sores

Intrinsic
  Paralysis
  Decreased sensation (reduced pain stimuli)
  Decreased attention (sedation, coma, depression)
  Diminished tissue turgor (dehydration, hypotension)
  Malnutrition
  Peripheral vascular disease
  Systemic disease
  Failure of vasomotor reflexes (recent cord injury)
  Endothelial cell disruption in ill patients (compared with
    healthy patients)

Extrinsic
  The application of pressure:
    Long periods on hard trolleys in A&E/X-ray/operating
      theatre
    Relative hardness of hospital beds
    Long periods up in a chair
  Macerated skin secondary to sweat and incontinence
  Shearing forces – in bed and during poor lifting/turning

Blood flow and oxygen

The mean capillary pressure (in healthy medical students) is approximately 25 mmHg. We have no measurements for elderly people let alone those who are ill. Beyond 25 mmHg the blood vessels are occluded and the surrounding tissues (including skin) become anoxic. Pressure loading studies show that healthy people can tolerate high pressures for short periods very well, their

oxygen-carrying capacity in the tissues recovering from the 'assault'. The equation appears to be damage = pressure × time for us all, but in the 'at-risk' groups (some elderly, the ill, spinal injury patients, etc.) the amount of pressure and duration of time before damage occurs is probably very short. A bed-ridden patient easily generates pressures in excess of 100 mmHg, especially over the sacrum, heels and greater trochanter (96 per cent of pressure sores occur below the umbilicus).

PATHOLOGY AND HEALING OF PRESSURE SORES

Eighty per cent of sores are superficial (type 1) and 20 per cent deep (type 2).

Superficial (type 1) (Fig. 24.1)

These sores occur mainly in dehydrated and incontinent patients exposed to sustained pressure (most

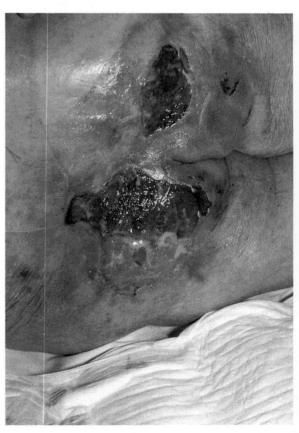

Figure 24.1 Superficial (type 1) pressure sores

commonly seen postoperatively). The majority of these sores are preventable. They will deepen if pressure is not relieved. Histologically the endothelial cell lining is swollen but remains intact.

Deep (type 2) (Fig. 24.2)

These are formed when localized high pressure cuts off a wedge-shaped area of tissue usually adjacent to a bony prominence (Fig. 24.3). Microthrombi block the capillaries and the endothelial cell lining separates, allowing extensive inflammatory damage to occur. The necrotic tissue breaks down over days to form a deep sore.

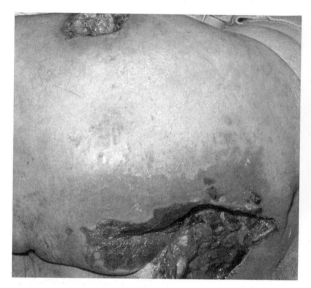

Figure 24.2 Deep (type 2) pressure sore

Healing

Once pressure is relieved and the blood supply to surrounding tissues restored most sores heal by the following processes.

Debridement. Over a few weeks the necrotic slough (often hardened to form a scab/eschar) separates from the wound. This occurs naturally and should rarely be interfered with. Large areas of necrotic tissue may need surgical debriding and specialist referral is necessary.

Contraction. Over the next month the wound contracts and this forms one of the most important aspects of the closure of the pressure sore. To contract fully the wound needs to be moist and free from infection.

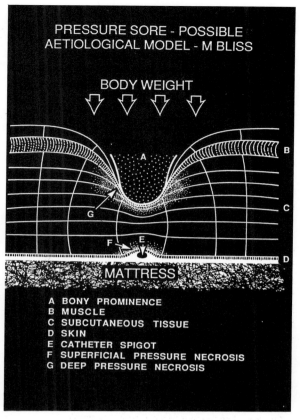

Figure 24.3 Possible aetiological model of a pressure sore (M. Bliss)

Epithelialization. Epithelial cells migrate from the ulcer margin (healthy skin), this is decreased by dryness, infection, systemic disease and by some topical agents.

Remodelling. There is early profuse growth of capillaries which diminishes as scar collagen matures and subsequent fibrosis leaves a depressed scar.

PREVENTION AND TREATMENT OF PRESSURE SORES

All patients in the 'at-risk' groups should have antipressure protection starting immediately a new illness or injury (at home or in hospital) occurs. Nurses use assessment scales (e.g. Norton, Waterlow) to try to predict potential risk. At home pillows can be used to protect bony prominences and the patient should be repositioned frequently. Alternating-pressure air mattresses (APAMs) such as the large-cell ripple mattress can be used for short-term protection.

Hospital admission (from A&E to discharge planning) requires at-risk patients to have their pressure areas actively managed. APAMs are proving to be highly effective in both prevention and treatment. These active systems range from the inexpensive to very expensive. Research indicates that for all bar the most at-risk patients the inexpensive APAMs are reliable and effective. An example of an APAM available in the UK is shown in Fig. 24.4. This system has a double bank of air cells that provide alternating pressure relief so that no area is subject to ischaemia for more than a few minutes. In most cases this mattress obviates the need for regular turning.

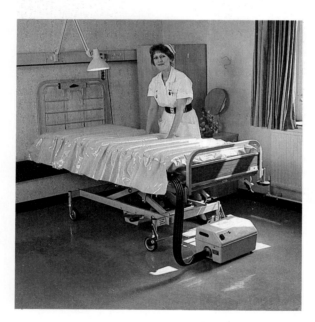

Figure 24.4 The Pegasus Airwave mattress

Static air mattresses, e.g. mattress overlays, flotation beds etc. have many disadvantages compared with APAMs. Patients should have bed cradles in place and may benefit from an anchored fleece at the end of the bed. Immobile patients should have a pillow between the knees. Ill patients should be nursed in bed and then, as they recover, sit out for gradually increasing periods.

Local treatment

Local hyperaemia is common as is a raised white cell count with associated mild pyrexia. Debridement should occur naturally, aided by cleaning the wound with saline (Normasol) and keeping it moist (with one of the numerous non-toxic dressings). Dressings need to encourage moist wound healing. Recent developments include a wide range of products including hydrocolloids, hydrogels and alginates. They have specific indications and contraindications so the help and advice from a clinical nurse specialist in tissue viability can be invaluable. The dressings should deal with exudate, be easy to put on and remove, and keep the wound moist yet encourage granulation and epithelialization. Antiseptics such as 'Eusol' should be avoided. Deep wounds should not be tightly packed.

There is a mounting interest in the use of growth factors as a future local treatment. Growth factors are peptides with mainly stimulating effects on cell proliferation and early research work indicates that they may have considerable potential in healing.

General measures

Other medical conditions need to be treated vigorously (e.g. diabetes, dehydration, etc.) and in the initial stages pain relief is usually necessary — some patients needing regular low-dose morphine. Patients may need catheterizing for a short while to ensure that the sore is kept clean and dry. Offensive odours should be tackled with increased frequency of dressings, charcoal-containing coverings and occasionally metronidazole (via suppository). This should help stop the patient becoming depressed and from being ostracized by other patients and staff. Pressure sores often appear infected but appearances can be misleading. Surrounding erythema may be due to pressure effects and slough and exudate may look like pus. Wound swabs generally reveal heavy mixed growth. If, however, there are systemic effects or local changes compatible with infection, cellulitis systemic antibiotics should be used (never topical). Broad-spectrum plus metronidazole are indicated though microbiology guidance is needed if a pure growth is obtained on culture or a wound is deteriorating.

A normal diet with supplements if necessary is sufficient, though some patients may require supplementary feeding and advice from the dietician and/or nutrition team. Subclinical scurvy is quite common in the elderly and vitamin C is necessary for wound healing (1 g a day in the healing phase). Other vitamin deficiencies should be sought and treated. Patients with chronic sores often develop an anaemia unresponsive to haematinics (chronic disease type) and the patient and the rate of ulcer healing benefit from a packed-cell transfusion. Drug therapy should be reviewed to try to stop or decrease corticosteroids and other anti-inflammatory drugs (NSAIDs etc.) which delay wound healing. There is some evidence that zinc-deficient people have poor wound healing and as zinc is difficult to measure it can be given empirically (as zinc sulphate 220 mg bd) in the healing phase.

As the patient improves and begins to mobilize, most sores heal rapidly. Mobility increases muscle bulk and blood flow, decreases oedema and all these measures enhance ulcer healing.

Surgery

A surgical opinion should be sought in all cases where a deep sore is present and not healing rapidly. Modern anaesthetic and plastic surgery techniques (myoplasty) have revolutionized the care in this type of case. Rapid surgery has the added advantage of allowing the elderly person to leave hospital quickly, avoiding months of slow medical treatment and possible further complications.

PREVALENCE OF LEG ULCERS

Leg ulcers are known to affect 1 per cent of the total population and 4 per cent of those over 65 years old — at least 100 000 active leg ulcers in the UK at any one time. Approximately 10 per cent are treated as hospital inpatients, 30 per cent as hospital outpatients and 60 per cent by community (district) nurses. Half of all community nursing time is devoted to the largely ineffective treatment of chronic venous stasis ulcers. The cost to the NHS in 1992 was estimated at between £300 and 600 million.

AETIOLOGY AND PATHOLOGY OF LEG ULCERS

Approximately 50 per cent of leg ulcers are due to venous stasis (Fig. 24.5), 10 per cent to arterial disease (a component of peripheral vascular disease) and 30–40

per cent are mixed. All patients with a leg ulcer need a full clerking, asking (where relevant) especially about pregnancies, venous thromboses and current drugs. Unusual causes of ulcers need to be considered — is the ulcer malignant, arteritic or secondary to the side-effects of drugs? If oedema is present the cause has to be ascertained, as well as a complete history concerning mobility and whether the person sleeps in bed or in a chair with their feet on a low and ineffective stool. This situation has often resulted from the effects of the swelling causing relative or absolute immobility. Salt and water retention with non-steroidal preparations can result in leg oedema.

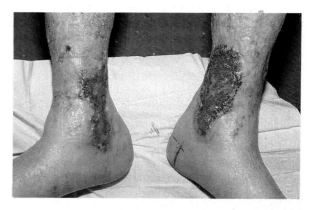

Figure 24.5 Venous leg ulcers

Examination should include feeling for pulses and the measurement of ankle blood pressure using a Doppler meter to determine whether the arterial circulation is adequate. The brachial pressure and ankle pressure measurements give the resting pressure index (RPI):

$$RPI = \frac{ankle\ pressure}{brachial\ pressure} \times 100$$

e.g.

$$\frac{120\ mmHg}{130\ mmHg} \times 100 = 0.9$$

An RPI > 1.0 is normal; 0.7–1.0 indicates some arterial component and care with compression bandaging is needed; < 0.7 indicates increasing ischaemia and a vascular opinion should be considered.

The ulcer needs to be accurately described, including any surrounding haemosiderin (evidence of regular small thromboses) and eczema. The size needs to be measured, which can be done using exposed X-ray films and an indelible marker.

MANAGEMENT OF LEG ULCERS

The presence of significant oedema requires a few days of bed-rest (with diuretics only if there are signs of heart failure). The ulcer should be cleaned with saline (e.g. Normosol) and systemic antibiotics only used if there is definite evidence of cellulitis. The effect of bed-rest can be dramatic, but the ulcer itself can be painful and analgesics should be given.

The correct management of venous ulcers (after Doppler assessment to exclude arterial insufficiency) is pressure bandaging (e.g. four-layer technique). This has to be effective, and so the type of bandage, its application and the role of exercise and elevation require a good level of skill and communication. Healing rates of up to 90 per cent can be obtained. In selected cases venous surgery to incompetent veins is helpful.

An arterial component to the ulcer is more common in elderly people (hence the need for pressure measurement) and the wrong use of pressure bandaging on an arterial ulcer can be disastrous. Arterial ulcers can be difficult to heal. The patient may have evidence of vascular disease elsewhere. Smoking is heavily implicated and benefit can still be obtained by stopping even at this late stage. Attention to detail (not elevating the foot, taking care of the surrounding skin with soft material and pressure area care) means that the ulcers may heal, but quite slowly. Large vessel disease may benefit from vascular surgery intervention and an opinion should be sought.

DIABETES MELLITUS

Diabetes mellitus affects 2 per cent of the total population and 16 per cent of those over 65 years old. In the diabetic population 10 per cent have foot ulcers and patients with diabetes mellitus get pressure ulcers on the feet very easily (secondary to the neuropathy) and they also suffer from small vessel disease. Sadly, some ischaemic foot ulcers require amputation to alleviate pain and infection.

If foot ulcers do develop, healing will occur if the blood supply is adequate, the blood glucose controlled and the pressure areas on the foot are relieved. This requires referral if possible to a footcare team where the podiatrist and orthotist especially can help correct high pressure and provide suitable footwear.

Key points

Pressure sores

- At-risk groups include the frail elderly, spinal cord injury patients, people with neurological disease and patients who are very ill or dying.
- Prevalence rates vary but approximately 8 per cent is a consistent 'norm'.
- Health districts spend about £1 million per year treating pressure sores.
- Aetiology includes both intrinsic and extrinsic causes.
- Damage = pressure × time.
- Pressure sores are either superficial (80 per cent) or deep (20 per cent).
- Healing comprises debridement, contraction, epithelialization and remodelling.
- Most pressure sores would be prevented if all ill elderly people were nursed on APAMs (alternating-pressure air mattresses) and had bed cradles in place.
- Local treatment measures involve moist wound healing. Dressings include hydrocolloids, hydrogels and alginates.
- General treatment measures include pain relief, infection control, nutrition assessment, the management of other medical problems and attention to continence and mobility.
- Pressure sores are as much a medical as nursing responsibility.

Leg ulcers

- Approximately 4 per cent of elderly people have a leg ulcer.
- Fifty per cent of leg ulcers are due to venous stasis, 10 per cent arterial and 40 per cent mixed aetiology.
- Assessment of leg ulcers must include Doppler pressure measurement to exclude an arterial component.
- Adequate compression bandaging (e.g. four-layer technique) is extremely effective in healing venous leg ulcers.
- Foot ulcers in diabetic patients can result in amputation; measure the blood supply, control blood glucose and refer to a footcare team if possible.

FURTHER READING

Bader D (ed.). *Pressure Sores. Clinical Practice and Scientific Approach.* Macmillan, London, 1990.

Barton AA, Barton N. *The Management and Prevention of Pressure Sores.* Faber, London, 1981.

Bennett GCJ, Moody M. *Wound Care for Health Professionals.* Chapman & Hall, London, 1995.

Kenedi RM, Cowden JM, Scales JT (eds). *Bedsore Biomechanics.* Macmillan, London, 1976.

Kosiak M. Etiology and pathology of ischaemic ulcers. *Arch Phys Med Rehab* 1959; **40**: 62–69.

25 ACCIDENTAL HYPOTHERMIA

- Introduction
- Regulation of body temperature
- Clinical features
- Management
- Anticipating and avoiding complications
- Preventive measures

Accidental hypothermia is defined as a core body temperature below 35°C. The core or central temperature is reflected accurately when measured with a low-reading thermometer in the oesophagus, the covered external auditory meatus or, more commonly, the rectum. Oral temperature readings are unreliable. The temperature of immediately voided urine can be used to reflect the central/core temperature but is approximately 1°C cooler. The hypothermia is termed 'accidental' to differentiate it from the carefully induced hypothermia of some surgical procedures. It is a medical emergency with a high morbidity and mortality.

INTRODUCTION

In the early 1960s reports began appearing in the medical press of isolated cases of accidental hypothermia. Researchers, including the Royal College of Physicians, studied this and found a true phenomenon occurring. One large study involving elderly people at home found few cases of actual hypothermia but almost 10 per cent with very low core temperatures just outside the definition range. This pre-hypothermic group appeared to have some social characteristics in common — including poverty. Extrapolation from this study indicated that nearly 750 000 elderly people were at risk of hypothermia, but large long-term follow-up studies have not been done to confirm the size of the problem or the extent of the risk.

The occurrence of accidental hypothermia is usually related to a low environmental temperature — hence it is especially common in winter. A common story is of an elderly person getting out of bed, falling, and remaining on the floor for several hours. They are usually poorly clothed with no heating in the room and are only discovered 24–48 hours later by friends, neighbours or statutory services. However, cases can occur when a person is in bed and although apparently well covered, not generating sufficient body heat, the insulation obviously being ineffective. Accidental hypothermia cases can therefore also be found in hospitals and residential homes.

REGULATION OF BODY TEMPERATURE

The maintenance of a constant central temperature of 37°C is under nervous system control with afferent and efferent pathways. On exposure to cold, heat is conserved by cutaneous vasoconstriction and increased heat produced by shivering. Appreciation of cold at a conscious level encourages movement away from the cold environment, the wearing of suitable clothing and occasionally exercise. Most elderly people have normal thermoregulatory mechanisms but there is an 'at-risk' subgroup where some degree of thermoregulatory failure occurs and where the mechanisms for conserving body heat are impaired. These subjects, while their deep body temperature is falling, have a poor shivering response, are less aware of the cold exposure and tend not to complain of the cold or alter their environment.

Drugs

Drugs can act on the nervous system and further impair the physiological mechanisms. Phenothiazines (e.g. chlorpromazine) affect temperature regulation by abolishing the shivering response and causing vasodilation. They also lessen the awareness to environmental changes and hazards. Alcohol, sedatives, tranquillizers, hypnotics and antidepressants have all been implicated in causing cases of accidental hypothermia. Nitrazepam (a benzodiazepine with an extremely long half-life) can have accumulation problems, causing drowsiness, ataxia and falls which in some circumstances can predispose to a hypothermic state.

Clinical disorders

The most severe cases of hypothermia usually have some underlying clinical condition (Table 25.1).

CLINICAL FEATURES

All organ systems of the body are affected in hypothermia and increasingly so as the core temperature falls (Table 25.2). The skin feels cold and may become mottled and feel like marble. If clinical examination reveals a cool/cold abdomen or inner thigh then always suspect hypothermia. Intense peripheral vasoconstriction gives extreme pallor to the skin and the face becomes puffy due to subcutaneous oedema. This and a husky

Table 25.1 Clinical conditions associated with hypothermia

Endocrine	Hypothyroidism
	Hypopituitarism
Vascular	Stroke
	Transient ischaemic attack
Neurological	Epilepsy
Immobility	Severe arthritis
	Parkinson's disease
	Paraplegia/hemiplegia
	Fractures
Psychiatric	Depression
	Drug overdosage
	Chronic confusional states, e.g. dementia syndromes
Severe infections/ circulatory disturbances	Bronchopneumonia
	Myocardial infarction
	Pulmonary embolism
Unconscious patient	Postoperative
	Sedated
	Diabetic

Table 25.2 Clinical features of hypothermia

Skin	Cold, marble-like, pallor, subcutaneous oedema (causing puffiness)
Neurological	Confusion, disorientation, drowsiness and coma. Ataxia, flapping tremor, extensor plantars. Reflexes slow and then become absent (inc. pupillary)
Muscular	Stiffen then hypertonic (can simulate meningism)
CVS	Poor volume pulse, slowing to atrial fibrillation or sinus bradycardia
Respiratory	Respirations get slower and shallower
GI	Paralytic ileus, gastric dilatation and acute pancreatitis can occur. Insulin is inactivated
Renal	Decrease in renal plasma flow, GFR. Oliguria occurs
Haematological	Venous blood pools and is unreliable for sampling. There is a decrease in arterial oxygen saturation

voice (if the patient is conscious) due to oedema and poor movement of the vocal cords often lead to a mistaken diagnosis of hypothyroidism. A body orifice such as the rectum or mouth may feel cold and shivering is absent.

As the core temperature falls so cerebration slows. Below 32°C there is usually confusion and disorientation eventually leading to drowsiness and coma. As body fat cools the abdomen takes on a 'doughy' feel. Muscles stiffen and become hypertonic (giving rise to neck stiffness simulating meningism). Ataxia is common, an involuntary flapping tremor may be seen and plantar responses become extensor. Reflexes are slowed and then absent (including the pupillary response), the knee jerks characteristically being the last reflexes to disappear. Respirations become slow and shallow and there is a fall in arterial oxygen saturation. The pulse is of poor volume and may be difficult to find. The rhythm changes to slow atrial fibrillation or sinus bradycardia due to the effect of the cold on the atrial pacemaker. The heart sounds eventually become inaudible. The blood pressure falls and is then difficult to measure. A pathognomic ECG feature is the J wave best seen in lead 1 (Fig. 25.1).

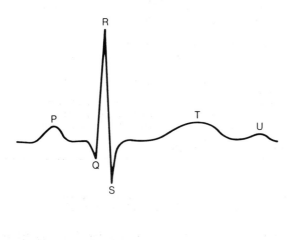

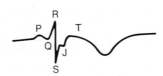

Figure 25.1 The top trace shows the normal PQRST complex; the bottom trace shows the J wave at the junction of the QRS and ST segments

Cardiac failure can occur as can gastric dilatation with the risk of aspiration. Acute pancreatitis is relatively common (the pancreas being very sensitive to the effects of the cold) though the diagnosis is difficult. Paralytic ileus occurs and a decrease in renal plasma flow and glomerular filtration rate with oliguria is common. Venous blood tends to pool and hence for accuracy arterial samples must be taken. Tissue metabolism and oxygen consumption are decreased. Insulin is inactivated by very low temperatures and hence glucose cannot enter cells. Abnormal glucose measurements are common; how-

ever, on rewarming glucose rapidly enters tissues and hypoglycaemia can result.

MANAGEMENT

Mild degrees of hypothermia (around 35°C) can occasionally be treated at home, but associated medical problems and adverse social circumstances usually preclude this. All other degrees of hypothermia require urgent hospital admission. Some doctors believe that practically all hypothermia patients should be managed in intensive care, others that most intervention is unwarranted and even dangerous. Intensive nursing can be, and for the majority is, performed on ordinary wards. The management must take into account the metabolic, cardiac and biochemical problems that can occur. An airway may need to be established, fluid and electrolytes or acid–base balance may need to be corrected and the heart and vital signs monitored. Most patients fall into one of four categories during rewarming (Table 25.3).

Table 25.3 Categories during rewarming

Favourable
  Rewarming spontaneously and rapidly at 0.5°C/hour
  No haemodynamic complications
  Consciousness steadily recovers
  Biochemical and haematological abnormalities correct
    themselves

Less favourable
  Unexpected hypotension ('rewarming collapse')
  Episodic sinus bradycardia or atrioventricular block
  Profound hypoglycaemia
  Persistent hypoxaemia
  Intercurrent infection

Poor prognosis
  Severe bronchopneumonia
  Circulatory/cardiac arrest
  Acute pancreatitis

Worst prognosis
  Core temperature fails to rise or rises only very slowly
  Evidence of 'shock'

The 'less favourable' category probably accounts for the largest number of patients seen clinically. A few points should be made concerning cardiac arrest. At low temperatures the decreased oxygen demands permit longer periods of arrest with theoretical eventual recovery; however, electrical defibrillation is usually unsuccessful at temperatures below 30°C and some patients have underlying disease of such severity that cardiac resuscitation is inappropriate.

ANTICIPATING AND AVOIDING COMPLICATIONS

A plain chest X-ray may detect pneumonia or pulmonary oedema (there can be marked fluid shifts from one compartment to another). Similarly, abdominal X-rays may show bowel dilatation or free gas indicating ileus or perforation. Blood sampling (arterial) may suggest infection, kidney disease, glucose intolerance, pancreatitis, hypothyroidism, etc. Blood gases (corrected for temperature) may be necessary. ECG or cardiac monitoring may show dysrhythmias etc.

Many of the complications (fluid shifts, hypoxia, hypercalcaemia, metabolic acidosis and hypoglycaemia) may correct themselves during the rewarming process. The rate and means of rewarming is controversial (slow peripheral, fast peripheral or central rewarming). The ambient temperature for those admitted should be between 25 and 30°C. At this temperature (most easily achieved in a side room with heaters) most patients rewarm spontaneously at about 0.5–1.0°C per hour if insulated against further heat loss (using a 'space blanket') (Fig. 25.2). The patient should be placed into the blanket (silver side up if only silver on one side) and swaddled, i.e. the head should be included to prevent the massive heat loss from this area. The rectal temperature should be monitored, ideally continuously with an electrical temperature probe.

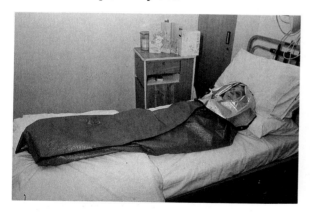

Figure 25.2 Space blanket

Maclean and Emslie-Smith have formulated the idea of a conservative management plan, a modified version of which is shown in Table 25.4. For most patients slow external rewarming is the best method despite the fact that it means prolonging the physiological abnormality for many hours. Hospital staff are conversant with it and, importantly, survival figures equate with those of the more complicated rapid rewarming techniques. 'Rewarming collapse' is severe hypotension, probably as a result of rewarming too fast causing a sudden fall in peripheral resistance. Cooling the patient again usually stabilizes the blood pressure and a slower rewarming regime can then be employed. Occasionally inotropes can be given to 'support' the blood pressure while more active rewarming occurs. Rapid central rewarming techniques (gastric/colonic lavage, warm intravenous infusions, mediastinal irrigation) have been used in specialist centres.

Table 25.4 Management plan for hypothermia

Nurse in ambient temperature 25–32°C
Ripple mattress/space blanket
Cardiac monitor, portable chest X-ray
IV loading dose prophylactic antibiotics (after urine, sputum and blood cultures)
Monitor rectal temperature, respiration rate and blood pressure
Monitor arterial blood gases (give oxygen if necessary)
Monitor blood glucose, electrolytes, acid–base balance
IV access but no routine infusions, steroids, vasoactive drugs or thyroid hormone
Disturb as little as possible

PREVENTIVE MEASURES

Many elderly people can be considered at risk from hypothermia (e.g. the confused, isolated, poor, recently bereaved, malnourished, those on medication, etc.). A pattern recognition should emerge among GPs, health visitors, district nurses and non-statutory workers, involving the social (poor financial resources, poor heating, inadequate accommodation, inadequate clothing, outside lavatory, poor lighting, dependent on statutory services, etc.) and the medical (undernutrition, chronic confusion, sedative medication, associated diseases, etc.) factors that indicate high risk.

General practitioners and district nurses must have adequate access to low-reading thermometers to diagnose cases early and, if possible, prevent hospital admission. Many local authorities or non-statutory groups such as Age Concern or Help the Aged run winter hypothermia schemes giving better access to warmer clothing, extra heaters and advice. Good neighbour schemes in very bad weather can help enormously by the provision of a hot meal/drink and a close eye kept on the situation.

Governmental responses have been inadequate. Many elderly people cite poverty for not spending extra money on heating, clothing and food. Elderly people should not be reliant on pitifully low (and complicated to assess) 'severe weather payments', or indeed have to take out loans from social services. An adequate pension would be all that most require.

General advice (from any source) on food, clothing, bedding and household features needs to be more widespread and comprehensive. For maximum comfort and warmth clothing needs to be light, loose and loosely woven with a few layers to trap air. The same applies to bedclothes (though duvets are extremely warm and useful). A hat and warm socks should be worn in bed. Electric overblankets are excellent but the use of heated underblankets is not advised if there is any problem with incontinence. If the bed abuts on an outside wall it should be moved. In severe weather consideration should be given to one-room living, even to the provision of a commode in that room if the passage to and from the toilet itself is unheated.

There should be a store of carbohydrate-rich foods for use in the event of an emergency, and some spare blankets on the floor in case a fall occurs. The person can then wrap themselves up in them if they are unable to pull down the bedclothes. Techniques of getting up off the floor after a fall can be taught. The true mortality statistics for hypothermia are difficult to assess because of low reporting (if written on a death certificate it implies neglect and hence a Coroner's inquest is necessary) and many cases are not found until many days after the event, making an accurate diagnosis impossible. Most cases could be prevented and a pre-winter assessment of medical and social factors could help considerably.

Key points

- Accidental hypothermia is defined as a core body temperature below 35°C.
- Core central body temperature must be measured with a low reading thermometer (oesophagus, external auditory meatus, rectum).
- The occurrence of accidental hypothermia is usually related to a low environmental temperature.
- Most elderly people have normal thermoregulatory mechanisms.
- Drugs can impair the physiological responses to cold and predispose to hypothermia.
- The most severe cases of hypothermia usually have some underlying clinical condition.
- All organ systems of the body are affected with some unique clinical features.
- Management of established cases requires rewarming in hospital.
- Rewarming complications, e.g. hypotension, are common.
- Preventive measures include assessing for the social and medical predisposing causes.
- General advice includes information on nutrition, clothing (many loose layers, wear hat and socks in bed), bedding, house heating and emergency measures.

FURTHER READING

Maclean D, Emslie-Smith D. *Accidental Hypothermia.* Blackwell Scientific, Oxford, 1977.

Maudgal D. *Hypothermia – Medical and Social Aspects.* Pergamon Press, Oxford, 1987.

Wicks M. *Old and Cold (Hypothermia and Social Policy).* Heinemann, London, 1978.

26 JOINT CONTRACTURES

- Common causes of immobility leading to contractures
- Prevention and management

This dreadful condition, though seen less frequently today, is still an all too common sight in units dealing with the chronically disabled. When putting elderly people to bed for long periods was a common treatment the sight of numerous skeletal figures in the fetal position with hips, knees and elbows contracted, and stress fractures and pressure sores on opposing limbs must have saddened everyone. It is hard to believe, but none the less true, that this state arose from putting sick elderly people to bed for too long. One of the slogans of the first generation of geriatricians was 'bed is bad'. This message has been taken up but often with too much zeal and too little thought. Being up in a chair when ill may be totally inappropriate; long periods immobile in a chair result in chair-shaped people and this is only marginally less of an evil.

Synovial joints must move to remain healthy, for immobility produces damaging effects in the joint and the surrounding tissues. Bone, cartilage, muscle, ligaments and synovium are all affected. It appears that the water and proteoglycan gel cushioning the collagen fibres is reduced, leading to friction between the fibres and the development of adhesions. Increased and abnormal collagen cross-linking at the molecular level also occurs, changing its tensile properties. The effects of immobility on joints has been studied using animal models. A prolif-eration of fibro-fatty connective tissue covers the entire inner surface of the joint within 30 days of immobility. During the second month the connective tissue becomes more dense and adherent with the surface cartilage becoming thin and irregular. The degree of cartilage damage depends on the rigidity of immobilization, the position and any compressive force. Compression results in erosion of cartilage and bone. If the immobilization is continued, the underlying marrow becomes hyperaemic as vascular connective tissue proliferates, penetrating the subchondral bone producing bone cysts. Similar changes are seen in neglected long-standing contractures in patients. The bones forming the joints may be shown on X-ray to have fused together.

COMMON CAUSES OF IMMOBILITY LEADING TO CONTRACTURES

Joint pain

Inflammation secondary to infection, rheumatoid disease, injury, osteoarthritis, gout, etc. leads to pain and muscle spasm producing immobility. If prolonged, this produces disuse muscle and bone atrophy, further compounding the immobility.

Spasticity

Following a cerebrovascular accident or in other neurological conditions (e.g. multiple sclerosis) hypertonic muscles of large bulk overcome their antagonists, producing a joint held in an abnormal posture. Prolonged spasticity is associated with derangement of muscle spindles and inappropriate inhibition of the antagonist muscles which may make the deformity worse. Eventually this situation leads to fixed shortening of the muscles involved.

Fetal posture

Patients with advanced dementia syndromes (and some people deprived of sensory input) may adopt a curled-up position in bed, obviously resenting all interference. Attempts to improve posture are usually resisted (with unexpected vigour) and fail.

Burns

The contractures resulting from burns involve a different aetiological mechanism to the previous causes. They are a result of wound healing and subsequent contraction involving contractile myofibroblasts (cells not present in the other causes). However, inadequate changing of position may result in oedema and pressure ulceration of the skin with subsequent infection. Management consists of firm pressure around healing/grafted burns to control oedema and prevent contractures.

PREVENTION AND MANAGEMENT

In 1843 W.J. Little gave a lecture and clinical demonstration entitled 'Deformities of the Human Frame'. He noted that spastic contractures are more difficult to treat than others, particularly in the upper limbs. He used springs and splints to aid deficient muscles and he instructed his nurses to endeavour to straighten the affected joints several times a day. Over 150 years later it is still possible for elderly patients to receive less attention than this.

Joint pain

The inflammatory process must be attacked with all the methods at our disposal. These include aspiration to confirm the diagnosis and also to relieve a tense 'hot' joint, drugs, physical methods (e.g. heat and ice) and, paradoxically, the temporary immobilization of joints in good functional postures by means of orthotics (splints), particularly at night. Active or assisted exercises are used to regain muscle power, encourage reabsorption of effusions and regain range of movement. Early contractures (when an elderly person has been confined to bed with an intercurrent illness) respond to energetic treatment with analgesics, active exercises and passive stretching (manually or with traction). Injection of local anaesthetic can help reduce pain and spasm and allow treatment programmes to begin. Rarely manipulation under sedation or anaesthetic is required (there is a real risk of fracturing bones during manipulation under anaesthetic and it requires expert assessment). Any gain in range of movement should be maintained and in some cases orthotics are used. Orthotics can be made of plaster of Paris, but increasingly light thermoplastic materials are being used. Velcro fastenings aid easy removal for active exercises

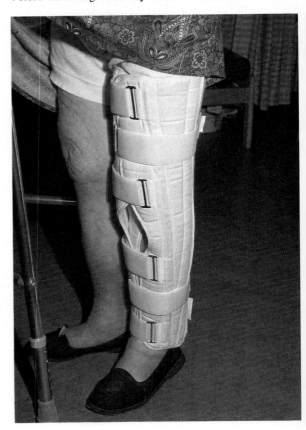

Figure 26.1 'Cricket-pad' type of orthotic splint

but strongly resisting joints may need serial splinting using the 'cricket-pad' type of orthotic with firmer side-straps and buckles (Fig. 26.1). Progress is often slow and can cause discomfort. Pressure sore formation must be assiduously avoided. However, serial splinting can result in improved function and the regained use of an otherwise painful, contracted and useless limb.

Spasticity

The prevention of spastic contractures depends on good positioning of the patient combined with frequent gentle exercising of the limbs through a normal range of movements. Physiotherapists are the 'experts' in this field and nurses and doctors should take their guidance from them. In the case of a stroke patient the limbs should be placed in the opposite position to the fully developed spastic posture (Fig. 26.2). Thus elbows and

wrists are extended, fingers are abducted and extended. A bed cradle should keep the bed clothes from actively extending the feet. During the initial flaccid stage of a stroke care must be taken not to stretch joint capsules (particularly the shoulder) by traction on the joint during lifting and positioning of the patient. The positioning diagram should be by the patient's bed so that the less experienced can refer to it. The shoulder or 'Australian lift' method is used to move the patient (Fig. 26.3).

After a few days spasticity begins to develop (the time scale is variable and in some cases the limbs remain flaccid) and all joints need to be put through a normal range of movements several times a day, i.e. whenever the patient is turned, cleaned and examined. Sudden or jerky movements can induce clonus (rhythmic beating movements) and should be avoided. Slow, sustained traction will reduce tone for several minutes and, by

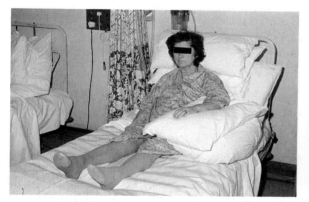
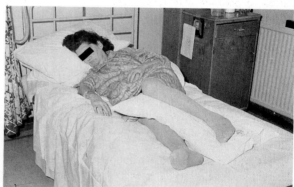
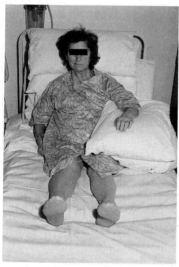
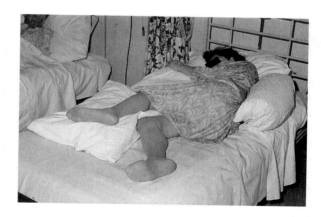

Figure 26.2 Correct positioning of a stroke patient (see text)

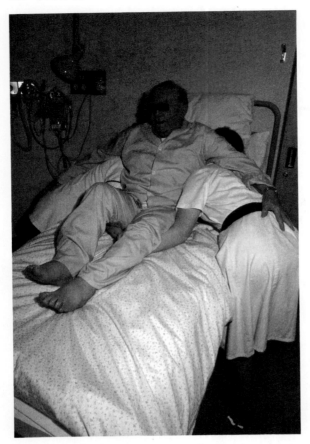

Figure 26.3 The 'Australian' lift carried out by two helpers

using postural reflexes involving the neck and trunk, tone in the limbs may be reduced to allow an improved range of movement. Ice, vibration or tapping may be used by the therapists to reduce tone during treatment. As soon as power begins to return, active movements, assisted if necessary by slings and counterweights, are used. Exercises involving symmetrical movements of the limbs (e.g. Bobath technique) which can be practised by the patient at any time are particularly valuable. The full range of therapy expertise is brought to bear to prevent poor posture and contractures (e.g. hydrotherapy). Drug therapy can play a role. Drugs specifically aimed at reducing excess spasticity are available (e.g. Baclofen/lioresal and Dantrolene/sodium dantrium), but confusion is a side-effect in frail elderly people. Analgesia plus low-dose oral diazepam (used as a muscle relaxant) is another useful combination.

Spastic contractures which have been present for months are very difficult to treat. Surgical treatment is only usually appropriate for a small number of patients with specific problems. For example, lengthening of the Achilles tendon may be necessary to overcome severe equinus deformity (if stretching under anaesthesia or intravenous diazepam has been tried).

Contractures, like other less glamorous aspects of disease, must become multidisciplinary areas of concern. Where interest leads to research, more resources and improvements follow.

Key points

- Synovial joints must move to remain healthy.
- Joint immobility affects bone, cartilage, muscle, ligaments and synovium with the development of adhesions and fibro-fatty connective tissue.
- In long-standing cases bone fusion around the joint can occur.
- The common causes of immobility leading to contractures are joint pain, spasticity, fetal posture and burns.
- Joint pain can be reduced by various methods (e.g. drugs, physical).
- Orthotics (splints) can be used to temporarily immobilize joints to decrease pain or to maintain gains in the range of movement (serial splinting).
- The prevention of spastic contractures depends on good positioning of the patient as well as assisted limb movements.
- Slow sustained traction will reduce tone for several minutes.

FURTHER READING

Johnstone M. *Restoration of Motor Function in the Stroke Patient*. Churchill Livingstone, Edinburgh, 1978.

Lee JM, Warren MP. *Cold Therapy in Rehabilitation*. Bell & Hyman, London, 1978.

Lehmann JF *et al*. Therapeutic heat and cold. *Clin Orthopaed*; 1974; 99: 207–247.

Nickel VL. Physical rehabilitation of the stroke patient with emphasis on the needs for integration into the community. In: *Stroke: Proceedings of the Ninth Pfizer Symposium*. Churchill Livingstone, Edinburgh, 1976.

27 DEPRESSION

- Signs
- Causes of depression
- Pathogenesis
- Occurrence
- Assessment of depression
- Management
- Prognosis for recovery

SIGNS

Depression is common but may be masked by physical symptoms in older people, leading to missed diagnosis. Typically the patient will have characteristic features of depressed mood, may be tearful, anxious, lack concentration, and may also suffer the more biological symptoms of weight loss, sleep disturbance and loss of libido. Depression is not a single diagnosis, but comprises several well recognized syndromes: major depression, minor depression, psychotic major depression, seasonal affective disorder, adjustment disorder with depressed mood, organic affective disorder, dysthymia, and bipolar disorders (manic depressive syndromes). Great progress has been made in producing explicit criteria for classifying patients into these diagnostic groups, and the criteria of the *Diagnostic and Statistical Manual of the American Psychiatric Association* are now widely used (Table 27.1). The treatment and prognosis of these different types of depression vary, so there is an increased emphasis on categorizing depression.

Table 27.1 DSM-III criteria of major depressive illness

A. Essential feature: dysphoric mood or loss of interest/pleasure in usual activities

B. Other symptoms: at least four of the following
   1. Appetite or weight change
   2. Sleep difficulty or hypersomnia
   3. Loss of energy, fatiguability or tiredness
   4. Loss of interest or pleasure in usual activities (including sexual drive)
   5. Feeling of self-reproach or inappropriate guilt
   6. Diminished ability to think or concentrate
   7. Recurrent thoughts of death or suicide or suicidal behaviour

C. Duration at least two weeks

D. Exclusions: patients with
   1. Schizophrenic symptoms
   2. Organic mental disorder
   3. Residual-type schizophrenia
   4. Simple bereavement

In old age, hypochondriasis and importuning behaviour may give the clue to an underlying depressive illness. Symptoms more typical of psychotic illness, such as paranoid delusions and hallucinations — particularly of disintegration and smelliness — may occur. Suicide is relatively common amongst elderly depressives, and much more often successful than among younger people, where attempts far outweigh suicides. Depression may be the underlying cause of any of the common presentations of illness in old age: confusion, immobility and falls, incontinence, and inability to cope.

Some elderly patients become severely withdrawn and are at great risk of dying from dehydration and malnutrition. It is vital to recognize their perilous state and ensure that vigorous treatment is given, both to resuscitate and to treat the depression. Often this may entail electroconvulsive therapy (ECT).

Rarely, patients present with non-specific symptoms, and have extensive investigations which find nothing. A trial of antidepressants may result in a dramatic improvement, and a presumptive diagnosis of depression is made.

CAUSES OF DEPRESSION

Life events

Old age may be seen as intrinsically depressing, associated with losses — job, status, abilities, bereavements. There is considerable evidence that major life events are associated with depression at all ages, and particularly in old age. People with supportive social contacts, with a confidante, tend to weather the storm of losses better than those without. It may be that it is not the losses themselves that are significant, but the elderly person's resilience to the changes induced by losses.

Loss of special senses

Loss of hearing and of vision are associated with increased risk of depression. It is likely that the reduced sensory input leads to disengagement — both within the family and the wider world. Over time the lack of social contact and intercourse may make the person less able to cope with changes, more withdrawn, and vulnerable to depression.

Associations with physical illness

Depressive symptoms commonly accompany physical diseases, particularly strokes, heart disease, Parkinson's disease and severe arthritis. Often the symptoms are relatively mild, and do not warrant a diagnosis of depressive illness or antidepressant drugs. Control of the underlying physical illness, particularly pain and immobility, may lead to improvement in mood. However, patients who do not improve during rehabilitation may be suffering with depression leading to poor concentration, negative feelings and 'poor motivation'. These patients often do respond well to antidepressants and the importance of diagnosing their symptoms is obvious (see Chapter 29).

PATHOGENESIS

The underlying biological changes in depression are not fully understood, but there is evidence that catecholamine (adrenaline and noradrenaline) levels in the brain are low. This theory is attractive because catecholamines are responsible for arousal, hence low levels might be expected to lead to depression. Further support comes from the antidepressant effects of drugs that increase the effective amount of catecholamines in brain nerve endings by reducing the activity of enzymes that destroy catecholamines — the monoamine oxidase inhibitors.

It is likely that the mechanisms of depression are multiple and complex. A more recently researched class of brain messenger, 5-hydroxytryptamine (5-HT), also seems to be involved in regulation of mood. Drugs designed to increase 5-HT activity are also potent antidepressants. The precise nature of biological damage that causes depression is still uncertain, but research using radioisotope-labelled neurotransmitters and positron emission tomography to define which parts of the brain and which messengers are active and inactive in depressed patients will help unravel the mystery.

OCCURRENCE

The prevalence of depressive illness is high in old age, and is more common amongst women than men (Table 27.2). In very old people the prevalence falls, suggesting that susceptibility is less in those who have greater survival potential. This may be related to the better social networks which are related to both survival and low risk of depression.

Table 27.2 Prevalence of depression

Age group	In the community M	F	Under Part 3 of the 1948 Act	Long-term care in hospital
65–74	6.0%	12.0%	16.6%	35%
75+	5.5%	10.5%		

ASSSESSMENT OF DEPRESSION

Depression is frequently missed by doctors and nurses, which is unfortunate because it is a treatable problem. Part of the problem is because of the altered, more physical presentation of the disease. In addition, there is a tendency to assume that depression is a normal response to the adversity of old age — 'I'd be depressed too if that happened to me'. Increased recognition of the problem is needed, but must be coupled with better management.

Simple self-filled rating scales are available, and give an easy means of picking up people who will require a more thorough assessment. The questions used in such scales may usefully be used by doctors and nurses as part of the routine assessment of an elderly patient (Fig. 27.1).

Several of the depression scales do not perform as well with old people as with younger adults. This is because many of them rely on physical markers of depression, that may easily be present in any older person with concurrent physical illness. Such scales tend to produce large numbers of 'false-positives', people incorrectly labelled as suffering with depression. However, provided it is accepted that simple rating scales are no substitute for proper psychiatric assessment, this should not be a problem since it is better to overdiagnose than to miss such a treatable condition.

Pseudodementia is depressive illness masquerading as dementia. It is easy to see how this happens since the patient may appear confused, lacks concentration and performs badly on tests of cognition. Poor self-care and psychomotor retardation combine to give a picture of moderate dementia. Unless thought is given to the possibility of depression, the patient may be inappropriately consigned to long-term institutional care.

Assessment of severity of depression

It is vital that careful assessment for suicidal risk is made so that appropriate management can be given. Severe depression in old people is associated with a high mortality, and admission to hospital is usually necessary so that effective treatment and monitoring may be given. Of great importance in such patients is daily weighing. This gives a good yardstick to monitor both the initial severity (provided that pre-illness weight is known) and response to treatment. Rapid losses in weight are usually due to dehydration and indicate the need for intravenous fluids.

MANAGEMENT

In primary care, even those patients who are diagnosed correctly often receive inappropriate treatment with hypnotics or anxiolytics — the 'Valium (diazepam) syndrome'. However, treating depression is more than simply giving a course of an appropriate antidepressant drug. As in every other aspect of health care for elderly people, a holistic approach is needed. This is best done by a psychiatry of old age team with direct access to occupational therapy, clinical psychology and community psychiatric nursing. This will ensure that the patient gets a multidisciplinary assessment, and attention will be given to other physical and social problems that may be aggravating the depressive illness. The general practitioner has a major role in this team as the person who probably knows the patient best, and the person who will be responsible for the continued monitoring of the patient's recovery. Some patients may not wish to be managed by a hospital-based team, particularly in areas where there is substantial stigma to visiting the local psychiatric hospital. In such cases, home visits by a consultant in conjunction with the GP are vital for assessing the severity of the depression, and also for ensuring that the patient does get access to services at home. For milder cases of depression, the GP may wish to manage the patient. Provided mood is monitored, and the patient is not experiencing problems with activities of daily living, and if a recurrent problem, previous episodes have been successfully treated, then this obviously saves resources. However, such patients are relatively uncommon.

Non-specific management

The hospital ward environment is often bleak with little source of stimulation besides the television or radio. Use of as much domestic (rather than institutional) furniture, lighting and paint finishes as possible can help promote a more homely environment. With a little imagination day rooms can be more like sitting rooms, and the rest of the ward more like a series of bedrooms. Emphasizing the identity of patients is necessary, and can be aided by providing space for cherished possessions from home. Many units have managed to obtain the authorization necessary to get a ward cat or dog. Such pets can be a remarkable source of interest and activity among patients recovering from depression.

Questionnaire

Your answers to the questions will help us in our research. We are interested in how you are feeling generally and all answers are *entirely confidential*. Some of the questions may seem strange but we would be most grateful if you would answer them anyway. Simply tick the box next to the statement that seems most appropriate for you.

There are 12 questions in all.

1. In general, how is your health compared with others of your age?
   (Please tick one box only)
   ☐ Excellent
   ☐ Good
   ☐ Fair
   ☐ Don't know what is meant by question

2. How quick are you in your physical movements compared with a year ago?
   (Please tick one box only)
   ☐ Quicker than usual
   ☐ About as quick as usual
   ☐ Less quick than usual
   ☐ Considerably slower than usual
   ☐ Don't know what is meant by question

3. How much energy do you have, compared to a year ago?
   (Please tick one box only)
   ☐ More than usual
   ☐ About the same as usual
   ☐ Less than usual
   ☐ Hardly any at all
   ☐ Don't know what is meant by question

4. In the last month, have you had any headaches?
   (Please tick one box only)
   ☐ Not at all
   ☐ About the same as usual
   ☐ Some of the time
   ☐ A lot of the time
   ☐ All of the time
   ☐ Don't know what is meant by question

5. Have you worried about things this past month?
   (Please tick one box only)
   ☐ Not at all
   ☐ Only now and then
   ☐ Some of the time
   ☐ A lot of the time
   ☐ All of the time
   ☐ Don't know what is meant by question

6. Have you been sad, unhappy (depressed) or weepy this past month?
   (Please tick one box only)
   ☐ Not at all
   ☐ Only now and then
   ☐ Some of the time
   ☐ A lot of the time
   ☐ All of the time
   ☐ Don't know what is meant by question

7. In the past month, have you been lying awake at night feeling uneasy or unhappy?
   (Please tick one box only)
   ☐ Not at all
   ☐ Once or twice
   ☐ Quite often
   ☐ Very often
   ☐ Don't know what is meant by question

8. Do you blame yourself for unpleasant things that have happened to you in the past?
   (Please tick on box only)
   ☐ Not at all
   ☐ About one thing
   ☐ About a few things
   ☐ About everything
   ☐ Don't know what is meant by question

9. How do you feel about your future?
   (Please tick one box only)
   ☐ Very happy
   ☐ Quite happy
   ☐ All right
   ☐ Unsure
   ☐ Don't care
   ☐ Worried
   ☐ Frightened
   ☐ Hopeless
   ☐ Don't know what is meant by question

10. What have you enjoyed doing lately?
    (Please tick one box only)
    ☐ Everything
    ☐ Most things
    ☐ Some things
    ☐ One or two things
    ☐ Nothing
    ☐ Don't know what is meant by question

11. In the past month, have there been times when you've felt quite happy?
    (Please tick one box only)
    ☐ Often
    ☐ Sometimes
    ☐ Now and then
    ☐ Never
    ☐ Don't know what is meant by question

12. In general, how happy are you?
    (Please tick one box only)
    ☐ Very happy
    ☐ Fairly happy
    ☐ Not very happy
    ☐ Not happy at all
    ☐ Don't know what is meant by question

Figure 27.1 The Selfcare (D) rating scale for depression (reproduced with permission from Bird, 1990)

The patient's day requires more thought than in the acute medical ward setting. Time needs to be given to physical activity that may lead to a faster recovery. Simple ball games — such as throwing a large beach ball around in a circle — may seem childish but help develop psychomotor skills. Mealtimes assume great importance, and are a focal part of the day. The social aspects of eating are used to increase engagement with other patients and staff. Inventiveness is needed to promote activities that engage patients, staff and family, and this is part of the challenge of nursing elderly people.

Many patients will require rehabilitation to resume normal activities of daily living. They need to be given time to practise kitchen skills, getting dressed, and restoring their mobility. Those with long-standing depression may have become physically very weak and stiff, simply through disuse. Active programmes of physiotherapy and occupational therapy are needed for most patients.

Clinical psychologists are often part of the team, and are extremely helpful in assessing the degree of cognitive impairment of depressed patients, and providing behavioural treatments for patients with phobias, and anxiety states that are associated with depression.

Social work is frequently needed by depressed patients. Often they have given little attention to paying bills, to maintenance of their homes, and have very limited social networks. Advice about finances, about local opportunities for joining clubs, day centres and lunch clubs, and organizing home care services are often of great value in aiding the patient's successful return home.

Psychotherapy for elderly people is such a rarity in the health service, and is quite scarce for those patients able to pay for private care, that its place in the management of depressed elderly patients is unclear. Much of the work of community psychiatric nurses is probably within the sphere of supportive psychotherapy, particularly during the recovery phase.

Antidepressant drugs

Antidepressants are powerful drugs, with potentially serious side-effects (Table 27.3). Care is required in their use, and as with most prescribing in older people, the rule is to start with very low doses and build up slowly. Side-effects are often avoided by using a single night-time dose of drug, and the hypnotic effects of some antidepressants can be useful if sleep disturbance is a problem.

These days, monoamine oxidase inhibitors are rarely used, as newer antidepressants are both safer and as effective. Occasionally psychiatrists will treat patients with these drugs if response to other drugs has been poor. Tricyclic antidepressants (so called because of the shape of the drug molecule) are most commonly used. Newer versions have fewer anticholinergic side-effects (dry mouth, constipation, postural hypotension, retention of urine, confusional state), but are not completely safe. Careful monitoring of side-effects is still needed. The newest drugs — 5-HT agonists — seem to have great potential, but experience among elderly patients is quite limited at present and they are expensive.

Lithium is typically used in manic–depressive psychosis, but may be useful as an adjunct in patients who do not respond to tricyclic antidepressants. Side-effects are frequent with lithium and regular monitoring of serum levels is necessary.

Electroconvulsive therapy (ECT) has an accepted place in the management of severe depression, and can be very effective in elderly patients, particularly those who are becoming very withdrawn and are refusing medication, food and drink. Because of some antipathy to the use of ECT it is sometimes not considered soon enough in patients who are resistant to other forms of treatment.

Table 27.3 Classes of antidepressants and their side-effects

	Sedation	Anticholinergic effects	Postural hypotension	Other effects
Tricyclic antidepressants				
Amitriptyline	+++	+++	+++	Heart block,
Imipramine		+	++	arrhythmias,
Nortriptyline	++	++	++	acute glaucoma
Lofepramine		+	++	mania (lofepramine)
Dothiepine	+++	+++	+++	confusion
Monoamine oxidase inhibitors				
Phenelzine	+	++	+++	Tyramine reaction to red wines, cheese
5-HT agonists				
Fluoxetine				Flushing, hypotension
Other drugs				
Lithium carbonate	++			Thyroid failure, diabetes insipidus
Carbamazepine				In toxicity: ataxia, visual disturbance

PROGNOSIS FOR RECOVERY

Depression in old age is not good news, and although the condition is treatable, patients die; up to 14 per cent die within a year of diagnosis. However, it is debatable whether death rates are higher than expected, since depressed patients frequently suffer with concurrent life-shortening diseases. Untreated depression may resolve, following a pattern of recurrent episodes. In general the results of treatment are better among older than younger patients. Up to a quarter of treated patients will enjoy a complete recovery within a year of diagnosis, but between a third and a half will still have symptoms.

Little information is available on the continued use of medication after symptoms have disappeared but drugs are often used for about a year, gently withdrawing treatment. In patients who have suffered relapse, routine 'maintenance' therapy is used.

Key points

- Depression is common in old age but may present atypically with non-specific symptoms. It is frequently unrecognized and can be a life-threatening disease.
- Depression is associated with adverse life events (losses), with hearing and visual impairment, and with physical illness.
- Depression can lead to poor performance on tests of cognitive function suggesting a dementia — this is sometimes termed 'pseudodementia'.
- Management of depression is multidisciplinary, involving the GP, hospital consultant, community psychiatric nurses, clinical psychologist and occupational therapist, as well as family and other carers.
- Attention to small details is a necessary part of non-specific management.
- Tricyclic antidepressant drugs have serious side-effects (anticholinergic: dry mouth, blurred vision, urinary retention, postural hypotension) and low doses must be used initially, building up the dose depending on response.
- Depression in old age has a better prognosis than at younger ages: up to a quarter of patients will get better, but between a third and a half will still have symptoms after a year.

FURTHER READING

Bird J. The use of the self-care (D) rating scale for depression. *Care of the Elderly* 1990; **2**(3).

Jenkins R, Newton J, Young R. *The Prevention of Depression and Anxiety. The Role of the Primary Care Team.* HMSO, London, 1992.

Murphy E (ed.). *Affective Illness in the Elderly.* Churchill Livingstone, Edinburgh, 1986.

Palmer RM. 'Failure to thrive' in the elderly: diagnosis and management. *Geriatrics* 1990; **45**(9): 47–50, 53–55.

Wattis J, Hindmarch I (eds). *Psychological Assessment of the Elderly.* Churchill Livingstone, Edinburgh, 1988.

28 PSYCHOTIC AND OTHER DISORDERS

- Hallucinations and delusions
- Paraphrenia
- Management of paranoid symptoms
- Mania
- Schizophrenia
- *Folie à deux*
- Diogenes syndrome
- Jekyll and Hyde syndrome
- Learning difficulties
- Substance abuse

HALLUCINATIONS AND DELUSIONS

Hallucinations are the experience or perception of phenomena that are not present in reality; delusions are false beliefs that are firmly held despite evidence to the contrary, that are not acceptable or normal within the society or culture, and may be supported by misinterpretations of real phenomena. For example, a hallucination is hearing voices or seeing little people walking around a room, whereas a delusion is believing that a partner is putting poison rather than sugar into the tea.

Hallucinations occuring on falling asleep and on waking are extremely common (hypnogogic and hypnopompic hallucinations) and have no pathological significance at all. However, they can be a source of concern to anxious people who may infer that they herald madness.

Hallucinations and delusions are quite common but may be difficult to uncover as patients may be understandably afraid of admitting to them, or may include the doctor, nurse or carer into a delusional belief system of persecution. A patient's behaviour may be the clue to these symptoms. For example, a patient may appear frightened, may scream or strike out, or may start up a conversation without anyone present.

The significance of hallucinations and delusions is much less clear-cut than in younger people. Auditory hallucinations and paranoid delusions are common in severe depressive illness, in mania, and may occur in people with long-standing deafness or visual impairment. Hallucinations also occur in organic brain disease, particularly in alcohol withdrawal (delirium tremens), dementias and after stroke. It is important to realize that medication (particularly L-dopa, opiates, antidepressants, steroids) can cause hallucinations, and to enquire whether this has occurred on prescribing such drugs. The delirium of acute illness may be associated with hallucinations and paranoid delusions, and the psychiatric symptoms may be much more florid than the underlying physical illness.

Commonly hallucinations occur after bereavement of a dead partner. These can be very vivid, and are often a source of comfort rather than a problem, although some people may fear that madness is not far away and require reassurance that this is normal. Hearing voices and seeing visions might lead some to belief that the diagnosis is schizophrenia, but first onset of schizophrenia in old age is highly unlikely.

PARAPHRENIA

This term is used to describe schizophrenia-like illness occurring for the first time in old age. Paranoia is the usual presenting symptom, but unlike chronic schizophrenia, the disease does not lead to deterioration in personality and emotions. The onset is insidious with increasing suspicion that neighbours are interfering with the patient's life. A patient may complain that a neighbour is spreading gossip about them, or is trying to irritate them with noise from the television. Often these delusions become more dramatic with allegations of use of magic rays, tunneling under the floorboards, use of the television for spying on the patient, and so on.

Sometimes such delusions occur in an isolated person who has always been the sort 'to keep herself to herself', and is frequently considered to be a little eccentric. Despite remarkably strongly held delusions, in a few patients the disease does not progress and the person continues to live a suspicious life without coming into contact with medical services.

More usually hallucinations develop along with the paranoid delusions and make life intolerable for the sufferer. The hallucinations are usually of voices that are critical of the person, and interfere with thinking and action. It is usually at this stage that help is sought by friends or neighbours because the person's ability to cope with day-to-day life breaks down.

It is essential to decide whether the acute breakdown is due to paraphrenia or to an organic brain syndrome (i.e. delirium from whatever cause, or early dementia). Such patients require careful medical and psychiatric assessment. Frequently underlying acute neurological signs will be found, and the diagnosis of cerebrovascular disease made. Up to a third of patients with a diagnosis of paraphrenia will develop obvious dementia within a few years, implying that the paranoid symptoms were an early manifestation of organic brain disease.

MANAGEMENT OF PARANOID SYMPTOMS

In general, it is not sensible to reinforce a patient's delusional beliefs or hallucinations; gentle explanation that what is happening is understandable but not real is the best line to take. The patient should be nursed in a well-lit room, with the minimum of extraneous noise, and avoidance of frequent changes of position in the ward and of nursing staff. Hallucinations and delusions caused by organic brain syndromes should be treated by controlling or removing the underlying cause. All patients with these symptoms should be assessed by a psychiatrist who will be able to advise whether the symptoms are part of a depressive illness, a secondary reaction to drugs or acute illness, or due to paraphrenia.

It is usually necessary to treat the symptoms themselves as they can be so distressing. Small doses of major tranquillizers are used: haloperidol or promazine may be useful if agitation is pronounced. Chlorpromazine (Largactil) is not recommended for elderly patients because of its hypotensive effects. Sometimes a hypnotic may be helpful if symptoms are relatively mild. Major tranquillizers may have serious Parkinsonian side-effects and it is essential to monitor the patient's mobility and tone, reducing the dose if side-effects occur. Routine use of anticholinergic drugs (e.g. benzhexol, orphenadrine) in an attempt to prevent Parkinsonism is not recommended because these drugs are potent causes of confusional states and postural hypotension in old age.

The longer term management of paranoid patients is likely to require psychiatric rehabilitation, re-engagement into usual activities, and social support. Correction of visual and hearing impairment should be given a high priority. The prognosis of paraphrenia is relatively good with over 90 per cent achieving some degree of recovery.

MANIA

Mania is usually encountered as part of a bipolar illness: one pole being depression and the other mania. The patient oscillates between the two, although the manic symptoms may be relatively mild (hypomania) and not lead to medical attention. A past history of episodes of depressive illness is frequent.

Manic patients are usually overactive, overtalkative, and may also have paranoid delusions. They are usually great fun to talk to as the flight of ideas and pressure of speech, together with grandiose ideas, are entertaining. Occasionally the mania will lead to extravagent acts such as spending large sums of money, or destroying the furniture in an effort to redecorate.

Mania can be due to underlying physical illness, usually a stroke or brain tumour, or to medication (tricyclic antidepressents, psychostimulants, anticholinergics). Treatment is then removal of the underlying cause, and use of major tranquillizers to control the manic symptoms. If the mania is part of a bipolar illness, then long-term control with lithium is the usual management.

SCHIZOPHRENIA

Schizophrenia is usually seen in its 'burnt out' form amongst long-term residents of psychiatric hospitals who have reached old age. The disintegration of personality, the loss of emotions, the thought disturbance are usually less apparent, and often it is only the lip-smacking and tongue writhing (tardive dyskinesia) due to treatment with major tranquillizers that sets a schizophrenic patient apart from other residents in a long-stay institution. However, the auditory hallucinations and paranoid ideas may remain and come to the fore from time to time.

FOLIE À DEUX

This is a rare, but rather delightful, sharing of a delusional belief by two people, usually husband and wife. The delusion is usually paranoid in nature and directed towards neighbours who are believed to be hostile to the couple. The delusion is extremely difficult to treat, as the couple reinforce each other's beliefs. Fortunately, it is not usually associated with other psychopathology, and the delusions are relatively mild. It is worth being aware of *folie à deux* so that delusions are not inappropriately believed and acted upon by doctors, nurses, police or others.

DIOGENES SYNDROME

Diogenes was a Greek philosopher who lived in an earthenware jar. By the end of his life the jar had presumably become pretty squalid and the syndrome refers to people who live in extreme squalor. Typical sufferers are reclusive men who are often hoarders of apparently useless material such as newspapers, empty jars and bottles. Usually the person will have held down a job until retirement age, but will have very few social contacts, and will have remained single. Sometimes the syndrome is associated with schizophrenia or alcohol abuse, although the majority are not ill, but simply eccentric. Some patients with paraphrenia may be wrongly suspected of having Diogenes syndrome if they keep their paranoid delusions and hallucinations to themselves. It is helpful for all these patients to see an experienced psychiatrist who will be able to elicit such symptoms. Cleaning up their places usually leads to a return to the orginal squalor within a matter of weeks, and is only possible if intercurrent illness has led to their removal from home, as most refuse all forms of help.

JEKYLL AND HYDE SYNDROME

The patient is admitted from home in an acute crisis of immobility, incontinence and acopia (an acute state of inability to cope with life — often applied to carers as well as patients). Once in hospital the patient becomes self-caring within a day or so. No acute illness is found, nor any psychiatric symptoms. All seems well so discharge is arranged. The patient usually returns to hospital in the same state as before within the week; hence the label Jekyll and Hyde syndrome. The prognosis for independent life at home is poor and most patients find themselves in institutional care.

LEARNING DIFFICULTIES (previously mental handicap)

People with learning difficulties (or mental handicap) are surviving much longer than in previous times and are now reaching old age in substantial numbers. Many of them have outlived their parents and many have spent the majority of their lives in long-term hospital care. As the long-stay psychiatric hospitals are closed, the care of these elderly people becomes ever more precarious and is a responsibility that falls between social services, learning difficulties services and geriatric services. People with learning difficulties are likely to be much more affected by changes in location, changes in main carers and by disease. Several schemes have been established to relocate older people with learning difficulties into the community in small residential units. Their medical care is then the responsibility of general practitioners. It always most helpful to ensure that a careful summary of their medical, social, psychiatric and behavioural background is prepared as a means of understanding and as a benchmark against which to evaluate the effects of new illnesses.

SUBSTANCE ABUSE

Alcohol

Alcohol abuse affects about 5–12 per cent of old people, depending on definitions used. Elderly drinkers fall into two main groups: those who have drunk all their lives and present with the long-term consequences of abuse, and those who start in late life, usually as a result of bereavement. The prognosis for the latter group is much better than the former.

A high index of suspicion is needed to make the diagnosis of alcohol abuse. Often drinking is an unrecognized cause of falls, hypothermia or confusion. The management of acute alcohol syndromes — delirium tremens and Wernicke–Korsakoff's syndrome — is the same as at younger ages. It is essential that high doses of thiamine are given to avoid permanent brain damage.

Frequently, long-standing drinkers have evidence of cirrhosis of the liver, unsteadiness on walking (due to degeneration of the cerebellum), and heart failure due to damage to the heart. The life expectancy for such people is not good, but both they and their families may gain support from Alcoholics Anonymous.

Tobacco

It is usually felt, by health professionals, that old people should be allowed to enjoy their cigarettes and not be lectured about giving up. Old people are more enlightened, and in surveys a majority of smokers claim to be interested in giving up, and would value help. The main forces for giving up are the health and example set to young grandchildren, and for a minority their own health. Since life expectation has increased so much after retirement age, and the benefits of stopping smoking are apparent within 4–5 years at younger ages, it is reasonable to support giving up smoking in any elderly person with a life expectation of over 10 years. The methods that are effective with younger adults (one-to-one counselling, hypnosis, substitute behaviour) are likely to be as useful with elderly people.

Key points

- Delusions and hallucinations may be caused by organic brain disease (dementia, stroke, acute confusional states, delirium tremens), and may be associated with depression.
- Paraphrenia — a schizophrenia-like illness — is quite common and may be due to an underlying dementia. Treatment with major tranquillizers is usually associated with a good prognosis.
- Mania is usually part of a bipolar illness, but can be caused by organic brain syndromes.
- Alcohol abuse is common and often occult. A high index of suspicion is needed, and treatment with thiamine should be started if there is any likelihood of alcohol abuse.

FURTHER READING

Barrios G, Brook P. Visual hallucinations and sensory delusions in the elderly. *Br J Psychiat* 1984; **144**: 662–664.

Boyd R, Woodman J. The Jekyll-and-Hyde syndrome. *Lancet* 1978; ii: 671–672.

Isaacs AD, Post F (eds). *Studies in Geriatric Psychiatry*. John Wiley & Sons, New York, 1978.

Kafetz K, Cox M. Alcohol excess and the senile squalor syndrome. *J Am Geriatr Soc* 1982; **30**: 706.

29 PSYCHOLOGICAL ASPECTS OF PHYSICAL DISEASE

- The experience of illness
- Responses to illness
- Factors determining psychological status
- Identification of psychiatric problems
- Approaches to treatment

It is not surprising that old people tend to think about, talk about and prepare for the end of life. This phase of life may be characterized by major life events and losses, particularly important being loss of a partner. The increased risk of physical disability, due to a wide range of chronic, degenerative diseases, is undeniable. Yet the majority of elderly people, when questioned about their health, rate it as 'good' or 'better than average'. The very heterogeneity of elderly people means that the range of psychological responses to physical illness will also be wide.

THE EXPERIENCE OF ILLNESS

The mechanisms by which people accept and come to terms with physical disability in old age are not understood in any empirical sense. The paradigm borrowed from the bereavement literature of a sequential move- ment from shock, denial, anger, despair, to acceptance may be applicable in some circumstances, but in many may not be, and evidence is lacking. A possible interpretation of existing evidence is that old people are most likely to respond to the onset of physical ill-health with depressive symptoms.

Shock and anger may be less likely to occur since old age is already so likely to be associated with ill-health and loss. The analogy with grief — a process triggered off by a particular event (bereavement) and capable of some satisfactory resolution — may be less relevant in old age, where illness tends to be a continuing burden.

The meaning of illness to the patient

Physical illness means different things to different people. Most obviously it poses a threat: of disability, of pain and suffering, or even of death. Illness is commonly associated with loss which might tangible (e.g. sight) or intangible (e.g. autonomy).

The response of those close to the patient

Illness means something not just to the sufferer, but to those around them. The ill person should be seen not just as an individual coping with an illness, but as somebody also needing to negotiate a new position in their personal network. The ill older person is often a peripheral member of the family rather than an integral part of its functioning. About a third of old people live alone, but even those who live in families will express the fear of being or becoming a burden on those who care for them when they are physically ill. By contrast, when the patient is young, family re-adjustment often increases their centrality with a new illness-focused network revolving around their needs.

Symptoms as stressors

Physical illnesses produce changes which are stressful: fatigue caused by anaemia, breathlessness from lung disease, pain or sexual dysfunction are all primarily distressing experiences. Changes in personal appearance such as obesity, pallor, visible scars or hair thinning are generally less troublesome to the older patient although they may still be relevant.

Social consequences of illness

The practical impact of illness on day-to-day life — handicap — may be most stressful. For example, the inconvenience of time spent travelling to hospital, learning how to use aids and appliances, or financial hardship. It is more expensive to live with a physical disability and yet, particularly in later life, the increased financial burden is rarely compensated.

Unusual or idiosyncratic meanings of illness

Sometimes illness may represent a real advantage or gain. This is most obvious when symptoms (pain, funny do's) are used to manipulate social occasions. Emotional blackmail may be a very effective way of getting the attention desired by an isolated, lonely older person. Chronic illness in one partner in a marriage can re-define a relationship over years so that a state of mutual interdependency replaces a more open and adult arrangement.

Coincidental life events and difficulties

A high proportion of physically ill people have experienced a life stress in the recent past which might be responsible for psychological disorder, either in its own right or by making the patient more vulnerable when faced with the stress of illness.

RESPONSES TO ILLNESS

Coping strategies

The central challenge of illness is its impact on autonomy and personal integrity. Successful coping allows the person to remain independent. It is important to remember that autonomy and dependence are related but distinct concepts. Autonomy is the exercise of choice and free will which is possible even for very disabled people.

The patient's view of their ability to control or influence matters is another factor which will determine ability to cope. This is often referred to as the 'locus of control'. A high personal or internal locus of control may be important in achieving successful coping.

A third element in coping is how active or passive the individual is as a problem-solver. Chronic illness generally requires an active, engaged approach from the patient which should lead to a partnership with doctors, nurses and therapists rather than a dependent relationship. In a partnership, goals are agreed through negotiation and responsibility is shared.

These three components of coping style (exercise of autonomy and independence, sense of personal responsibility or locus of control, activity or passivity) can be seen to varying degrees in the commonly described strategies for coping. One typical coping style is an active engagement in treatment with seeking of information, sensible monitoring of symptoms and progress, and resistance to unnecessary dependence on others. A strikingly different style is passive dependence on others, often associated with social withdrawal and unhealthy focusing on physical symptoms.

However, it would be wrong to suggest that there is only one appropriate coping style. Lack of interest in seeking information and self-care may not be maladaptive. For example, stoical acceptance of disability coupled with minimizing of symptoms and downplaying of their impact on day-to-day life is a common and successful illness response. Every clinician will know an ill old person who responds like this, perhaps to the extent of stubborn refusal to accept an obvious need for help.

FACTORS DETERMINING PSYCHOLOGICAL STATUS

A patient's psychological status is a reflection of the response that people make to the experience of illness, and an indication of how psychologically adaptive their response has been.

Characteristics of the individual

Elderly people are prone to develop depression in response to disease events and health difficulties although this may occur in younger people as well. There is no evidence that women respond worse than (or even differently from) men when the stressor is a physical illness.

Social class, wealth, intelligence and educational level are assumed to influence the individual's capacity to cope with a physical illness. However, these characteristics may merely act as markers for an ability to get the best out of the system.

Previous and recent experiences of illness and other stress are likely to be of great significance. Life events are so common that most older people have some direct experience of coping with them which will help.

Nature of the illness

Diseases with a sudden onset or a life-threatening course will have more profound effects than those with a gradual or remitting prognosis. The underlying aetiology may also be relevant. Smoking-related diseases may lead to a feeling of guilt in the sufferer. In some cases patients assume that an event was caused by specific activities (e.g. sexual intercourse and stroke) which may lead to avoidance of the activity and resultant problems.

Specific problems, such as loss of vision, deafness, communication difficulty, urinary incontinence and falls, may lead to a disproportionate impact on lifestyle and social engagement and consequently on mental state.

Some diseases may lead to psychiatric disorder as a result of their pathology. For example, anxiety may be associated with thyrotoxicosis, delirium associated with hypercalcaemia, hypoxia or uraemia and emotionalism provoked by steroid medication or stroke.

Adaptation

It is important to distinguish between psychological states which are abnormal by virtue of being unusual and those which are abnormal by virtue of being maladaptive, that is, which lead to disability or handicap. For example, a few years ago the dependent coping style of retreating to lie in bed for long periods during physical illnesses was not unusual. Recent medical practice, however, is based on the belief that it is probably maladaptive and best discouraged.

Successful adaptation is perhaps most likely to occur when patients themselves have sufficient autonomy to select the activities that they wish to do, when optimal performance of these activities has been achieved, and treatments and environments have been specifically tailored to compensate for those tasks and activities that patients can no longer do for themselves (see Chapter 13).

IDENTIFICATION OF PSYCHIATRIC PROBLEMS

Simple self-filled questionnaires may be useful to uncover psychiatric symptoms. They generally identify the presence of mood symptoms and physical symptoms associated with states of personal distress. However, the inclusion of physical symptoms may lead to false positives in physically ill older people, as symptoms become commoner with age and physical illness may explain a high score. This may be dealt with by raising cut-off points or using a scale that avoids physical symptoms. In clinical practice questionnaires are rarely very useful because patients are often unable to complete a form due to visual impairment, language impairment or global intellectual impairment.

A way round this practical problem is to adopt simple screening interviews as an alternative. There are a number now available which are similar to brief screening tests for intellectual impairment and are designed to identify mood disorder on the basis of responses to a structured list of questions. The enthusiasm with which screening questions for intellectual impairment have been adopted by geriatricians suggests that with appropriate education, this approach could be adopted to help in the identification of mood disorders (see Chapter 27).

Atypical psychological states

Many people do not suffer with a clear-cut depressive illness or an anxiety state but with much vaguer distress that defies diagnosis. This is nevertheless unpleasant and contributes to their suffering. An example would be the patient who is apathetic, inert and socially withdrawn and who cooperates poorly with efforts at physical rehabilitation. Such people are often described as poorly motivated and the question is raised whether they are 'depressed'. They rarely, if ever, have the more usually recognized symptoms of depressive illness.

Another common presentation is of the ill older person who has physical symptoms which cannot be explained by physical pathology; sometimes these somatic symptoms are accompanied by hypochondriacal ideas. In the past it has been suggested that hypochondriasis and related disorders are invariably manifestations of mood disorder, and certainly they can be in elderly people. None the less, it is an oversimplification simply to regard all somatizing elderly patients as suffering from depressive disorders and attempts to do so limit the scope of both of our descriptions and of our interventions.

It is necessary to be aware of the trap of falsely identifying psychological barriers to rehabilitation when it is the very severity of physical impairments that is preventing successful rehabilitation. Equally important is to recognize when a patient's goals conflict with those of the rehabilitation team, leading to apparent difficulties. Physicians must learn to live with their failures as well as to enjoy successes, and not simply treat every disaffected patient with antidepressants.

APPROACHES TO TREATMENT

Drugs

Antidepressants are helpful if the patient suffers typical depressive symptoms. Their role in the more common atypical states is not clearly defined and the preceding discussion of the underlying factors and aetiology of atypical states indicates that they are not indicated. Apprehension about side-effects, particularly confusion, postural hypotension and impairment of mobility, should lead to caution in prescribing antidepressants.

The practice of giving patients who are apathetic amphetamines to 'perk them up' is widespread in some units, and has no rational basis. There are anecdotal suggestions that emotionalism in the absence of depressive symptoms responds to low-dose antidepressants.

The psychotherapeutic approach

A psychological approach based on talking and behavioural change would seem to be theoretically desirable. However, orthodox psychotherapies are difficult to deliver in this setting. The patient rarely has the stamina or attention span for a sustained therapeutic session. Cognitive impairment often makes talking therapies unsuitable. The other practical demands of illness and its treatment (especially for inpatients) compete with and can disrupt time-consuming psychotherapies.

It is possible to offer psychological help based on a counselling educational model. Sessions need to be short and frequently repeated and they need to be focused on the issues outlined above. Where at all possible they should involve 'significant others', because of the importance of the personal network in determining the patient's response. The issues are best dealt with through discussion of practical aspects of the current situation: the 'here and now' approach.

As an example, visiting time and mealtimes often provoke strong emotions which can be observed and responded to immediately by ward staff. Photographs of patient and family can be used as a starting point for discussion of isolation and belonging, fears of being a burden, behaviour of other people and so on.

The milieu as therapeutic

The negative effects on morale of being in an atmosphere of disinterest, impersonality and passivity should be obvious, but many acute medical wards are just like this. In general, once an acute ward has thrown in the towel by asking for the transfer of a patient to a geriatric ward it is best to accede to the request speedily. A patient who is not wanted on a ward knows it, but lacks advocates to ensure that his or her needs are considered. Transfer of elderly patients from acute to rehabilitation wards can make all the difference and play a big part in psychological recovery from illness. More subtle and difficult to guard against is the creation of a relentless over-enthusiastic jollity in which the patient has no 'space' to express feelings of grief or apprehension.

Teamwork is a further essential element in the therapeutic milieu. The sharing of information about how patients respond to different members of staff or how they behave with relatives and other patients is crucial in achieving an informal understanding of the psychological impact of disease for the individual.

It is common to hear of patients breaking into tears on seeing their homes on a home visit after a long spell in hospital. It is at this point that the full implications of the disease for the patient become obvious, and counselling is needed to develop adaptive coping mechanisms.

Family conferences are a useful but time-consuming means of exploring what illness means to both patient and family. They are probably an underused counselling device. Even a single session of working with families on ways of coping with stress, disability and change is rewarded with improved family dynamics, and, usually, a happier patient.

Specialist psychiatric care

Just occasionally the patient needs to be transferred to a specialist psychiatric facility, perhaps for ECT or for specialist nursing care of difficult behaviour. Under these circumstances, the physical illness is usually of less importance.

Key points

- The meaning of physical disease and thereby the psychological response will depend on a number of factors: the response of others; the nature of the symptoms; social consequences; and previous experience.
- Coping with physical disease requires strategies that reduce dependency, maintain control and require active engagement. However, some individuals cope by alternative mechanisms, such as denial.
- The psychological states experienced by patients will depend on the individual's age, socio-economic status, the natural history of the disease and the degree of adaptation possible.
- Identification of psychological suffering is important and may be best done by structured interview. Most patients do not have clear-cut depressive illness or anxiety states. Most commonly, patients have a combination of apathy, disengagement and poor cooperation.
- Treatment with antidepressants is not the answer. A psychotherapeutic approach is best and this should be combined with an appropriate, supportive environment, and good communication between team members.

FURTHER READING

Adams GF, Hurwitz LJ. Mental barriers to recovery from stroke. *Lancet* 1968; ii: 533–537.

Berkman LF, Berkman CS, Kasl S *et al.* Depressive symptoms in relation to physical health and functioning in the elderly. *Am J Epidemiol* 1986; **124**: 372–388.

Feldman E, Mayou R, Hawton K, Ardern M, Smith EB. Psychiatric disorder in medical inpatients. *Quart J Med* 1987; **241**: 405–412.

Goldberg D. Identifying psychiatric illness among general medical patients. *Br Med J* 1985; **291**:161–162.

House A. Mood disorders after stroke: a review of the evidence. *Int J Ger Psych* 1987; **2**: 211–221.

Lipowski ZJ. Physical illness, the individual and the coping processes. *Psychiat Med* 1970; **1**: 91–102.

30 PALLIATIVE CARE

- Living wills
- Euthanasia
- Good medical practice
- Pain control
- The general practitioner

In most people's minds the words 'palliative care' (preferred to 'terminal care') mean the last few days of a person's life, the use of drugs to control pain and an image of separateness, the dying person being outside of and excluded from conventional health care. This image has not arisen recently. Dying and death have remained taboo subjects for many centuries but socio-culturally current generations are legitimately avoiding 'dying' until maturity, many adults only being exposed to the situation when a very elderly parent dies.

The diagnosis of a condition that is irreversible and will cause the person to die within a definable short period is never easy to make. Some conditions are more predictable than others, the certainty of death may only come within hours or days of the event. Despite the universal fact that we will all die there has been an awesome failure to understand this event, compared to say birth. Cultural and religious views have moulded our attitudes to those of fearful avoidance.

This professional neglect has been acknowledged and slowly the accumulated knowledge base is being disseminated. As health care workers we are becoming aware of the art and skill needed to break and explain bad news, to expect and understand the reactions of disbelief, denial, anger and resentment. We are learning about how different societies react to death and comparing this to our own attitudes. The time scale of caring in this situation is changing, for in some disease states we must allow for the process of care to last years. We have only begun to evaluate the role of psychological approaches, counselling and holistic/alternative medicine.

The hospice movement has been our impetus towards change with the pioneering work of Cicely Saunders and others. Recently, however (especially in the USA), there has been the impact of AIDS in this area. The fact that death was suddenly confronting a large, articulate and questioning number of younger people in society placed the topic of palliative care under critical scrutiny. Unfortunately the subject and whole process was found to be lacking in many fundamental aspects. The American gay movement has led the way in support and counselling schemes and information networks. They have stressed the important fact that we live until we die and how we live during this time is what matters. The gay movement has also spawned numerous effective pressure groups trying to ensure adequate funding and a high public profile over the issue of dying.

LIVING WILLS

Attitudes are certainly changing. There is a small but increasing interest in information that might help the individual avoid a protracted illness. One such scheme is known as a living will. This refers to a document whereby a person while still mentally competent specifies the health care they wish to receive should they ever become mentally incompetent due to brain damage or dementia. Such a document has no legal validity in the UK but has been adopted by most of the States in the USA. In addition to the living will an enduring power of attorney (for health care) allows the competent person to appoint an advocate to act on their behalf and act as the 'fine tuning' to the whole mechanism. The belief is that the living will returns autonomy to an otherwise disenfranchised adult and is a departure from a very paternalistic area of medicine.

Views in this area are often polarized from the concept of it being morally wrong, through the premise that 'good medical practice' already allows people to die in certain circumstances, to the notion that this form of legislation (if adopted) falls short of the ultimate upholding of autonomy and dignity, that is the right to die at a time of one's own choosing (i.e. euthanasia). Living wills (generically called 'advance directives') are usually in a prescribed form of declaration, but can vary as to complexity. An example is given below.

- If the time comes when I am incapacitated to the point when I can no longer actively take part in decisions for my own life, and am unable to direct my physician as to my own medical care, I request that I be allowed to die and not be kept alive through life-sustaining measures if my condition is deemed irreversible. I do not intend any direct taking of my life, but only that my dying not be unreasonable prolonged.
- It is my express wish that if I should develop
  - (a) brain disease of severe degree, or
  - (b) serious brain damage resulting from accidental or other injury or illness, or
  - (c) advanced malignant disease, in which I would be unable or mentally incompetent to express my own opinion about accepting or declining treatment, and if two independent physicians conclude that, to the best of current medical knowledge, my condition is irreversible, then I request that the following points be taken into consideration.
    - (i) Any separate illness (e.g. pneumonia, or a cardiac or kidney condition) which may threaten my life should not be given active treatment unless it appears to be causing me undue physical suffering. Cardiopulmonary resuscitation should not be used if the existing quality of my life is already seriously impaired.
    - (ii) In the course of such an advanced illness, if I should be unable to take food, fluid or medication, I would wish that these should not be given by any artificial means, except for the relief of obvious suffering.
    - (iii) If, during any such an illness, my condition deteriorates and, as a result, my behaviour becomes violent, noisy, or in any other ways degrading, or if I appear to be suffering severe pain, any symptom should be controlled immediately by appropriate drug treatment, regardless of the consequences upon my physical health and survival, to the extent allowed by law.
    - (iv) Other requests. The object of this declaration is to minimize distress or indignity which I may suffer or create during an incurable illness, and to spare my medical advisers and/or relatives the burden of making difficult decisions on my behalf.

EUTHANASIA

An even more controversial area of debate surrounds the subject of euthanasia — the deliberate taking of life. This issue has aroused intense debate and in some countries (e.g. the Netherlands) it has been incorporated into a semi-legal framework under clearly set-out guidelines. The criteria include issues around competence, certainty of near death and/or unrelieved distress and suffering. The doctors taking part certainly see it as an extension of their caring role — indeed caring up to and including death. The client chooses the time and place and sleep is induced by an intravenous drug and death occurs by the same route (potassium chloride can be used). The procedure is explained beforehand and verbal refusal at any stage cancels the 'agreement'. This subject needs to be debated away from the glare of publicity and, together with advance directives placed in a correct perspective. In the UK there has been an increased awareness of the topic with a wide diversity of opinions. The House of Lords has upheld the current status quo.

GOOD MEDICAL PRACTICE

It is stated that there is an interest in both euthanasia and advance directives because currently medical practice is deficient in certain key areas and hence these options are seen as desirable. In the care of the terminally ill, those who are chronically disabled and those with dementia of severe degree it is important to ask and attempt to define what constitutes good medical practice. Many of these people are elderly. There are no clearly defined guidelines apart from what is permissible by law and many people are unhappy at certain aspects concerning the care of these groups in both institutional and community settings. In the case of long-stay and terminally ill patients, nurses have more frequent, prolonged and personal contact with patients and relatives than have the medical team, and so the opinions of the nursing staff are vitally important in assessing the medical and ethical problems of patient care. The management of a clinical dilemma which involves ethical considerations should be decided upon by a process of open communication between the patient (where possible), doctors, nurses, relatives and other carers and important conclusions should be recorded in the case notes. The notion of 'quality of life' is essential in this process of assessment and decision-making. It is an elusive concept, but various attempts have been made to define it.

In the context of frail elderly people, Denham feels that measures of quality of life must include health (mortality and survival), health perception, function and mental health. He also stresses the importance of the quality of the environment. Fear of growing old with mental frailty is usually accompanied by a 'mind's eye' image of slovenly and dirty clothes, uncontrolled incontinence, disruptive behaviour or a dulled 'twilight' life of drug-induced stupor in a Victorian workhouse setting. This image is uncomfortable because it has an unpleasantly realistic basis. What can and does happen where imagination and resources are combined is a very different picture.

In the areas of intensive care and the role of cardiopulmonary resuscitation on patients with terminal malignant disease and dementia, several attempts have been made to develop valid systems for quantifying jointly the stage of the disease, its prognosis, and the burdens on the individual in such a way to allow an objective evaluation of the quality of life. Well-designed studies have an important place in setting standards in these areas of care.

Hospices, despite their rapid growth, still only care for about 5 per cent of those dying per year. Yet in their teaching role they are exerting a far greater influence by raising the standards of palliative care of those people dying in hospital or at home. The science of symptom relief and the art of nursing care are integral and well matched. Dying should occur in the absence of distressing symptoms and distressed patients. However, research shows that relatives are highly critical of the care given in the last stage of a person's life. This brief summary only focuses on particular areas. It is meant to be a guide and stimulus to further reading and to illustrate that it is ignorance that leads to health care professionals dealing badly with the dying — reinforcing prejudices and fear in the lay public.

PAIN CONTROL

Pain can be a significant problem in advanced cancer yet the majority of patients can be relieved of it without specialist intervention. It is argued that there is often hesitancy to ensure adequate pain relief because of the fear of being seen to hasten the end of life. The goal is full pain relief, no breakthrough pain and as few side-effects as possible. Only in the later stages should dosages impinge on consciousness and then the relief of pain is part of the dying process not the cause of it. However, it is not only a matter of analgesia: pain is an emotion altered by fear, weakness, tiredness — hence the broad approach needed. Patients often have more than one pain and the management is a detailed affair (Table 30.1).

Table 30.1 Assessment and treatment of pain

Assessment
Identify individual pains (pain chart) and for each pain determine
    History
    Severity
    Diagnosis (cause)
    Response to previous treatment

Treatment
General
    The affective component of pain
Specific (for each pain)
    Adequate dose of analgesic for the individual patient
    Continuous pain needs continuous medication
    Co-analgesics as necessary
    Consider non-drug treatments

Objectives (discussed with the patient)
Pain free at night
Pain free at rest
Pain free on movement

Monitor
Review progress soon and often

Analgesics

As a general guide, use paracetamol or aspirin for mild pain, a weak opioid (dextropropoxyphene) for moderate pain, and morphine for severe pain.

With morphine most patients need a 4-hourly regime. Doses should start low (2.5–5 mg 4 hourly) increasing as necessary, some patients eventually needing more than 30 mg 4 hourly. Elderly and frail patients should always be started on the smaller doses and the response assessed. Pain relief is the aim, and not a fast route to unconsciousness. Using an aqueous solution of morphine the dosage can be increased without increase in the volume of liquid taken. For many patients a controlled release preparation of morphine (MST) is available in tablet form in various dosages. Rectal administration of drugs can be used if a patient is unable to take oral drugs (morphine and oxycodone suppositories). In some cases prolonged parenteral administration is needed and a syringe pump is used. The side-effects of opioids (constipation, nausea and vomiting) are amenable to treatment if they occur. Indeed, constipation is so common that laxatives should be given routinely.

Co-analgesics

These are drugs or devices which may not have intrinsic pain-relieving activity but when used with conventional analgesics will aid pain relief. Examples are diazepam, psychotropics, corticosteroids and muscle relaxants, etc.

Non-drug measures

Flowtron (pneumatic compression sleeve) for lymphoedema (swollen limbs), radiotherapy, chemotherapy and hormone treatments, palliative surgery, nerve blocks, neurosurgery, massage, aromatherapy, relaxation hypnotherapy, acupuncture, diet, transcutaneous nerve stimulation and biofeedback techniques may all have a place in management. The multiplicity of methods suggests that specialist help is needed in guiding choice of management in those not helped by single treatments.

Other major symptoms of the terminally ill can be assessed and treated similarly. Cough can be suppressed, dyspnoea (shortness of breath) relieved, nausea and vomiting controlled. Weakness and confusion are perhaps harder to treat. Confusion can result from polypharmacy, comparatively minor intercurrent infections and other causes which when found and treated may reverse some of the confusion.

The art of nursing the terminally ill requires communication, listening and responding to anxieties. It involves helping to maintain dignity and some independence until death. Prevention of other complications such as pressure sores by adequate support mechanisms is essential. When mobility is limited (as in weakness) a wheelchair is a useful adjunct. Continence aids sometimes require expert assistance from the continence adviser. Catheters/penile sheaths can make a patient comfortable and less exhausted, while leg bags mean that dignity is maintained.

THE GENERAL PRACTITIONER

The GP is the resource centre both practically and often emotionally to a person and their family in a pre- and post-bereavement situation. The GP often makes the diagnosis or is involved on discharge from hospital. The GP acts as the 'key worker' to all the primary health care services, the social services as well as specialist groups such as psychiatrists (in the treatment of depression), bereavement counselling, home palliative care schemes, pain relief clinics, inpatient hospice care, etc. Other support groups are often part of this network: neighbours, friends, church and self-help groups.

Death and dying are obviously difficult issues, concerned as they are with the emotions and attitudes of all parties including the patient, doctor, relatives and other staff and carers. Areas of concerned interest such as euthanasia, the role of cardiopulmonary resuscitation guidelines and the issue of whether we should try to keep many frail elderly people alive at all costs are issues for urgent and effective debate.

Key points

- Many people do not experience a death situation of a close relative until reaching mature adulthood.
- Death and dying are still taboo subjects surrounded by myth and ignorance.
- The impact of AIDS is changing the way the subject of palliative care is being addressed.
- Living wills (generically called advance directives) are statements of wish with reference to health care in the case of the subject becoming mentally incompetent.

- Living wills plus an enduring power of attorney (for health issues) are valid in the US, allow some autonomy of an incompetent patient's wishes and are the subject of intense debate.
- Euthanasia is an entirely separate issue from living wills, it is the deliberate taking of life. Controlled access is available to people in the Netherlands where some doctors view it as an extension of their caring role. Strict guidelines are enforced there and euthanasia can only be carried out on mentally competent individuals.
- Quality of life measures include health (mortality and survival), health perception, function, mental health and the quality of the environment.
- Hospices only care for about 5 per cent of those dying per year.
- The science of symptom relief and the art of nursing care are integral and well matched.
- In pain control the goal is full pain relief, no breakthrough pain and as few side-effects as possible.
- Assessment of pain includes identifying individual pains with a pain chart.
- Treatment should result in the subject being continuously pain free, will involve dose monitoring and the use of various analgesics, co-analgesics and non-drug measures.
- The GP is the key worker in palliative care at home.

FURTHER READING

Age Concern Working Party Report. *Living Wills (Consent to treatment at the end of life)*. Edward Arnold, London, 1988.

Kubler-Ross E. *On Death and Dying*. Tavistock Publications, London, 1970.

Parkes CM. *Bereavement: Studies of Grief in Adult Life*. Penguin, Middlesex, 1980.

Rachels J. *The End of Life (Euthanasia and Morality)*. Oxford University Press, Oxford, 1986.

Saunders C. A therapeutic community: St Christopher's Hospice. In: *Psychological Aspects of Terminal Care*. Columbia University Press, New York, 1972.

Update Postgraduate Centre Series. *Terminal Care*. Update Siebert Publications, Guildford, 1986.

31 BETTER PRESCRIBING

- Adverse drug reactions
- Reasons for adverse reactions
- Compliance

Elderly people are frequent users of prescribed medication. Over the years, they are the only age group that has had an increase in the amount of medication prescribed. In 1977 the average pensioner received about 11 prescription drugs a year, but by 1985 this had risen to about 15 drugs per year, almost three times the national average. This increased prescribing for older people is because they suffer with multiple diseases which need treatment, and in part is because doctors tend to respond to every symptom by prescribing a medication. The common drugs used in the old age group are more commonly prescribed the older people get, certainly up to the age of 80 years (Fig. 31.1).

It is debatable whether so many elderly patients really require treatment with diuretics, benzodiazepines, and non-steroidal anti-inflammatory pain killers.

ADVERSE DRUG REACTIONS

If drugs were free of side-effects then it might not matter too much, but all the commonly used drugs can have major adverse effects. Measuring the occurrence of adverse drug reactions is complicated, because of the wide range of different drugs used, the different durations of use, and the range of adverse effects which may be trivial to life-threatening. Consequently many studies of adverse drug reactions report data that are difficult to interpret.

All the evidence points to older people being at greater risk of adverse reactions. For example, fatal reactions occur about four times more often in patients over 70 than at younger ages. Adverse effects of hypnotics are more common in older patients, even at low doses.

REASONS FOR ADVERSE REACTIONS

Inadequate clinical assessment

The greatest danger to the patient is the knee-jerk response doctor: joint pain equals non-steroidal anti-inflammatory pain killer; ankle oedema equals diuretic. Poor assessment of the need for therapy is a major preventable cause of adverse reactions.

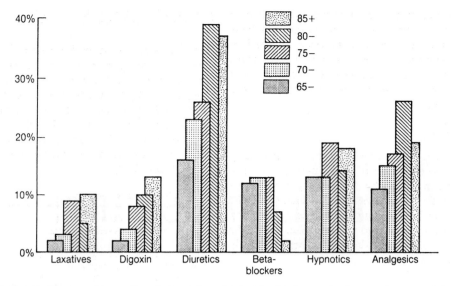

Figure 31.1 Variations in drug use with age (from A Cartright and C Smith, *Elderly People, their Medicines and their Doctors.* Routledge, London, 1988)

Excessive prescribing

Both the dose of drug and the number of drugs used are related to risk of adverse effects. A general principle with elderly patients is to start with the lowest possible dose and work up gradually. This is, of course, time-consuming but is essential for safe prescribing. A case where elderly patients differ is the use of L-dopa preparations (i.e. Sinemet, Madopar) in Parkinson's disease, where some neurologists will start patients on large doses to demonstrate an effect and then work the dose downwards. Another example is the use of antidepressant drugs, which are often given in very high doses in younger patients, but are usually effective in much lower doses in old age.

The number of drugs given should be tempered by a sense of what is reasonable. Treatment schedules, particularly in hospital, seem quite unreasonable, with many different medications prescribed. It is useful to set priorities and aim to examine the effects of treating a single problem, rather than treating every disease process simultaneously. Many patients avoid excessive prescribing by simply not taking all their medications!

Inadequate supervision of long–term medication

Beware of the repeat prescription. In many general practices it is usual to insist that repeat prescriptions are only issued without review for a fixed time, say six months. Further problems can arise when different doctors treat the patient and are not aware of each others' actions. This can happen easily when patients attend clinics and day hospitals. It is wise to have a policy that all prescribing is done by one doctor, usually the general practitioner.

Altered pharmacokinetics and pharmacodynamics (Table 31.1)

These aspects of prescribing in old age usually receive far too much emphasis, as most of the age-related changes in drug handling (with the exception of reduced renal excretion — see below) are not very important. Very limited information is available about pharmacodynamic changes (i.e. in receptor sensitivity

Table 31.1 Changes in pharmacokinetics

Drug absorption
 Unchanged

Drug distribution
 Increase in distribution volume of lipid-soluble drugs
 Decrease in distribution volume of water-soluble drugs

Hepatic metabolism
 Reduced liver mass
 Reduced phase I pathways

Renal excretion
 Decreased glomerular filtration rate and tubular secretion

to drug molecules) with age. However, elderly people appear to have a greater sensitivity to the effects of benzodiazepines, and perform tasks less well at a given dose than younger subjects. By contrast, beta-blocker drugs are less effective in old age. This may be because elderly people have fewer active receptor sites for the drug molecules to occupy.

Drug absorption

Absorption of drugs is generally unchanged in elderly people, with the exception of drugs that are metabolized to active compounds by the liver (e.g. major tranquillizers, tricyclic antidepressants). In such cases, the absorption of the drug is greater than expected, leading to a greater bioavailability and greater effect. Hence the usual advice to give small doses of drugs to elderly patients should avoid problems.

Drug distribution

The volume of distribution of a drug depends on whether it is a water- or lipid (fat)-soluble. With age, the ratio of fat to lean muscle increases, leading to fat-soluble drugs having more space to spread around, thus exerting their effects for a longer time. For example, benzodiazepines have a prolonged elimination time, leading to prolonged effects, because they are fat-soluble and more widely distributed. Water-soluble drugs tend to have a smaller volume of distribution, leading to rapid peak effects following a dose. Examples include alcohol, digoxin and cimetidine. None of these effects has great clinical significance beyond the golden rule of low doses for old people.

Hepatic metabolism

Liver metabolism involves the oxidation, reduction and hydrolysis (phase I pathways) and glucuronidation, acetylation, and sulphation (phase II pathways) of drugs. The phase I pathways tend to be reduced in old age, leading to reduced elimination of some drugs, such as benzodiazepines.

Renal excretion

Reduction in renal excretion is an important aspect of pharmacokinetics. Many drugs are excreted in urine, and reduced glomerular filtration and tubular secretion can lead to serious accumulation. The best examples are aminoglycoside antibiotics, lithium, chlorpropamide and digoxin, all of which can build up to dangerous levels.

COMPLIANCE

It is traditional to blame the patient for poor compliance — not doing what the doctor says. However, several factors can lead to poor compliance. The patient must know why the medication is needed and should understand the expected effects and the instructions for use. Doctors seldom spend sufficient time explaining, and make limited use of tablet cards and drug information leaflets to aid understanding and medicine taking (Table 31.2).

Table 31.2 Rules of prescribing

Make a careful clinical assessment
Know your drugs: side-effects, doses
Use low starting doses
Simplify dose and drug regime
Review the medication regularly
Maintain good compliance — check for problems
Communicate with general practitioner, patient and family
Remember about adverse drug reactions: notify all of them
When in doubt do not prescribe

There is a wide range of pill holders that can be of some help in reminding patients when to take their medication and, as importantly, what they need to take (Fig. 31.2). In general, the simplest devices are the most useful. They consist of a plastic box for each day of the week, divided into morning, lunchtime and evening. A relative, or the patient, places the correct drugs for the week in the correct positions. However, the patient must be sensible enough to remember that they need to take medication.

Labelling of bottles and the type of container can give elderly patients problems. The increasingly popular 'blister' packs can be extremely difficult for arthritic fingers to open. It is always worth looking at medication

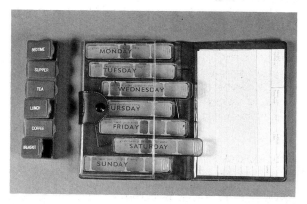

Figure 31.2 Boxes to aid compliance

with the patient so that both you and the patient can see what is being given, and go over the reasons for the prescription (Table 31.3).

Table 31.3 Aids to better compliance

Explain why the drug is needed
Give information about the drug's effects and side-effects
Make use of tablet cards and pill holders
Label bottles with clear instructions in large type
Avoid blister packs and childproof containers
Review medication at each encounter

Always remember that the prime function of doctors is to treat the patient and not their own anxieties: 'I feel that when my doctor writes me a prescription for Valium, it's to put him out of my misery'!

| Key points |

- Up to 80 per cent of women over 75 years are on at least one prescribed medication. Much treatment with diuretics, benzodiazepines and non-steroidal anti-inflammatory drugs is unnecessary.

- Adverse drug reactions increase in frequency in old age. Adverse reactions and unnecessary prescribing can be avoided by improved clinical assessment, using low drug doses, reducing the number of medications, and by regular review of patients on long-term medication.
- The most important change in pharmacodynamics is reduced renal excretion of drugs such as digoxin, aminoglycoside antibiotics, oral hypoglycaemics and lithium.
- Compliance with medication can be improved by careful explanation of reasons for treatment, expected drug effects and side-effects, use of tablet cards, pill holders, and by better labelling of bottles.
- If in doubt, don't write a prescription!

FURTHER READING

Cartwright A, Smith C. *Elderly People, their Medicines and their Doctors*. Routledge, London, 1988.

32 ELDER ABUSE AND INADEQUATE CARE

- The 'abused' and the 'abuser'
- Prevalence
- Recognition
- Social assessment
- Management and intervention
- Prevention and legislation

The 1980s saw the recognition of the phenomenon of elder abuse. Eastman defines it as 'the physical, emotional and psychological abuse of an older person by a formal or informal carer. The abuse is repeated and is the violation of a person's human and civil rights by a person or persons who have power over the life of a dependent'.

Eight major categories of abuse have been identified (Table 32.1).

Table 32.1 Major categories of abuse

Physical/assault
Emotional and verbal abuse (psychological)
Financial
Deprivation of nutrition
Involuntary isolation and confinement
Sexual abuse
Administration of inappropriate or deprivation of prescribed
  drugs
Deprivation of help in performing activities of daily living

Research in this field (mainly in the US) is now widening the scope of the debate and some people feel that the previous definitions have been limiting and stigmatizing. Professionals especially have been reluctant to report suspected cases. They feel that cases of abuse and neglect can be better described as 'inadequate care', defined as the presence of unmet needs for personal care. The needs include all basic requirements as well as those of supportive relationships, the opportunity to define an acceptable lifestyle and the freedom from all forms of violence. Thus elder abuse can be defined as the 'actions of a caretaker that create unmet needs for the elderly person'. Neglect is defined as 'the failure of an individual responsible for caretaking to respond adequately to established needs for care'. It is easier to agree on what is adequate or inadequate care than what is acceptable or unacceptable behaviour.

THE 'ABUSED' AND THE 'ABUSER'

Much attention has been placed on the characteristics of the victim (Table 32.2). These characteristics are vulnerable to the view that they are based on early inadequate research. Recent work indicates that a significant number of men are abused and that an abused person does not necessarily have to be dependent. In surveys in the USA one of the most common forms of abuse is physical violence from husband to wife (spouse abuse) that has continued into old age. Victims of sexual abuse, however, are chosen because of their communication difficulties, e.g. dementia or stroke.

Table 32.2 Victim characteristics

Elderly (over the age 75)
Female
Roleless
Functionally impaired
Lonely
Fearful
Living at home with an adult son or daughter
In addition the person is often heavy, immobile, incontinent
  with negative personality traits.

Research on abusers indicates that they tend to be sons, with psychological abuse predominating over physical abuse. The abusers were likely to be dependent on the victims for finances, led stressful lives and had health and financial problems. One-third had psychological difficulties and even more a history of mental illness and alcohol abuse. It needs to be stated, however, that there is considerable debate surrounding this issue. One school of thought advocates that anyone is a potential abuser if inflicted with sufficient stress. Others feel that abuse is much more likely from individuals with a long history of sociopathic behaviour involved in a caring role, emotionally let alone practically unable to cope.

Factors leading to the identification of abuse and inadequate care have been defined (Table 32.3).

Table 32.3 Factors in identification (after Eastman)

Physical and mental dependence on a key family member
Poor or breakdown of communication
Marked change in carer's lifestyle
Poor perception by carer towards dependence of the older
  person
Frequent visits to GPs by carers to talk about their problems
Role reversal
History of falls and minor injuries
Triggering behaviour — incident that acts as a catalyst
  inducing loss of control
Cramped or substandard living conditions
Isolation of the household

Other risk factors include people with chronic progressive disabling illnesses (e.g. dementia syndromes, severe arthritis, Parkinson's disease, stroke) that impair function and create care needs that exceed the carer's ability to meet them. Two-way abuse is being recognized in situations where a carer is subject to physical or verbal abuse from the elderly person they are caring for, which may or may not lead to retaliatory abuse.

PREVALENCE

Research work in the USA and Canada has indicated a prevalence rate of between 2.0 and 5.0 per cent. This is probably an underestimate in view of the difficulty in obtaining the information and the sensitivity of the subject. If frail and physically and mentally dependent elderly people are high-risk groups then underestimation will continue to be a problem in research surveys of victims, as these groups will have difficulties cooperating with the research process. In the UK in 1992 Ogg and Bennett carried out the first national prevalence survey on elder abuse. They found that 5 per cent of a random group of elderly people (household survey) admitted to verbal abuse, 2 per cent physical and 2 per cent financial abuse. Of adults surveyed who had close contact with an elderly person 10 per cent admitted to verbally abusing an elderly person and 1 per cent admitted physical abuse. Though small percentages these translate to hundreds of thousands of cases.

RECOGNITION

This can be extremely difficult because some ageing processes can cause changes which are hard to distinguish from aspects of physical assault (skin bruising can occur easily in the elderly due to blood vessels becoming very fragile). Fulmer and O'Malley's outline of manifestations of inadequate care is shown in Table 32.4.

Table 32.4 Manifestations of inadequate care

Abrasions	Dehydration
Lacerations	Malnutrition
Contusions	Inappropriate clothing
Burns	Poor hygiene
Freezing	Oversedation
Depression	Over/under medication
Fractures	Untreated medical problems
Sprains	Dangerous behaviour
Dislocations	Failure to meet legal obligations
Pressure sores	

Indications of physical violence can include bruises, welts and fractures. This occurring in the genital area accompanied by vaginal or rectal bleeding (with or without venereal disease) may indicate sexual abuse.

The presence, however, of one or more items from the list of manifestations of inadequate care obviously does not establish a diagnosis of abuse or neglect as the same findings can occur in ill frail elderly people as part of a chronic disease process. In spite of this the presence of these signs should alert the attending doctor to the possibility of inadequate care. The most common presentations usually involve combinations of features such as poor hygiene, poor nutrition, inadequately managed medical problems, frequent falls and confusion. Thus the GP, district nurse, health visitor and casualty officer will often be the first people to be presented with the diagnostic dilemmas. Less commonly legal, social services or the police are the agencies first involved because of financial or housing problems.

SOCIAL ASSESSMENT

This aspect may require many interviews over a period of time and can be extremely time-consuming. As much information as possible should be obtained, including financial details. Asking about a client's typical day involving all aspects of daily living as well as any recent crises (both carer and client) may be very revealing. The person's current mental status is very important, because the most difficult situations involve clients with memory loss. The most sensitive area of questioning is that of actual abusive episodes detailing verbal and physical incidents. Interviewing the carer is also an emotionally difficult situation.

Formal protocols (screening instruments) for use in suspected cases of elder abuse are being developed in the USA. They can be very lengthy to complete but are thorough and likely to provide conclusive information. Currently the only way this important information can be disseminated and an exchange of views obtained in the UK context is at a case conference — the mainstay of multidisciplinary exchange. Guidelines for health and social service staff are now becoming available. These are developed locally and often jointly written enabling the staff concerned to use a procedure to deal with cases.

MANAGEMENT AND INTERVENTION

Access to an elderly person who is receiving inadequate care can be very difficult. Access can mean both the physical as well as the more psychological barriers that people put up around themselves. Three clearly defined groups are the elderly living alone, the elderly in institutions, and the elderly living with the family/carer.

Those living alone may not cooperate through fear of losing all independence, embarrassment or simple stigma or distrust. Clients who are cognitively impaired may need evaluating by a range of professionals. The complex issues of the elderly living with family involve not only the elderly person concerned but the carer. One approach is to focus first on the needs of the carer. A non-judgemental approach implying an acknowledgement of an ongoing difficult job may then allow the needs of the elderly person to be identified. The elderly in institutions should in theory be less of a problem in that all institutions (be they continuing care wards, old people's homes, private residential or nursing homes) should have regular visits by the statutory authorities. However, numerous reports document the scale and range of institutional abuse.

PREVENTION AND LEGISLATION

In order to develop and use prevention strategies it is useful to discuss some of the current theories and hypotheses concerning abuse.

Theories

Impairment of the older person

The presence of physical and mental impairment makes the older person dependent and hence vulnerable.

Psychopathology of the abuser

Abusers often have personality defects/disorders.

Transgenerational violence

Children (often abused themselves) observe adult violent behaviour in the family and internalize it as acceptable. This can lead to spouse abuse/child abuse and later eventually to parental abuse.

Stressed carer

Carers, especially if subject to their own life crises, react to the stressful situation and dependent person with violence or inadequate care.

Exchange theory

The abuser will continue to abuse as long as he or she gains from it. When the 'exchange' becomes unfavourable (guilt, professional 'knowing', etc.) the abuse ceases.

Discussion

Prevention of inadequate care involves analysing our current patterns of health and social care delivery. Issues such as housing, pensions, payment of a family carer, and voluntary initiatives are raised. If inadequate care results from impairment of an elderly person or a stressed caregiver then hopefully health and social services can be mobilized to try to help both parties. If the carer is psychologically or psychiatrically disturbed then the prevention strategy must protect the client as well as seek trained help for the carer.

The US experience has been to endorse the legal route vigorously. Many States have passed mandatory reporting laws for elder abuse. This means that health care professionals who fail to report cases can be subject to fines or rebuke from their professional organizations. This has led to the setting up of teams of social workers (Adult Protective Services) to deal with the cases. In the UK Age Concern favour the setting up of a Charter of Rights to protect the needs of all elderly people. In 1993 the Law Commission entered the debate with its proposed reforms for the mentally frail. The Commission specifically addressed elder abuse and proposed an emergency assessment order. This would give statutory obligations to assess a client's mental state and if found incompetent to address the issue of possible abuse. The Law Commission's recommendations need urgent implementation by government.

Whatever the motivating force for change, change must occur. Elder abuse/inadequate care is another iceberg phenomenon. Elderly people have an absolute right to expect to be protected from poor care by every means at our disposal. This will need education, research, reallocation of resources and perhaps legislation. An organization called Action on Elder Abuse was launched in 1993 to specifically address these issues. Ignoring the problem will not make it go away. Facing it and using expertise developed elsewhere is a positive way forward.

Key points

- There are many types of abuse (physical, emotional, sexual, etc.) but all can be described as inadequate care, defined as the presence of unmet needs for personal care.
- The typical victim is an elderly woman, functionally impaired and living at home with an adult son, daughter or husband, but men can be abused and indeed any elderly person is a potential victim.
- US research on abusers indicates that they tend to be sons with psychological/emotional abuse predominating.
- Abusers tend to be dependent on victims for finances, lead stressful lives and have health (especially alcohol and psychological difficulties) and financial problems.
- Risk factors include chronic progressive disabling illnesses, breakdown of communication, isolated or substandard living conditions.
- Factors in identification include frequent visits to GPs by carers with their problems, marked changes in a carer's lifestyle inducing extra stress, and the poor perception by a carer toward the dependence of the older person.
- Recognition of cases is made difficult by the physiological and pathological changes that can occur with ageing (e.g. senile purpura).
- The presence of some of the usual manifestations of inadequate care (abrasions, pressure sores, malnutrition, etc.) should alert to the possibility of the condition.
- Assessment includes not only a physical examination but a full social history, including a sympathetic questioning of the carer's role. The client's mental state must be assessed and recorded.
- A diagnosis of suspected inadequate care must not be made hastily; expert help and advice (social work, psychiatrist, clinical psychologist) may be necessary.
- Aetiological theories are impairment of the older person, psychopathology of the abuser, transgenerational violence, stressed carer and exchange theory.
- The US response to the problem has included legislation (mandatory reporting laws) and a separate social service division (Adult Protective Services). In the UK the Law Commission has recommended changes to the law for the elderly mentally frail.
- Action on Elder Abuse, Astral House, 1268 London Road London SW16 4ER. Tel no: 0181 679 2648.

FURTHER READING

Bennett GCJ, Kingston P. *Elder Abuse: Concepts, Theories and Interventions.* Chapman & Hall, London, 1992.

Eastman M. *Old Age Abuse,* 2nd edn. Grosvenor Press (Age Concern), Portsmouth, 1994.

Fulmer TT, O'Malley TA. *Inadequate Care of the Elderly.* Springer, New York, 1987.

Kosberg J. Understanding elder abuse: an overview for primary care physicians. In: Ham R (ed.), *Geriatric Medicine Annual.* Medical Economics, Oradille, NJ, 1987.

Tomlinson S. *Abuse of Elderly People: an Unnecessary and Preventable Problem.* Public Information Report, British Geriatrics Society, London, 1989.

Wolf RS, Pillemar KA. *Helping Elderly Victims: The Reality of Elder Abuse.* Columbia University Press, New York, 1989.

33 ETHNIC ELDERS

- A brief history of migration
- Demography
- Health and social needs
- Ethnic myths
- Providing sensitive services
- A checklist for ethnic elders

Many countries are now home to people who were not born there, and are growing old in a second homeland. Each country has its unique pattern of migration and links with other countries. Britain is a multicultural society representing people from many different parts of the world. Many of these people have settled in Britain and consider themselves to be British. Some, particularly more recent arrivals such as Vietnamese and Bangladeshi, although living in Britain, do not identify strongly with British culture. A unifying factor is that all ethnic minorities have contributed and continue to contribute to the economic wealth of the country. The majority pay their taxes and are increasingly concerned by the white ethnocentric bias in the services that they are paying for.

A BRIEF HISTORY OF MIGRATION

The first major movements of 'visible' (i.e. black and Asian people) migrants to the UK occurred shortly after World War II. Active recruitment policies were used to bring labour from the Caribbean and from India to help with rebuilding post-war Britain. Many of these migrants held the belief that they would be returning to their home countries and the stay in Britain would be but a short sojourn, and an opportunity to accumulate some wealth. These migrants have mostly given up this dream, and once their families followed, they became residents.

These early migrants are now ageing, and many are of pensionable age. Because of recruitment practices, many of them lied about their true ages, giving ages up to 10 or 15 years younger. Consequently, many men of pensionable age are unable to claim their pensions because of their younger 'passport' age.

During the mid-1970s, two further waves of migration occurred: one from East Africa, particularly from Uganda (associated with the Idi Amin regime of terror), of East African Asians, and another wave from a newly independent country, Bangladesh (formerly East Pakistan). The two groups of migrants could not have been more different. The East African Asians were mostly from the Gujarat region of India (around

Bombay), and were a sophisticated, well-educated class of merchants and professional people. The Bangladeshi migrants had mostly left because of the religious civil war between Hindu and Moslem, and were from the rural areas of Sylhet. Most were landless farmers with little formal education and virtually no money.

Their fortunes in Britain have been shaped by these origins. The East African Asians have found a secure niche in British society, often running corner shops, or returning to professional occupations. The Bangladeshi are concentrated in inner-city slums, particularly in the East End of London, occupying the traditional migrant territory that used to belong to a former generation of Jewish people. Unemployment is high, and opportunities are to be found only within the restaurant and clothing manufacture trades.

It is important to remember that there are many ethnic minorities in Britain: for example, Irish, Eastern European, Mediteranean, and white South African. Some of the considerations that apply to visible groups may apply to an extent to those minorities that are able to 'blend into' the host culture.

DEMOGRAPHY

Black and Asian people make up less than 4 per cent of the total population of Britain, numbering some 2.5 million people. Yet as an island race, Britons display remarkable xenophobia, feeling overrun by hordes of foreigners. Because of the patterns of migration, the density of minority groups in some parts of the inner-city turns them into the ethnic majority.

The numbers of pensioners are still comparatively small. A city the size of Nottingham (around 400 000) had only 300 Asian and 300 Afro-Caribbean pensioners according to the 1981 census. However, all that is set to change quite rapidly. Most ethnic pensioner groups are going to increase by between two- and seven-fold over the next 20 years. This is demonstrated by recent data from the 1991 census (Figure 33.1).

HEALTH AND SOCIAL NEEDS

The 1991 census enquired about long-standing chronic ill-health and from this data it is possible to compare the self-reported health status of different ethnic groups in Britain. With the exception of Chinese people, all ethnic groups show an increase in ill-health with age as does the indigenous white British population. However, at every age, ethnic minorities have an excess of ill-health (Fig. 33.2). The reasons for this excess may be found in the environment in which a majority of ethnic elders live: poverty, poor housing, limited education and prospects, prejudice and hostility.

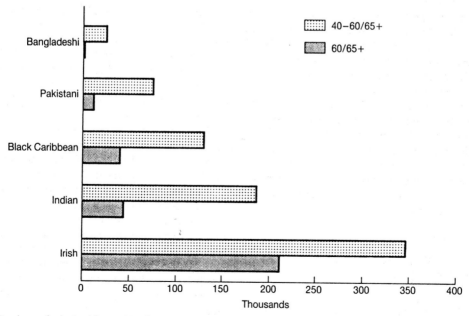

Figure 33.1 Numbers of ethnic elders, 1991 (from OPCS Census, 1991)

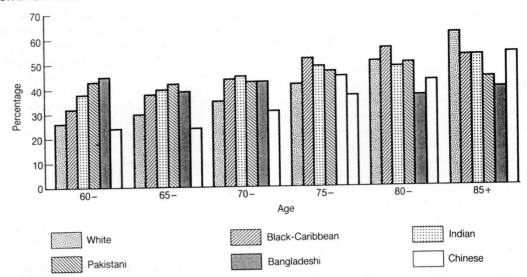

Figure 33.2 Prevalence of long-standing illness in different ethnic groups (from OPCS Census, 1991)

Traditionally Britain has adopted a policy of assimilation to cope with the needs of ethnic minorities. This means that with time the minorities will adapt to British ways and customs and no special services will be needed. This is a wonderful way of avoiding having any real policy at all!

In practice, those who work in inner-city areas are already confronted by the lack of suitable services for black and Asian elderly patients. Very few hospitals have a reliable interpreter service, and few hospitals and general practices go out of their way to recruit staff from ethnic minority groups. Consequently it is difficult for patients to get access to services, and even when they do, the standards of practice are likely to be poor because of poor communication and inappropriate or unavailable services.

The health problems of black and Asian elders are shown in Table 33.1. Although ethnic minorities do suffer with 'exotic' diseases such as sickle cell anaemia, and tropical infections, the greatest burden of disease is caused by common conditions: heart attacks, strokes, diabetes, cataracts. This suggests that the health and social needs should be similar to those of the host community.

Table 33.1 Health problems of ethnic elders

Tuberculosis
Diabetes
Ischaemic heart disease
Asthma
Stroke
Cataract

However, sick black and Asian elders face serious problems in getting the services they need. The problems have been described as a series of jeopardies: the first jeopardy is to do with being a visible ethnic minority — racial prejudice; the second is to do with being old — ageism; and the third is caused by limited access to services.

For example, for a white stroke victim, it is possible to arrrange a day centre, meals on wheels, a home help, a stroke club. For a Bangladeshi stroke victim there are no day centres, no attempt is made to provide Halal food (meat slaughtered according to Moslem requirements) and stroke clubs do not cater for Bangladeshis because none of the staff speak the language. If the Bangladeshi patient is so disabled that residential home care is needed, most boroughs have decided not to provide Moslem old people's homes. Moreover, because the Bangladeshi person is from a different culture they are frequently denied places on the grounds that the homes are culturally unsuitable. A real 'catch-22', and yet these people have paid their taxes and are British citizens.

ETHNIC MYTHS

Part of the reason why so little is provided for ethnic minority groups is because of some popular myths. Myths will always exist because they help both the ethnic minority and the host community to come to terms with each other.

The extended family

This is a most popular myth, which like all good myths has some basis in reality. The myth is 'All black and Asian elders live in extended families who provide all the care that is needed'. This is an extremely useful myth because it means no money has to be spent on ethnic minority services, it almost compliments black and Asian people for their devotion to their elders, and it is sustainable because so many black and Asian people seem to live in very large family groupings.

A study from Birmingham showed that 1 in 3 West Indian male pensioners lived alone, and that 1 in 5 Indian pensioners lived alone or in husband/wife households. The myth is partly true, but a substantial minority of ethnic elders do not live in well-supported large families.

In addition, although the family may wish to support a dependent elder they frequently do not get the sort of help from health and social services that is needed and expected by the white community. For example, it is common to find that incontinence is not managed but ignored by health care professionals. Respite admissions are not arranged, and day care is non-existent.

Learning English

It is tempting to think that communication in the same language would reduce all the problems of service provision. This too is a myth. Caribbean elders all speak excellent English, but services have not been forthcoming that help with their needs.

Health and social services are just beginning to realize that they will have to appoint staff with appropriate skills if they are to make any headway. The most appropriate skill in an inner-city area may well be the ability to speak a local minority language.

Assimilation

Linked to the learning-English myth is the assimilation myth, which says that in time everything will be all right because the ethnic minorities will become much more like the white community. Interestingly, the Jewish community have retained their cultural identity and have stopped waiting for local services to meet their needs. Jewish homes and hospitals are frequently set up to provide appropriate care.

No demand for the service

This is frequently said by service managers: 'What is the point in trying to provide Halal meals on wheels? There are not enough customers to make it worth while.' Provision of Chinese meals on wheels in Tower Hamlets, inner London, only occurred because a Chinese social services manager decided to give it a try. The demand has been huge, even though they cost more than the 'meat and two veg' meals on wheels. Unless an appropriate and sensitive service is provided, demand for it will not emerge.

PROVIDING SENSITIVE SERVICES

The key to a better deal for ethnic elders lies in three directions: ethnic monitoring, positive discrimination, and self-help and voluntary sector organizations.

Ethnic monitoring counts both the numbers of service users and providers that come from ethnic minorities. Such information should alert managers to problems with the services they run. It will also help ensure that equal opportunities legislation in employment of black and Asian people is not ignored. Positive discrimination of people from black and Asian groups to fill senior managerial positions has been highly successful in the USA in producing a better and wider mix of services in multicultural areas. Strengthening the existing self-help and voluntary sector organizations that work with ethnic elders will enable such organizations to take a major role in some aspects of social service provision.

A CHECKLIST FOR ETHNIC ELDERS

It is worth considering the following questions:

1. Are there any interpreters available in your workplace?
2. Does your workplace employ any senior staff from black and Asian backgrounds?
3. Is it possible to get Halal, Chinese and Kosher meals on wheels in your district?
4. Are signposts, outpatient information, health education material translated in appropriate languages?
5. There any ethnic elder patients/clients using your service?

This may be the first step to improving the state of affairs.

Key points

- Many towns and cities have people from a wide range of ethnic groups, all of whom contribute to social and economic productivity. Ethnic populations are ageing rapidly.
- Services, particularly social, provided for ethnic elders are generally non-existent. This is partly because of a desire, in Britain, for assimilation to occur, and because of an assumption that the extended family will cope with the majority of problems.
- The health problems experienced by ethnic elders (with the exception of tuberculosis) are similar to those of the indigenous population: heart attacks, strokes, diabetes, cataracts.
- Health services would be more sensitive to the needs of ethnic minorities if emphasis was placed on the following: employment of staff from ethnic minorities; use of interpreters and advocates; better signposting; provision of health education material in appropriate languages.

FURTHER READING

Ebrahim S, Hillier S. Ethnic minority needs. *Rev Clin Gerontol* 1991; 1: 195–199.

Norman A. *Triple Jeopardy: Growing Old in a Second Homeland.* Centre for Policy on Ageing, London, 1985.

34 AGEING IN DEVELOPING COUNTRIES

- Fertility and mortality decline
- Dependency ratios
- Health implications
- Health services
- Cross-sector collaboration

Ageing is an international issue. In 1980, just over half of all old people lived in developing countries — 198 million people. By 2000, this will have risen to 362 million people. By then about two-thirds of the world's elderly people will be living in developing countries, and 1 in 12 of the people in developing countries will be over 60 compared with 1 in 16 now (Fig. 34.1).

The World Health Organization's Health For All by 2000 target was for all countries to achieve an average life expectancy of 60 years by 2000. Africa, particularly sub-Saharan Africa, is not going to make it.

FERTILITY AND MORTALITY DECLINE

Why have these major changes come about? The major cause of the rapidly ageing population of Japan

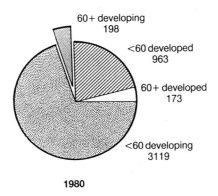

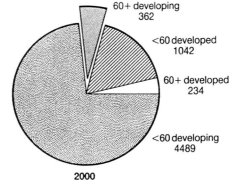

Figure 34.1 Population of the world (millions), 1980 and 2000

is not the improvement in living standards and not increased usage of medical care. The reduction in fertility has been the most potent factor, accelerated by population control programmes in many poorer countries.

The other major forces causing population ageing are the reductions in infant mortality and death rates at older ages. The joint forces of public health engineering (clean water, sanitation, housing), maternal and child health (breast feeding, immunization, and nutritional monitoring), and socio-economic development (maternal education, money for food) have all contributed to reductions in infant death rates.

The very rapid ageing, particularly in Asia, may be seen as a measure of the success of development policy that has focused much more on economic development, public health and family planning than on curative health services.

These demographic changes are very similar to those that have occurred in the UK over the last century. The difference is the speed with which they have occurred.

As illustrated by Fig 34.2, initially all countries start out with high birth rates and high death rates — this is nature's way. Death rates then decline, leading to net growth of populations as the birth rates stay high. The decline in death rates also leads to increased life expectancy. Then birth rates decline, leading to an increased proportion of elderly people. Finally a new equilibrium point is reached of low birth rates and death rates. The remarkable thing about Asia is the speed at which these changes have occurred — the European experience of a century has been compressed into about 30 years.

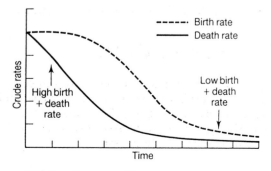

Figure 34.2 Population transition

DEPENDENCY RATIOS (Fig. 34.3)

Paying for support of old people is one of the things that keeps politicians awake at night and terrifies them. Population dependency is made up of children and older people. The child support ratio is the number of children divided by the number of adults aged 20–64, i.e. those that are potentially economically productive.

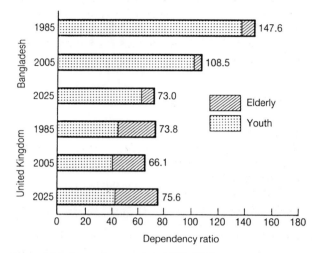

Figure 34.3 Dependency ratios, 1985–2025

Old people over 65 form the other half of the support ratio. The child and old age parts are usually added together to give a total support ratio.

It is worth stating that child support ratios are of little public or policy concern because the support is privately funded by the family. By contrast, old age support is more often from the public sector and leads to increased public spending which is never popular.

Interestingly, dependency ratios do not get out of hand that rapidly as developing country populations are relatively young. Provided that economic prosperity can be achieved, there is no reason for us to be alarmed that too few younger people will have to shoulder too heavy a burden for many older people.

HEALTH IMPLICATIONS

It is often said that the infectious diseases have been beaten and as causes of death this is true in many countries. Reductions in fertility give smaller family sizes, better child nutrition and better maternal and child health with greater host resistance to chronic infections such as TB, leprosy and malaria.

However, as causes of morbidity they are still very much around. Acute infections are common causes of ill-health and lead to considerable health services expenditure.

Chronic diseases add to the overall burden. Many developing countries have high levels of hypertension, diabetes and smoking which are sure to add to the toll of cardiovascular disease and common cancers over the next decades. Already in Bangkok teaching hospitals the problem of the old bed blocker is talked about by surgeons and physicians. It is certainly true that old people stay in hospital beds longer and tend to be there for non-essential reasons more often than younger patients.

HEALTH SERVICES

In poor countries that have only a small hospital sector the development of British-style geriatric medicine is not an option. However, many countries aspire to have geriatric medicine.

The hospital is a cul-de-sac down which it is easy to delude yourself that you are having a major impact on the burden of suffering — all you see all day is suffering and you must be doing some good. The World Health Organization has deliberately placed an emphasis on primary care as being the appropriate level of health care for most common problems.

Old people's homes are becoming common in Asian countries. This is a reflection of the changing society and reduction in opportunities for extended family support of older and dependent people. Indeed the tyranny of the extended family is now being mentioned by the middle classes in developing countries. There is some resentment of the way in which the oldest person in the household decides what is spent, what is eaten, what religious practices occur. Preserving existing social and family support is the only policy option that makes sense in a developing country. This should not be seen as a free option but will have training, respite and backup support costs.

CROSS-SECTOR COLLABORATION

Collaboration between housing, transport, education, welfare, taxation, civil engineering and health services is necessary to achieve better environments which will lead to better health. For example, public transport is often impossible for frail elderly people to use in busy cities because of the overcrowding and the athleticism required to board a bus. New housing is often designed with a nuclear, rather than extended family in mind. Treating older people as resources for teaching skills that are being lost and using them as contributors to verbal history projects emphasizes a positive role and provides an opportunity for old and young to get to know each other better.

The need for collaboration is recognized in Britain where the Government's white paper, Health of the Nation, requires multisector collaboration for development of a health policy.

Key points

- Ageing is occurring more rapidly in developing than developed countries. The bulk of the world's elderly people live in developing countries.
- The reasons for rapid population ageing are population control (family planning) and declines in death rates at all ages, but particularly amongst infants.
- The dependency ratio of the population will shift only gradually and there should be sufficient economically productive people to support an aged population.
- Infectious disease has not disappeared but is added to the increased burden of disease due to non-communicable chronic diseases affecting older people.
- Conventional hospital geriatric medicine services are unlikely to provide a suitable option in poorer countries. An emphasis on prevention and primary care will be most effective.
- Collaboration between different sectors of society is needed to ensure that environments, knowledge and attitudes towards older people are positive and do not add to the problems associated with ageing.

FURTHER READING

Jitapunkul S, Bunnag S, Ebrahim S. Health care for elderly people in developing countries: a case study of Thailand. *Age & Ageing* 1993; **22**: 377–381.

Tout K. *Ageing in Developing Countries.* Oxford University Press, Oxford, 1990.

35 LEGAL ASPECTS

- Wills
- Refusal to go into hospital
- Mental Health Act
- National Assistance Act
- The person who can no longer manage
- Litigation

Many elderly people and carers who have lived blameless lives untouched by legal affairs, find themselves confronted with legal aspects of old age that can be bewildering. Professionals should be able to provide some guidance.

WILLS

The death of a partner is often a cause for review of finances, and this can be particularly difficult if the dead partner did not leave a will. As part of a preventive approach to old age, ensuring that wills have been drawn up is a very practical task. Sometimes it may seem difficult to broach the topic of death with elderly people, but it is often surprising how easily it can be talked about.

REFUSAL TO GO INTO HOSPITAL

Many elderly people have an understandable dread of going into hospital. At best it will be difficult to cope in

unfamiliar surroundings; the treatment will be unpleasant; at worst it will end in death or herald the beginning of a terminal phase of severe disability. Confronted with a rational patient who refuses hospital admission, what should be done?

The first step is to discuss the patient's fears. Old workhouse hospitals have almost all disappeared and the patient can be reassured that the care will be up to date. The length of admission can be estimated, and plans made to look after pets, spouse and the home. The fear of being a burden, of not wanting to cause bother, is often not recognized. The desire to avoid being labelled a 'geriatric' is also strong, and fortunately many departments have changed their names to less derogatory terms such as 'Medicine of Old Age', or 'Health Care of the Elderly'.

The next step, assuming the patient continues in not wishing to go into hospital, is to reassess the purposes of admission. Frequently, the patient's needs are not the prime motive for admission. If nursing care is required, the extent to which family and friends, together with district nurses can manage needs to be considered. The level of staffing on most medical wards is now so low that it is quite feasible to provide as much one-to-one care at home. If the patient requires specific medical treatment, such as an antibiotic, it may be feasible to give it at home. Far too often, family doctors, relatives and other carers place far too high a judgement on the ability of hospitals to alter the outcome of disease in elderly people. A home visit by a consultant can often clarify the virtues and risks of hospital admission.

It is important to ensure that the patient is aware of the implications of refusal of admission. It is essential to be clear that refusal of admission is not the same as refusal of treatment, and that the patient can change his or her mind about admission. Patients with dementia are a special case when it comes to deciding whether they are competent to decide on management, particularly when this involves hospital admission or institutional care. A demented patient who is presenting major problems in the community (e.g. leaving gas unlit, wandering, not eating, aggressive behaviour) does not usually wish to be removed from home.

Social workers and solicitors often ask doctors whether a patient is competent to manage their own affairs, and to make valid decisions for themselves. Precise definition of how demented a person has to be before they are considered incompetent is not possible. The best a doctor can do is to make a personal judgement following a full history and examination of the patient, preferably on more than one occasion. The point of history and examination is to ensure that the patient is not suffering from an acute or subacute confusional state, or a depressive illness which may recover, and to assess the severity of any cognitive impairment. A history should be sought of cognitive decline and of behaviour that indicates mental incompetence (e.g. over financial matters). The examination must test orientation in time, place and person; short- and long-term memory; insight into problems surrounding the patient; reasoning ability; speech, writing and calculation. In cases where there is any doubt or controversy it may be helpful to ask a clinical psychologist, or another colleague, to carry out a full cognitive assessment and repeat it several months later to demonstrate decline.

MENTAL HEALTH ACT

Often attempts are made using the Mental Health Act 1983 to admit the person to an institution against their will. The Act was not intended to be used for patients with organic brain disease — dementia is not classed as a treatable mental illness for the purposes of the Act — so strictly should not be used for that purpose. However, in practice there are sections of the Act that can be useful in supporting a common-sense approach to management (Table 35.1). The Mental Health Act is based on a common law principle: the duty that we all have to help someone who appears to be unable to make an appropriate judgement of their own needs for care.

Table 35.1 Some sections of the Mental Health Act 1983

Section 2
Admission for assessment or assessment and treatment for up to 28 days. A relative or a social worker together with two doctors (GP plus a psychiatrist usually) must make the recommendation.

Section 3
Admission for treatment for up to 6 months. A relative and social worker must agree that treatment is necessary and the same medical recommendations as in Section 2.

Section 4
Emergency admission for up to 72 hours. A relative or social worker together with one doctor (usually GP) must make the recommendation.

Section 5(2)
Allows a patient already receiving treatment in hospital to be kept for up to 72 hours. Recommendation made by the hospital doctor.

Section 5(4)
Allows a patient already receiving treatment in hospital to be kept for up to 6 hours until a doctor can be found. Recommendation usually made by the ward nurse.

Section 136
Allows a police constable to remove a person presumed to have mental illness from a public place to a place of safety for up to 72 hours.

Section 136 is intended to be used by the police if they find someone who they suspect is mentally ill and in need of assessment. It allows the person to be taken to a suitable place, usually a hospital, for up to 72 hours. Section 4 is also used for emergency admission for 72 hours, but requires a relative or social worker and a doctor to make the recommendation. It is seldom necessary to use these sections, and since dementia is not a classed as a treatable mental illness, it is a questionable practice.

NATIONAL ASSISTANCE ACT

Section 47 of the National Assistance Act 1948 is sometimes used to admit elderly people who refuse to come into hospital. The section is specifically for a person who is unable to care for themselves, and is not receiving care at home, is suffering with a grave chronic disease (no definition given in the Act), and is living in insanitary conditions. The Act is not specific about whether the person has to be both suffering a grave chronic disease *and* living in insanitary conditions. Different parts of the country vary markedly in their use of this means of admitting elderly people. The safeguards to protect the autonomy of elderly people are weak in this section, and it may be misused to deal with 'difficult' elderly people, rather than those for whom it was intended.

More often the problem is a long-term decline in a demented person's ability to cope, together with behaviour that makes them either neglectful of themselves or unwilling to accept care and attention, that provokes the 'something must be done' phenomenon. It is not usually a good idea to respond to this type of pressure in the middle of the night, since it is likely to be frightening for the patient and the appropriate line of action is usually clearer the next morning. Talk and reassurance that although the situation has been going on for 'years' you will personally deal with it is often sufficient.

However, sometimes an alternative used by hard-pressed family doctors is the medical admission of demented patients with a label of 'toxic confusional state'. While this may solve the family doctor's problem, it is seldom good for the patient. Such patients usually require some form of sheltered accommodation, and inevitably institutional care unless they have relatives who are willing to look after them. The appropriate action is to contact the duty social worker (phone numbers are available in Accident & Emergency departments and police stations) and request an emergency Part 3 place, provided the person is not acutely sick or too behaviourally disturbed to live in Part 3. In the latter case, admission to a joint psychiatric–medical unit is the best option if available as this allows a full assessment of the patient's mental and physical status.

Institutional care is in short supply in many places, and is not the first choice of many demented people. Persuasion to accept institutional care is not easy, and until dementia becomes severe is almost always inappropriate. However, if a relative or social worker can take the patient to visit the intended home regularly, say for tea, the transition from home to institutional care can be made much more smoothly.

THE PERSON WHO CAN NO LONGER MANAGE

The prime consideration is whether a person's affairs are being managed in their interests, or in the interests of someone else. Although the legal mechanisms may seem long-winded, they provide a measure of protection both for the incapable person and for the person acting on their behalf.

Court of Protection

The Court of Protection was set up as an office of the Lord Chancellor's department to manage the finances of those who cannot do this for themselves. The majority of people under the Court's protection are elderly people living in institutions. It is usual for a relative, or sometimes a social worker, to apply to the Court for the appointment of a 'receiver'. This is a person nominated to act on behalf of the demented person, and may be a relative.

The procedure for application is time-consuming, taking several months to complete, and the expense is relatively high, often running into thousands of pounds, depending on the wealth of the person. If the person has only limited resources, the Court need not always appoint a receiver, but may permit assets to be converted into cash for the care of the person, for example to pay nursing home bills. The advantage of using this system is that it protects relatives, and others, from allegations of not acting in the interests of the demented person. Whenever there is conflict (e.g. between relatives) about the use of a person's money, it is sensible to consider application to the Court of Protection for the appointment of an unbiased receiver.

Power of Attorney

This permits an appointed person to act for another on his or her behalf. The appointee may be able to act in all financial aspects, or may be limited to particular tasks. It is possible to appoint more than one person as an attorney, which may help ensure that the person's wishes are respected. The document is very straightforward, and only has to be signed and witnessed.

However a Power of Attorney cannot be used if a person is mentally incapable of understanding its implications. It becomes invalid once a person becomes incapable and so must be replaced by a Court of Protection application.

An Enduring Power of Attorney has now been accepted as a means of permitting an attorney to continue to manage the affairs of a person who has become incompetent. This power of attorney works in the same way, but once the person does become incompetent, the attorney must register enactment of enduring powers with the Court of Protection.

Clearly, enduring powers are open to abuse. If it is thought that an attorney is not acting in the person's interests it is wise to discuss this with the attorney, and if necessary report matters to the Court of Protection. It is relatively common for Power of Attorney to be arranged by a solicitor who has not seen the person (nor assessed their competence), and for arrangements to be made for a relative to manage the person's money. Some relatives are more interested in getting their hands on the money than the care and protection of a dependent person — fortunately there are not too many of them.

Guardianship

The Mental Health Act 1983 permits local authority social service departments to provide guardianship to persons suffering from a 'mental disorder' to ensure the welfare of the person, or the protection of others. Guardianships are rarely used for elderly people, and are most widely used for people transferred from long-term hospital care back to the community. Usually the guardian is either a social worker or a relative.

In practice guardians have very little power. They cannot manage a person's affairs, they cannot impose treatment on a person, and they place a duty of ensuring adequate care on the local authority. A further difficulty is the definition of 'mental disorder'. The most common reason for seeking this sort of help for an elderly patient is dementia, but some authorities will not recognize dementia as a 'mental disorder'. Not surprisingly they are not much used. However, they are a means of ensuring that vulnerable people's needs for care are met, provided that the person is compliant with advice and support (which is usually the case).

LITIGATION

It is an avoidable fact that the number of litigation cases (doctors being sued) is increasing. The expectations of patients have never been higher and this may lead to an increase in verbal complaints of a comparatively minor nature. These are usually dealt with on the hospital ward by the staff at the time of the complaint. Apologising for mistakes and misunderstandings is not wrong; preventing them is better practice.

More serious complaints should always be treated properly and the complainant encouraged to put the details in writing. All hospitals now have sophisticated complaints procedures and personnel to deal with them quickly. Always record the complaint in the notes with a dated account of the alleged incident. In addition alert senior medical and nursing staff to the complainant's problem list.

Where appropriate, a meeting should be organized and encouraged to explore the complaint and hopefully resolve it, perhaps at a later meeting after some investigation of issues has taken place. It can be very difficult to use good communication skills and not become defensive.

Some complainants are not satisfied; they need to be told that they can pursue the complaint via the Health Service Ombudsman who may decide to take matters further and initiate further meetings. Serious complaints can go by this route, or the legal system is invoked and a solicitor for the complainant contacts the doctor concerned. In any serious complaint it is imperative to contact the relevant defence society or association for expert advice and help.

| Key points |

- Everyone should be encouraged to make a will. Have you made yours?
- When a patient refuses to go into hospital try to allay any fears, reassess the need for hospital admission, consider a home visit by a consultant, and ensure that the patient understands that a change of mind is permissible.
- The Mental Health Act 1983 does not recognize dementia as a 'treatable mental illness' and therefore the Act is not properly used for the compulsory admission of patients with organic brain disease.
- Section 47 of the National Assistance Act 1948 may be used to remove to hospital a person who is unable to care for themselves, is not receiving care at home, is suffering with a grave chronic disease, and is living in insanitary conditions. It offers very little safeguard for the person with none of the review procedures built into the Mental Health Act 1983.

- The Court of Protection will manage the finances of any elderly person who is no longer able to do this for themselves, usually setting up a 'receiver' to act for the person.
- A Power of Attorney can only be instituted if the person has a full understanding of its implications at the time it is made. An Enduring Power of Attorney can be applied for which is still valid if the person becomes mentally incompetent.
- Guardianships under the Mental Health Act 1983 can be used to ensure the welfare of the person or the protection of others but are rarely used for elderly people.
- Litigation is increasing. Any complaint deserves attention. Serious ones demand documentation in the notes and a meeting of all concerned to endeavour to resolve the matter.

FURTHER READING

Brahams D. Involuntary hospital admission under Section 47 of the National Assistance Act. *Lancet* 1987; **ii**: 406.

Briscoe M, Harris B. Compulsory detention in hospital under the Mental Health Act 1983. *Br Med J* 1987; **294**: 1141–1144.

Greengross S (ed.). *The Law and Vulnerable Elderly People*. Age Concern, London, 1986.

36 STROKE

- Diagnosis
- CT scanning
- Acute management
- Rehabilitation
- Long-term follow-up
- Prognosis

DIAGNOSIS

A stroke is defined as the sudden onset of a focal or global neurological impairment of over 24 hours' duration or, leading to death, of presumed vascular causation. Typically it causes weakness down one side, may cause speech impairment, or may lead to loss of consciousness and rapid death.

Haemorrhage or thrombosis?

Strokes are caused by two distinct mechanisms: the first is through the blocking or interruption of the blood supply to the brain (thrombosis or embolus); the second is through bursting of blood vessels (haemorrhage). It is possible to subdivide this crude classification further into lacunar stroke (due to blockage of small perforating vessels), cerebral haemorrhage secondary to a bleeding disorder, and stroke secondary to hyperviscosity (e.g. in myeloma or polycythaemia) but the mechanisms remain essentially bleeding or blockage. Over 70 per cent of all strokes

are due to thrombosis of arteries, most often the middle cerebral artery. Around 15–20 per cent are due to cerebral haemorrhages, and the remainder are due to rarer causes.

It is impossible to tell which type of stroke has occurred just by looking at the patient because the signs and symptoms are very similar. Management and prognosis of stroke occurring by different mechanisms differ.

Errors in diagnosis

When the impairment is weakness down one side of the body there is usually little problem with making the diagnosis; most patients can do it for themselves. However, even here it is possible to be wrong. Table 36.1 shows the common problems that can masquerade as stroke. Errors in diagnosis are common, with up to 15 per cent of admitting doctors wrongly diagnosing a stroke, and an even greater number of primary care doctors getting the diagnosis wrong. Such errors do matter because the treatments for many of the problems that mimic stroke are very different.

Table 36.1 Misdiagnosis of stroke: problems that can confuse

Intercurrent illness with previous stroke
Epileptic fit
Brain tumour: primary or metastases
Brain abscess
Meningitis
Neurosyphilis
Subacute bacterial endocarditis
Subdural haematoma
Hypoglycaemia
Fractured hip/humerus

Occasionally the presentation of stroke is masked. For example the patient may appear to be suffering with a toxic confusional state with no signs of weakness. Or the patient may have a speech problem (a dysphasia), without any weakness. These presentations frequently cause confusion in the admitting doctor, and may even lead to a false diagnosis of psychiatric illness. The clue is the sudden onset of the problem with previously normal mental function.

Subtle signs of brain damage can be helpful in supporting the diagnosis of stroke. One of the best tests to use is the clock drawing. The examiner draws a large circle and asks the patient to put the numbers in to make it appear like a clock face (Fig. 36.1). The patient is then asked to put the hands in to tell the present time. This is a global task testing cognition, comprehension, vision, hearing, psychomotor skill, writing, use of symbols, and spatial awareness. Inability to perform the task may be due to problems in any of the areas mentioned. Typically this test picks up patients with parietal lobe damage leading to

perceptual impairments — difficulty with spatial awareness, inattention on the hemiplegic side, and hemianopia (Fig. 36.2).

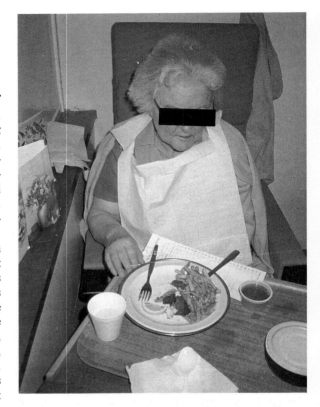

Figure 36.2 This patient shows neglect of the left side of her plate

CT SCANNING

CT scanning is now widely available in a majority of district general hospitals and is increasingly used in stroke, although in up to a third of cases nothing is found. CT scanning may be helpful if the presentation is atypical or if there is real doubt about a possible diagnosis of a tumour, haematoma or abscess in the brain. Many hospitals are now involved in multicentre randomized controlled trials of new therapies targeted at reducing damage caused by thromboembolic stroke. In these circumstances, it is mandatory to carry out a CT scan to exclude cerebral haemorrhage.

Any patient who has an unusual course to their illness merits consideration for a CT scan. The typical patient who improves over the course of several weeks does not need scanning to confirm the diagnosis. If it is

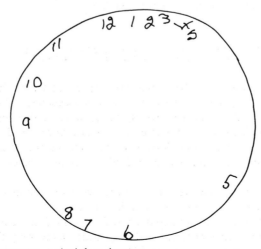

Figure 36.1 A clock face drawing

anticipated that the patient will be started on aspirin to prevent recurrent stroke, it is wise to arrange an early CT scan to exclude cerebral haemorrhage.

ACUTE MANAGEMENT

During the acute phase of a stroke a patient is at risk of complications that may hinder recovery or even cause death. The emphasis initially is to protect the airway if the gag reflex has been lost, maintain hydration, avoid pressure sores, and regularly turn and position the patient to prevent contractures and orthostatic pneumonia. Patients frequently suffer later because these basic principles are ignored.

There is no medical treatment that will reduce the extent of brain damage or have any beneficial effect on recovery, although the search for new drugs goes on.

REHABILITATION

Stroke recovery occurs over at least three months, and in some cases goes on for over a year. This spontaneous recovery is due to resolution of cerebral oedema surrounding the damaged brain, and relearning of skills. Rehabilitation should start from day one, although often this will be mainly concerned with putting joints through a passive range of movements, giving advice on handling and lifting the patient, and helping with positioning of trunk and limbs both in bed and in a suitable chair.

Swallowing difficulty after stroke may affect up to a third of patients, and it is vital that this is recognized. Often it recovers within two weeks or so, and all that is needed is careful feeding with thickened liquids. In more severe cases it may be necessary to use a nasogastric tube, or even a gastrostomy if the problem lasts a long time. Speech therapists are able to give useful advice on management and prognosis.

Speech impairment is devastating to most patients, and it is necessary to use whatever modalities of communication that remain. Gesture, noises and communication aids all have a role, and speech therapists are able to advise staff and relatives about how best to communicate and maintain a patient's morale. It is worth remembering that many patients were deaf or had poor sight before the stroke and that correction of these impairments can often aid communication.

Later on, therapy is directed towards achievement of specific goals which tend to recover in a fairly ordered way. The first step is to achieve reasonable sitting balance, and from this the patient moves on to standing and transfers, and then to walking. The usual approach in the UK is based on Bobath methods which encourage bilateral use of the body, rather than the 'natural' tendency for hemiplegic patients to walk in a crab-like unilateral way.

Obviously, some patients get stuck along the way, making only a poor recovery. When this occurs it is worth considering whether the patient has made an appropriate recovery in the light of pre-stroke ability and severity of the stroke (Table 36.2). If the patient seems to have got stuck, then it is essential to work out why. This always calls for a thorough reassessment.

Table 36.2 Markers of stroke severity

| Unconscious during first 24 hours |
| Incontinence of urine |
| Perceptual impairments |
| Loss of proprioception |
| Cognitive impairment |

The first question to reconsider is the diagnosis. Has the patient really got a stroke, or is the underlying problem a brain tumour? A CT scan may help resolve the diagnosis at this stage. Other questions to ask are: Was the patient fully independent before the stroke (e.g. any evidence of dementia pre-stroke?)? Is the patient deaf or blind? Is the patient depressed or dementing secondary to the stroke? Does the patient have unrecognised perceptual difficulties or performance problems (e.g. apraxia of dressing)? Does the patient have an intercurrent illness (e.g. heart failure, urine infection)? All of these barriers to rehabilitation are common and most are treatable.

LONG-TERM FOLLOW-UP

After the acute phase many stroke patients are not followed up and are left to their own management. They are at risk of further strokes, and the main medical priority is to prevent recurrence. The best treatment is to give aspirin (at least 300 mg on present evidence) which reduces the chances of a further stroke by about a quarter.

A major task is the prevention of complications of stroke. These are listed in Table 36.3.

Further management should be aimed at maintaining independence and if possible increasing the range of daily activities. Many families try to insulate stroke patients from everyday stress and do far too much for them. This hinders their chances of making a full recovery and encourages them in living a 'sick' role. Any fall in ability should be carefully assessed, and this is usually best done by the day hospital or rehabilitation staff. Any intercurrent illness will make the signs of a stroke much worse, and may fool the doctor into thinking a further stroke has occurred.

Table 36.3 Complications of stroke

Depression
Fractures
Subluxed, painful shoulder
Pressure sores
Contractures
Urinary incontinence/catheter problems
Constipation

PROGNOSIS

It is easy to be misled by the sight of so many hemiplegic patients living out their last years in long-stay hospital wards. The prognosis of stroke is not as bad as it might appear at first (Fig. 36.3). Death is, of course, possible, and up to half of all people suffering a stroke are dead within six months of onset. Stroke deaths are concentrated within the first few weeks of onset, with primary brain deaths occurring in the first week and subsequent deaths caused largely by complications of stroke (i.e. infections, pressure sores, dehydration, heart failure, pulmonary embolus).

A difficult problem is deciding how intensively to treat an unconscious stroke patient. Many of these patients are destined to die because of the severity of their strokes, but it is not possible to predict who with any accuracy. Doctors vary in the extent to which intravenous infusions and antibiotics are given to such patients. In general it is necessary to take the severity of the stroke, the person's previous ability and the relatives' view of what should be done into account when making such decisions.

The majority of survivors do get back home and lead reasonable lives, and a minority return to work and a virtually normal life. However, often there are problems of impotence, poor self-image, difficulty concentrating, and the persistent worry of a further stroke that make life much less enjoyable.

Key points

- Strokes are most commonly thrombotic, and the middle cerebral artery is most often affected. Discriminating thromboembolic from haemorrhage stroke is not possible clinically.
- Diagnostic errors are common, with up to 15 per cent of patients falsely diagnosed as suffering from a stroke. Among the diseases that mimic stroke are epilepsy (secondary to a previous stroke), space-occupying brain lesions, neurosyphilis, subacute bacterial endocarditis and hypoglycaemia.
- CT scanning is not essential in every patient with a stroke, but those with an atypical course may be more likely to have non-vascular pathology causing their symptoms and signs.
- No drugs will alter the natural history of an acute stroke. The trend is for patients either to die within the first few weeks of onset or to make a steady spontaneous recovery.
- Rehabilitation should start from day one and should be goal-directed. Patients who appear to get stuck require careful reassessment to detect problems (such as depression, cognitive impairment, hemianopia) that may have been overlooked.
- Long-term follow-up is needed. The aims are: to prevent further strokes by giving aspirin and controlling blood pressure; to prevent complications of stroke (depression, contractures, etc.); and to avoid the sick role and overdependency.
- Recovery is most rapid during the first three months, but can continue for over a year. About a third to half of all stroke patients die, most within the first six months. About half of all survivors make a reasonable recovery, and only 10 per cent end up in a long-stay hospital ward.

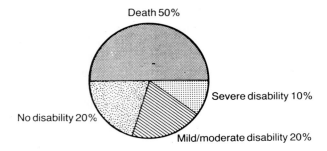

Figure 36.3 Outcome of acute stroke at six months

FURTHER READING

Dennis M, Langhorne P. So stroke units save lives: where do we go from here? *Br Med J* 1994; **309**; 1273–1277.

Ebrahim S. *Clinical Epidemiology of Stroke.* Oxford University Press, Oxford, 1990.

Wade DT, Hewer RL, Skilbeck CE, David RM. *Stroke: A Critical Approach to Diagnosis, Treatment and Management.* Chapman & Hall, London, 1985.

37 DIAGNOSES NOT TO BE MISSED

- The high ESR
- The hot joint
- Subacute bacterial endocarditis
- Head injury

THE HIGH ESR

The erythrocyte sedimentation rate (ESR) is an indirect measure of acute-phase plasma proteins. Plasma fibrinogen is probably the most important and this is known to rise in older people. There is no agreement as to 'normal' level with increasing age and indeed the ESR measurement is affected by many factors including room temperature and probably physiological changes due to the ageing process. Accepted normal ranges have increased and now span from 0 to 35 for men and 0 to 53 for women.

The ESR is used less and less as a 'screen' to aid the clinician and its value in the range 30–70 is limited because it is non-specific and not always an accurate marker of a disease process. It does have a place, however, especially in those most difficult of cases, the non-specifically unwell patient. The heartsink reply 'I feel anyhow' and the absence of major signs should lead to the use of the ESR as part of the investigation process. An ESR >100 should always ring alarm bells and lead to the active exclusion of tuberculosis, temporal arteritis/polymyalgia rheumatica, rheumatoid arthritis and myeloma.

The diagnosis of rheumatoid arthritis is usually obvious, whereas the other three groups of conditions can be notoriously difficult to diagnose, especially in the elderly frail person.

Many other conditions can also cause a high ESR, including blood dyscrasias, malignancies (e.g. occult carcinoma of the head of the pancreas), renal disease, connective tissue disorders and occult infection (e.g. pelvic abscess).

Tuberculosis

The recent resurgence of this once comparatively rare condition is well known. In younger people (though not exclusively) the weakened cellular defence mechanism secondary to HIV infection is one cause. There has also been an increase in cases in older people, however, and especially in those living in poor conditions (the homeless, overnight hostel dwellers, etc.) are particularly at risk. A lowered threshold to consider the diagnosis should also extend to people living in institutions in general, where an index case (resident or staff member) can rapidly cause a serious outbreak.

Most cases in older people are post-primary, i.e. reactivation of 'old' tuberculosis. The calcified foci of previous TB contact are extremely common on chest X-rays of older people. The debate continues about the reactivation process, the role of steroids with their immunosuppressive properties and whether or not impaired immune function with ageing increases risk.

The diagnosis of pulmonary tuberculosis can be difficult. The key is often to include it in the original differential diagnoses. Many elderly people have chronic lung disease with acute exacerbations, while others present acutely with chest complaints. In the absence of specific alerting features such as weight loss, night sweats, recent TB contact, cavitation on chest X-ray, it is best to treat the main condition diagnosed (e.g. acute or chronic bronchitis, chest infection, etc.). An ESR may be high due to an acute infection (indeed some clinicians do not measure ESRs until the acute illness is over or not responding). A lack of response to conventional therapy or a diagnosis of carcinoma of the lung but without histological confirmation should always suggest the possibility of pulmonary tuberculosis.

The chest X-ray is essential (especially with a high-risk client group). Apical shadowing and/or cavitation are almost diagnostic but other changes are often difficult to interpret, especially with pre-existing lung disease. Cases of clinical doubt should always be discussed with a radiologist and referral to a chest physician considered for further advice. Sputum staining for acid–alcohol fast bacilli (AFBs) and sputum for culture should be routine in all doubtful cases. Obtaining good sputum samples can be a difficulty in itself, so communicate their importance to the physiotherapist. Where sputum cannot be obtained, try early morning laryngeal swabs or gastric aspirate (AFBs are a gastric irritant and the patient may complain of indigestion which can be helpful). It is occasionally necessary to resort to bronchoscopy and biopsy and bronchial lavage to obtain specimens.

The Mantoux test is an intradermal injection of usually 10 tuberculin units (a purified protein derivative). A positive result is 5 mm or more of induration measured at 48 and 96 hours. Many older people are tuberculin-negative, indicating decreased recent exposure and possibly some immune paresis with age. However, older people with active tuberculosis can also have a negative reaction especially in severe cases and in people with malnutrition or immunosuppression.

Unless a patient is confused and spitting out sputum indiscriminately, pulmonary TB is not a highly infectious condition in normal circumstances. Strict isolation is therefore not required (certainly not after the commencement of treatment) unless special conditions apply (e.g. immunocompromised patients share the ward). Each department will have specialist infection control staff to give advice and implement local policy.

In cases of high clinical suspicion but without microbiological confirmation it is essential to involve a chest physician and often a microbiologist. The clinical state of a patient may require treatment to start whilst the results from sputum culture are awaited, as this can take six weeks. Treatment regimes are similar to those for younger people (with dosage adjusted for weight and any metabolic impairment) and in the very ill and frail special care should be taken with the condition of the skin to avoid pressure sores. Nutrition experts should be involved as malnutrition is almost invariably present.

Temporal (cranial) arteritis/ polymyalgia rheumatica

Temporal (also known as cranial or giant-cell) arteritis is a panarteritis affecting the temporal arteries and their branches, especially the ophthalmic. More general evidence of a multisystem disease is often present: normochromic normocytic anaemia, abnormal liver function tests, etc. The classic presentation is of a worsening headache with painful or tender temporal arteries which are non-pulsatile. In addition the scalp may be tender, there can be discomfort on combing the hair and even jaw claudication (an aching angina-like pain in the jaw with talking and eating). The most urgent symptom for treatment with steroids is visual disturbance heralding sudden total visual loss unless the vasculitis and tissue infarction are stopped. An ESR >100 completes the clinical picture though in obvious cases steroids should be given immediately and in high doses (e.g. prednisolone 60 mg per day) initially.

The diagnosis is confirmed by the histological features obtained by a temporal artery biopsy as well as the dramatic improvement in symptoms within 48 hours. Occasionally the biopsy report is not diagnostic with incomplete histological evidence. At least 2 cm of artery should be excised as the arteritis may not be uniformly distributed. The ESR may remain low in the face of a totally convincing clinical picture. In these circumstances it is best to use the clinical features to decide on treatment and err on the side of giving steroids.

Arteritis is not confined to the head, and within the spectrum of this process is the condition known as polymyalgia rheumatica. Once again the classic presentation usually presents no diagnostic problems. The patient complains of a short history (week to months) of an aching pain associated with muscle and joint stiffness, especially in the proximal muscles. There is an increasingly reduced ability to raise the hands above the head (when dressing and combing hair) and difficulties getting out of chairs, climbing stairs, etc. Rest worsens the feelings of stiffness and aching so that mornings are often described as being particularly bad, especially getting out of bed. Examination does not usually reveal any significant muscle weakness with pain restricting movement. On close questioning, however, up to a quarter of patients will have symptoms suggestive of temporal arteritis as well. A high ESR completes the diagnosis, as well as the not uncommon findings of a mild anaemia. EMG studies and muscle enzymes and biopsy are all normal. There is an equally dramatic effect to the use of steroids and in those cases without coexistent temporal arteritis a dose of 10–20 mg of prednisolone results in marked improvement within 48 hours.

Unfortunately, aching limbs, restricted movement, general malaise and a high ESR are not uncommon combinations in elderly people and the diagnosis of polymyalgia rheumatica can be difficult in these non-classic cases. To avoid the use of long-term steroids in this group of patients many rheumatologists (from whom advice or referral should be sought) recommend the use of a therapeutic 'sandwich' trial to aid diagnosis. This consists of the following regime:

Week 1	Placebo
Week 2	Steroids (15–30 mg day)
Week 3	Placebo

This is combined with both subjective and objective assessment of the patient's condition. This is usually in the form of a self-administered questionnaire and physiotherapy/occupational therapy assessment with graded exercises relating to any pain relief. Marked improvement in symptoms in week 2 combined with objective changes establishes the diagnosis.

Rheumatoid arthritis

This multisystem disease has usually been diagnosed many years previously and the complexities of the condition are known to the patient and their general practitioner. Occasionally new cases come to light: the patient who has endured 'arthritis' for many years and has not sought medical attention, the arthritis may have been misdiagnosed or is a late-onset presentation. An ESR >100 should encourage the clinician to fully reassess and examine the patient to positively exclude rheumatoid arthritis from the differential diagnosis. This may prove to be quite difficult in older people who may have associated osteoarthritis in many joints. The diagnosis may be hard to differentiate from polymyalgia rheumatica (PMR) in the early stages as some patients with rheumatoid arthritis (RA) develop synovitis late and patients with PMR can have synovitis. Seropositivity for rheumatoid factor plus erosions of affected joints will help make the diagnosis, whereas seronegativity does not exclude it (seronegative RA, non-erosive, usually affecting large joints with stiffness). Other possible seronegative arthritides include psoriatic arthritis, connective tissue disorder arthritis, crystal synovitis and arthritis associated with malignant disease. The other seronegative arthritides are very uncommon in older people.

Multiple myeloma

This diagnosis is still missed in elderly people despite highly suggestive symptoms, signs and biochemical results. Multiple myeloma is the neoplastic proliferation of immature plasma cells within the bone marrow. In this condition the affected plasma cells synthesize abnormal amounts of monoclonal immunoglobulin (e.g. IgG, IgA, IgM macroglobulinaemia, IgD, IgE), kappa or lambda light chains.

General malaise, weight loss, frequent infections and bone pain are common. Pain on pressing the sternum (be careful!) is a helpful clinical sign. There is usually a mild to moderate anaemia, often signs of thrombocytopenia (purpura, epistaxis and ecchymoses) as well as renal impairment and hypercalcaemia in patients with bone lesions. An ESR >100, a normal alkaline phosphatase and a reversed albumin/globulin ratio (i.e. albumin <globulin) indicate myeloma. Blood should be sent for plasma immunoelectrophoresis and urine for a single type of light-chain Bence-Jones protein. Discussion with a haematologist will decide over the relative merits in each case of proceeding to a bone marrow examination. The skeleton should be X-rayed for osteolytic lesions, the skull X-ray often providing the classic punched-out holes appearance. Absence of any bone lesions, Bence-Jones protein and small amounts of monoclonal gammopathy may indicate a benign monoclonal state which may later progress to the malignant form.

Further evaluation including renal function, calcium status and general health (mental and physical) needs to be performed and expert advice sought on the options for treatment.

THE HOT JOINT

The hot joint is by description at least warm if not 'hot' to the touch. It is usually painful (sometimes exquisitely so) and usually has an effusion present. The differential diagnoses include infective (septic) arthritis, crystal arthropathy (gout and pyrophosphate), trauma (haemarthrosis), osteoarthritis and rheumatoid arthritis.

The cardinal rule is to perform a diagnostic aspiration using careful aseptic technique. It is imperative to rule out an infective cause. The fluid obtained must be sent for urgent microscopy as well as culture. Any inflammation will produce turbid fluid so do not assume that this is evidence of septic arthritis. A sample also needs to be sent for crystal analysis. Blood cultures should be taken at the same time (there is often a coexistent septicaemia). Infective arthritis is common with a whole range of organisms being responsible (e.g. *Staphylococcus* (most common), *Streptococcus*, *Pneumococcus*, *E. coli* and *Salmonella*). Pre-existing damaged joints predispose to the development of infections, especially in elderly people with rheumatoid arthritis and those receiving oral steroids. All joints can be affected, though there appears to be a predilection for the knee joint. A less acute presentation and especially if there is X-ray evidence of bone destruction and cartilage preservation should suggest the possibility of tuberculous arthritis. Shoulder joints can be sites of occult infection. Aspiration of the joint generally helps relieve pain in these situations though local measures including a short period of immobilization with orthoses and hot or cold packs are recommended. Analgesics are needed and the most commonly used are the non-steroidal anti-inflammatory drugs (NSAIDs). There is now sufficient evidence to conclude that elderly people (especially frail elderly women) should receive some form of gastric protection with the NSAID. This can be in the form of an H_2 blocker or via a combination NSAID plus a gastric proton pump inhibitor.

If the patient has gout, NSAIDs plus gastric protection are useful. However, colchicine is very effective in the acute attack and as a prophylactic agent when allopurinol is introduced later. One limitation is its tendency to cause diarrhoea which is occasionally severe. Allopurinol (a uricosuric agent) cannot be used in the acute phase.

SUBACUTE BACTERIAL ENDOCARDITIS (SBE)

A few decades ago all medical students could recite the symptoms and signs of SBE practically in their sleep.

The condition was comparatively common and seen in younger people who were susceptible because of rheumatic heart disease. Nowadays students are more likely to be familiar with the acute form of bacterial endocarditis associated with intravenous drug use. The subacute form still occurs, however, and is more common in elderly people. Bacteraemia following dental (or other invasive procedures) is still the most usual cause, the severity of the bacteraemia being directly related to the level of periodontal disease. The classic presentation is shown in Table 37.1.

Table 37.1 Presentation of subacute bacterial endocarditis

Low grade fever
General malaise
Sweats and joint pains
Mild anaemia (normochromic/normocytic)
Weight loss
Clubbing
Café au lait pigmentation
Osler's nodes (tender red systemic emboli in the finger pads)
'Splinter' haemorrhages
Red cells in the urine
Retinal 'boat-shaped' haemorrhages
Splenomegaly
Purpura (chest and neck)
Valvular heart lesion (occasionally varying)
Raised ESR
Valvular vegetations
Heart failure

Many elderly people present atypically with non-specific complaints and neurological features including confusional states and focal neurological signs. A high index of suspicion must be kept. It is extremely important that blood cultures are taken before any antibiotics are given. The most common organism remains *Streptococcus viridans* though staphylococcal endocarditis occurs more frequently with prosthetic valves. Echocardiography of heart valves in elderly people often appears abnormal and the ECHO may not exclude vegetations unless they are large. Intravenous antibiotic treatment is the rule, with microbiologists providing the necessary expertise. Prophylactic antibiotics for dental treatment may be required for elderly people with heart murmurs and hence they should be told to report their murmur to their medical and dental clinicians.

HEAD INJURY

Falls and subsequent head injury are common occurrences in older people. A full history and examination usually alerts the clinician to the patients that need either admission for further monitoring or urgent CT/MRI scanning. It is obviously neither feasible nor appropriate to scan every head injury. The clinician must be alert, however, to the special features of head injury in elderly people. Table 37.2 lists those features obtained either from the history or on examination that usually require a scan to be performed urgently to exclude a subdural haematoma.

Table 37.2 Features following head injury indicating a scan to exclude subdural haematoma

---

External signs of head injury sufficiently severe to warrant a
    skull X-ray with or without skull facture demonstrated
Fluctuating conscious level
Drowsiness
Confusion
Personality or behaviour change
Headache (especially if associated with vomiting)
Demonstrable limb weakness, dysarthria, dysphasia
Complaints of visual disturbance
Incontinence of urine or faeces
Seizures

Progressive neurological focal signs usually dominate the clinical picture. Evidence of hemiplegia, deteriorating Glasgow Coma Scale and abnormal pupillary responses are late signs. The fact that a subdural haematoma can occur after even a minor head injury means that most elderly people that sustain a fall and have old or new neurological signs will need to be scanned. In a deteriorating patient the scan should be obtained immediately, alerting the neurosurgical team at the same time. There is no ignominy in a scan report indicating 'no acute changes', a cerebrovascular cause (infarction/haemorrhage) or more rarely another cause of a space-occupying lesion, e.g. primary or secondary tumour presenting following a head injury. These diagnoses help the clinician plan management and aid the communication process with relatives and carers. Clinicians who boast that they always get the diagnosis of subdural haematoma correct are probably missing more cases than they diagnose — a low threshold of suspicion is essential. In most cases a positive diagnosis will result in surgery. Results vary from poor to excellent with numerous factors influencing the outcome. These include any pre-existing disease, delay in diagnosis and post-operative complications. If a patient is deemed suitable for urgent scanning there should be few in whom an operable subdural haematoma is not acted upon.

Key points

- Single men, the homeless, hostel dwellers and those in institutions are at particular risk of pulmonary TB.
- Send sputum for AFB screening and culture in all clinically suspect cases.
- Temporal arteritis can cause blindness; treat with high dose steroids at presentation.
- A quarter of patients with polymyalgia rheumatica will also have symptoms of temporal arteritis.
- Both temporal arteritis and polymyalgia rheumatica respond rapidly and dramatically to steroids.
- Rheumatoid arthritis can mimic polymyalgia rheumatica and vice versa.
- The alkaline phosphatase is normal in multiple myeloma (the opposite to what you would expect).
- Think about multiple myeloma with a high ESR and a reversed albumin/globulin ratio.
- Always aspirate a hot joint to make a diagnosis and exclude an infective cause.
- Do not use NSAIDs in older people without gastric protection.
- Blood cultures (before antibiotics) are helpful in numerous conditions, especially SBE.
- A minor head injury can result in a subdural haematoma.

FURTHER READING

Cohen HJ. Multiple myeloma in the elderly. *Clin Geriatr Med* 1985; **1**: 827–855.

Fitzcharles M-A, Esdaile JM. Atypical presentations of polymyalgia rheumatica. *Arthr Rheum* 1990; **33**: 403–406.

Friedlander AH, Yoshikawa TT. Pathogenesis, management and prevention of infective endocarditis in the elderly dental patient. *Oral Surg, Oral Med, Oral Pathol* 1990; **69**: 177–181.

Vandenbrand P, Pelemans W. Radiological features of pulmonary tuberculosis in elderly patients. *Age & Ageing* 1989; **18**: 205–207.

PART THREE
SERVICES FOR ELDERLY PEOPLE

38 THE MULTIDISCIPLINARY TEAM

- The patient as a team member
- Aspects of teamwork
- Communication
- Key workers
- Team building
- Principles of rehabilitation
- Indicators of success
- The team in primary health care

One of the hallmarks of health care for elderly people is its reliance on teamwork as the main method of working. Working in a team implies that a common purpose is agreed, and that roles, responsibility, accountability and communication are clear.

THE PATIENT AS A TEAM MEMBER

It is essential to remember that the most important member of the team is the patient. This is so easily forgotten when professionals get together, and yet the patient is the focus of the activity. Surely patients should be able to determine their own fate and set their own goals? There can be a tendency for professionals to think they know best. Whenever there is conflict between what the patient wants and what the team decide to do, rehabilitation is highly unlikely to proceed smoothly or successfully.

ASPECTS OF TEAMWORK

Elderly people often have a multiplicity of medical and social problems. Acute illness requiring straightforward drug treatment (e.g. pneumonia) frequently leads to a realization that the patient has other problems that need attention before a safe return home can be arranged. The patient may have difficulty with activities of daily living because of long-standing physical or mental problems. The patient may live in a flat in a block without a lift, and no longer be able to climb the stairs. The patient may be lonely and in need of company.

One response to multiple needs has been for a group of people with different skills to assess the patient in their own ways, and then to share the findings and decide on a plan of action. A *doctor* may help by diagnosing previously unrecognized depression. A *social worker* may help with management by counselling patient and relatives, arranging attendance at a day centre, and home care services such as a home help and meals on wheels. An *occupational therapist* may make assessments of the patient's self-care abilities and institute a programme of practice, together with aids and appliances if necessary. A *physiotherapist* may improve the patient's mobility by improving muscle strength and balance. A *clinical psychologist* may assess the patient's cognitive ability and mood, and set a behavioural management regimen to aid the rehabilitation process. A *nurse* may discover that the patient is incontinent because of poor mobility and depression, and by counselling and bladder training, help the patient to regain self-respect and continence.

No one discipline possesses all the skills that a single elderly patient may require. Teamwork has arisen directly out of the needs of patients.

Teamwork is not always necessary

In some cases, extended teamwork, as described above, may be unnecessary for an elderly patient. A patient with a single-organ disease, and without any other problems, probably does not require the full range of assessments carried out by a multidisciplinary team. Medical and nursing assessments and management are often all that is required. However, amongst the oldest old, this is very rarely the case. By the time people reach their high 80s, most have some element of disability, and a team approach is most appropriate.

Who does what and who is in charge?

Effective teamwork is only possible if each member has has a clear idea of what their colleagues do (it is to be hoped that team members know what they are meant to do themselves!). In Chapter 47 an outline of the skills of various health professionals is given.

In many circumstances some overlap of tasks is both necessary and desirable. Increasingly physiotherapists and occupational therapists share a role of promoting overall independence in activities of daily living rather than focusing on, say, mobility and dressing respectively. Nurses also have a major role in maintaining practice regimens set up by occupational and physiotherapists. Equally therapists should be prepared to help with nursing management, for example toileting a patient if it is necessary when they are working with the patient. Doctors and nurses have to be prepared to carry out some of the information gathering that is considered 'social', because they are in the best position to speak to relatives visiting the patient.

'But that's not my job!'

A team where members start saying 'But that's not my job' is starting to fall apart, and probably lacks good leadership. The question of who should lead the team has sometimes been confused with ideas of the leader telling people what to do. This will never work. A good leader knows what team members are capable of, and respects their professional opinions, but should ensure that the team has a clear idea of its goals. The leader must ensure that there is a consensus on tasks, and that any disagreement over who does what is tackled, not avoided.

The doctor as team leader

Many doctors will assert that because of their longer training and high professional status, they should lead the team. Many claim to be trained to be the leader, although in practice this is more likely to mean that they have watched several other consultants be in charge of team meetings.

More important than professional status and number of years at university is the question of continuity and experience. Teams that are run by consultants usually work well because the consultant has a long-term investment in making the team work. Teams run by senior nurses in health care of older people work well if the same conditions apply. Teams will never work well if the team leader changes every six months.

COMMUNICATION

In any organization, good communication is essential to efficient and effective working. Teams are no different. The usual method is a regular team meeting. Often this is sufficient, but if patients are changing rapidly more frequent communication is needed. A means of exchange between night and day staff is needed, and between staff who cannot possibly come to every team meeting on every ward—for example, speech therapists, dieticians and clinical psychologists.

Team records

Increasingly, hospital teams are sharing a single, unified record. Professional boundaries and conflicts have not yet been completely submerged, so all too often the unified record is held along with medical case notes, nursing case notes, occupational therapy and physiotherapy records, and a social work file! A single record, preferably held by the patient and carer would be the ideal model to follow. Staff would communicate face to face, or by telephone as often as possible, but would also write a note to alert others to what they are thinking and doing.

Case conferences

For complicated patients there may be a need to organize a case conference meeting with people from the local community in attendance, the family and the patient. Such occasions can be very stressful for the patient and family and should not be organized without a very clear purpose. The most common reason for needing a case conference is where there is serious conflict between family and the team about the future prospects for the patient, usually their ability to manage on their own at home after discharge from hospital.

A case conference may reveal previously unknown information that alters the whole perspective of the case. Family members may feel happier when they see that the hospital and community services are working together. They may, however, feel that the professions are closing ranks and conspiring against them. Running a case conference requires a great deal of preparation; it is usually disastrous if the first meeting between consultant and family is at the case conference.

Case conferences should not be used simply to communicate information about a patient's complex needs to community staff. This is a waste of everyone's time. It is usually much wiser to ask district nurses, family doctors and community psychiatric nurses to come in to visit the patient and speak with the ward staff at a time that suits them. Provided everyone is working towards the same goal, with an agreed time scale, this is usually all that is needed in even the most complicated disability.

KEY WORKERS

The idea of a 'key worker' for every patient has grown very popular in some places. Who is a key worker? This person may be a relative or a professional, or sometimes is even the patient. Their task is to coordinate the care and treatment that the patient receives, and sometimes to act as an advocate on the patient's behalf.

In practice, the key worker turns out to be the ward sister or charge nurse far too often. This is a reflection of the multiple roles of the nurse, and the amount of

contact they have with patients. This tends to make the key worker idea less useful in a hospital setting. In the community it may be a more useful idea where a key worker might be a home help, a social worker, a district nurse, a spouse, or a family doctor, depending on the patient's problems.

Most hospitals now operate a 'named nurse' system where each patient's care is supervised by a single nurse. This requires good communication at handover times and the absence of the named nurse can be a source of some frustration to staff visiting the ward. The system does have advantages in ensuring that coherent and consistent messages are given to patients and relatives. The quality of information is generally far higher but greater effort must be taken in ensuring that good records are maintained.

TEAM BUILDING

Teams are like families if they are working well. They have their ups and downs, but somehow they struggle on. Like a family, the team members work best if they get on with each other. The team leader has an important role in ensuring that new team members are accepted, that personality conflicts are not allowed to get out of hand, and that the team develops a measure of self-respect and mastery of its tasks. This may mean substantial time is required for talking through problems. It may be helpful to examine the style of the team from time to time. Persuading other members to 'play' team leader from time to time may be useful in increasing mutual understanding. Changing the means of sharing information — for example, using standardized or computerized records — may increase enthusiasm if the team has hit a low spot.

In general, the best boost for any team is a steady stream of successfully managed patients. Team leaders should ensure that this results in a steady stream of praise.

PRINCIPLES OF REHABILITATION

Setting goals

The purpose of multidisciplinary assessment is to identify problems, and then to define a series of goals that will overcome these problems. For example, a patient with osteoarthritis of the knees may be found to have difficulty climbing stairs, be unable to get into the bath, and have unacceptable side-effects from analgesic medication. The goals may be defined to achieve independent stair-climbing up a full flight, to provide a bathboard, and to provide adequate analgesia by alternative, possibly non-drug, means.

Setting priorities

Whenever there are several interventions to be carried out for a single patient it is necessary to decide what to do first. This is where the team needs to get together and work out a plan of campaign. In the example given, it might be best to sort out the analgesia first so that the patient is not in pain, or suffering side-effects. This will permit the physiotherapist to then concentrate on improving mobility without pain limiting progress. The bathboard should wait till last because, although the occupational therapist is probably right in thinking it will be needed, it is possible that with increased mobility and better pain relief, the patient may not need one.

Monitoring progress

Having set goals it is essential to decide what rate of progress is acceptable. Team members should define in terms of days or weeks how long they think it will take to achieve a goal. If progress appears delayed, this should prompt a reassessment of the patient. Often a previously unidentified problem comes to light, most commonly mild cognitive failure, a small stroke, or depression. Having set appropriate goals, lack of monitoring and failure to reassess are the commonest reasons for rehabilitation failure.

INDICATORS OF SUCCESS

Increasingly rehabilitation teams are required to justify their existence, and some yardstick to measure success and failure is clearly desirable. It is quite difficult, however, to decide what to measure, particularly when patients are so different.

An obvious choice is the patient's ability in activities of daily living. Successful rehabilitation will lead to patients returning to full ability. However, amongst elderly people this approach is too simple. Many have chronic, progressive diseases that will not permit complete restoration of function. Successful rehabilitation may mean some degree of acceptance of disability by the patient, and provision of some alternative means of achieving the task that cannot be done independently. This may mean a wheelchair for a bilateral amputee, or a good neighbour scheme for a socially isolated housebound person.

The yardstick of success or failure is the extent to which the patient is able to return to a normal lifestyle. Rehabilitation aims to reduce the handicap caused by disease (see Chapter 1 for definitions).

THE TEAM IN PRIMARY HEALTH CARE

Primary health care deals with patients that are quite different from the hospital ward. The vast majority of a family doctor's patients are well, requiring very little attention from anyone. Furthermore the autonomy of people in their own homes is much more readily respected than in the hospital. Elderly people in their own homes really do know best what it is that they need; they are their own 'key workers'. They may define their needs in general rather than specific terms, and may focus on the family doctor as the route to specific help. A further difference is in time scale. Old people are in hospital for only a short time, and activity is intense. Old people are living in their own homes for most of the time, and the pace of activity need not necessarily be so brisk.

For these reasons, teamwork in primary health care has evolved in a different sort of way. It is possible for problems to be defined over a period of weeks. The family doctor may see an incontinent patient in surgery, and then ask the continence nurse to drop in the following week. The nurse may recommend that as the patient has severe urgency incontinence, a trial of bladder drill be started. The nurse may also ask the community occupational therapist to provide a toilet raise, and a bedside commode. A referral may also be made to the community physiotherapist who may help coexistent mobility problems. This sort of teamwork can take place over several months, and does not require regular face-to-face meetings.

When problems start to collect together, and more and more people seem to be involved, that is usually the time to refer the patient from primary care for a specialist opinion. Whenever everything seems to be going wrong, it is vital to get a complete overview. This takes time and is a skilled job, best done by a specialist with the resources of a team and the training and interest to ensure it is done properly.

Key points

- Elderly people benefit from multidisciplinary teamwork because their multiple medical and social problems require the skills of many different professionals. Never forget that the patient is the most important member of the team.
- Effective teamwork requires shared purposes and philosophy, good communication, a willingness to blur professional boundaries, and leadership.
- Rehabilitation comprises the following: multidisciplinary assessment, setting goals and priorities, treatment, and monitoring progress. Success should be measured in terms of the extent to which the patient returns to a normal lifestyle.

- Teamwork in primary health care has evolved in a different way to hospital teams. The time scale is longer, and face-to-face meetings of members of the team less often needed.

FURTHER READING

Andrews K. *Rehabilitation of the Older Adult.* Edward Arnold, London, 1987.

Ebrahim S. Rehabilitation. In: Brocklehurst JC, Tallis RC, Fillit RM (eds). *Textbook of Geriatric Medicine and Gerontology,* 4th edn. Churchill Livingstone, Edinburgh, 1992.

39 COMPREHENSIVE HEALTH CARE

- The role of the generalist
- Organization of health care of elderly people
- Age-related, integrated and needs-related services
- Links with old age psychiatry services
- Misconceptions

The health and social circumstances of elderly people commonly lead to multiple sources of help being required: neurologist, rheumatologist, psychiatrist, social worker, dietician, and therapists may all be involved in providing aspects of management. Elderly people, as they become frailer, are often required to attend several different places, at different times, which can be confusing.

Communication between different specialties, community services, the patient and carers also becomes more complicated the more people are involved. Furthermore, unless a single person is responsible for setting priorities and monitoring progress, conflicts can arise.

As a result of the multiple pathology suffered by elderly people, and the inherent divisions in hospital practice, health services for elderly people aim to provide comprehensive care. This means that each patient is assessed as an individual, a plan of action is decided, and organized by a single team of professionals. Much of the management required is within the competence of the multidisciplinary team, some is not.

THE ROLE OF THE GENERALIST

Health care for elderly people is a specialty for the generalist. With increasing super-specialization in many medical and surgical specialties, elderly people are at risk of not finding their way to the right professional; or worse, seeing a succession of super-specialists, each of whom gives an opinion on their own bit of the body, leaving the question of who puts all the information together and plans treatment unanswered.

For example, an elderly woman was admitted to a private hospital for a period of bed-rest to reduce her dependent oedema, at the recommendation of her vascular surgeon. This treatment is itself questionable! On the first night she fell on her way to the lavatory, fracturing her femur. This was repaired by an orthopaedic surgeon and the operation was pronounced a success. However, the patient was not well and her relatives were worried. She slipped into renal failure which prompted a referral to a renal physician who diagnosed dehydration and inappropriate treatment with diuretics, which were stopped. She then suffered with vomiting of altered blood, and a gastroenterologist was called in. He performed an endoscopy, and found multiple small ulcers in her stomach. He recommended treatment with drugs to reduce acid secretion. The patient remained confused, bedfast, and was developing pressure sores.

Each specialist had given a thorough assessment of their own organ system, but none had looked at the whole patient. At this stage a geriatrician was called in. The patient had subtle signs of a right hemiparesis, had nominal dysphasia, and was disorientated — she had suffered a stroke. She was transferred to a rehabilitation ward and subsequently made a fair recovery.

Elderly patients need doctors who have had a general and wide training, and enjoy the role of the generalist. Hovever, the main danger of generalists is that they tend to think they can do everything! Knowledge of limitations and the need to refer to specialist colleagues is vital. In Britain very few people in their 70s are referred for renal dialysis, yet renal physicians feel that such patients should not be denied access to life-saving treatment on the basis of age alone. In countries where geriatric medicine has not developed as a major specialty, rates of 'high-technology' medical and surgical treatment (e.g. surgery for stroke, use of heart pacemakers and replacement valves, renal dialysis) are much higher than in Britain. Generalists must ensure that access to appropriate (often high-technology) care is not denied to elderly people.

ORGANIZATION OF HEALTH CARE OF ELDERLY PEOPLE

Primary health care

Comprehensive health care starts with the primary health care team, which for most elderly people means their family doctor. Many elderly people have the good fortune to be looked after by a doctor who has known them for many years, and has a understanding of how the individual has responded to illness in the past. The family doctor also knows much of the background relationships in the family, about the health of a spouse, and about the local services and environment.

Family doctors are not the only primary health care resource. It is possible to arrange community nursing support in the patient's home. Nursing equipment, including anti-pressure sore mattresses, can be provided at short notice. Community physiotherapists can be asked to assess and treat the patient at home. Social services can be asked to arrange home care services, and a community occupational therapist can provide aids, appliances and home modifications. However, all of this takes time to organize and some family doctors do not do it well.

The most important element in primary health care is appropriate training in health care of elderly people for family doctors and community nurses. Most family doctors now accept that special training in child health is essential for competent treatment of babies and children. Training in obstetrics is legally required before family doctors are allowed to manage pregnancy. Increasingly trainees in primary health care, community nurses, and health visitors are gaining experience in health care in old age.

Primary care and hospital

Another essential for comprehensive health care is a good working relationship with local hospital services for elderly people. The interface between community and hospital is always a source of potential communication and responsibility problems. Easy access to the hospital departments is essential — this means high-quality secretarial staff who understand the constraints on family doctors, liberal use of phone answering machines, and accessible consultant staff and general practitioners with 'bleeps' when they are on duty. Equally, modern primary health care has to invest in good communication systems. Economizing by manning telephones for only three or four hours a day, and heavy use of deputizing services is not compatible with good communications.

Increasingly, geriatricians are experimenting with styles of practice that take them into closer contact with primary health care teams. Using a borrowed model from psychiatric practice, some geriatricians are carrying out clinics in health centres. Many geriatricians have links with local authority old people's homes, giving an informal service to the home and advice to family doctors about residents. Other possibilities are for geriatricians to conduct 'problem case' discussion groups with primary health care teams regularly, or to appoint liaison nursing staff to hospital teams who visit patients known to the hospital service, as well as visiting the patients' family doctors and nurses.

AGE-RELATED, INTEGRATED AND NEEDS-RELATED SERVICES

The relationship between geriatric medicine and general (internal) medicine has to be clear within the hospital. When elderly patients are admitted it is necessary to decide which service should look after them. In the past, geriatric medical services operated in isolation, taking those patients referred to them as the supply of beds determined. Often geriatricians did not have access to district general hospital beds, which limited the types of patient they could admit safely. Old style services frequently had long waiting lists, and this led to a feeling among both primary health care and the rest of the hospital that geriatric medicine was not working efficiently.

To combat this style of practice several different models of care have arisen. One of the earliest attempts to rationalize the services was the use of an age cut-off, usually set at 75 years. Everyone over 75 is referred to the geriatric medical service and those under 75 are referred to the general medical service. For many services, this was the best means of obtaining beds on a district hospital site and increasing the amount of acute work done. Obviously, some patients under 75 had multiple pathology and needed the teamwork approach adopted by geriatric medicine. By contrast, some people over 75 were 'biologically' young with single problems that might be equally well, or better, managed by general medicine. Age-related services always run the risk that they will offer a second-rate service to elderly people, managing them in worse wards, with fewer medical and nursing staff. Furthermore, age criteria are unpopular with the general public and suggest a form of ageism. In addition, hospitals using this model are committed to having a double complement of staff on call — geriatric and general medical.

An alternative model is that of integration. Here geriatricians are part of the general medical service. In the same way that most general physicians have a subspecialty interest, the geriatrician is considered to be a general physician with an interest in elderly people. This model ensures that geriatricians have full access to high-technology medicine, and more importantly use similar wards and junior medical and nursing staff as other physicians. A two-tier service cannot occur.

Another model is based on the 'needs-related' approach. Geriatricians take those patients who most need their style of practice, and those elderly patients who have single problems are managed by general medicine. This type of arrangement can end up providing a service to only the most difficult patients, which puts extra pressure on nursing and therapy staff. The image of the service may become that of a 'takeaway service', with the geriatrician simply viewed as a convenient disposal route for difficult patients.

However, this approach ensures that the scarce skills of the geriatrician are not diluted by the time spent managing the relatively more straightforward clinical problems of acute internal medicine.

In practice, the type of relationship with general medicine will be dictated by local circumstances and the interests and training of geriatricians. In smaller district general hospitals it makes good sense to adopt an integrated pattern of care, sharing resources between the small number of physicians and geriatricians. In large hospitals an age-related model may be more feasible, provided adequate medical and nursing staff can be allocated to the geriatric service, and physicians are willing to forego much of the general medical acute work.

The needs-related service is often in place where relationships between geriatric and general medicine have been poor in the past. To ensure that those acutely ill elderly patients who need to be managed by a geriatrician are dealt with appropriately, some form of limited integration can be organized. This usually involves the pairing of general medicine teams with a geriatrician. The geriatrician then provides the care for some or all of the elderly patients admitted acutely, using the general medical wards and staff. There is no research to indicate which service provides the best outcome measures for patients.

LINKS WITH OLD AGE PSYCHIATRY SERVICES

Old age psychiatry has blossomed as a separate subspecialty in psychiatry over the last two decades. This can be seen as a deliberate response, similar to geriatric medicine, to provide services for a growing patient group with specific problems requiring a different style of management.

An ideal model of collaboration is for combined departments of geriatrics and old age psychiatry — departments of comprehensive health care of elderly people. Primary health care, hospital colleagues, and other agencies are never in any doubt about where to refer. A single department acts as the entry point into the service. Thereafter care may be supervised by whichever specialist is most appropriate, or if necessary, by both.

However, this model is the exception rather than the rule. Old age psychiatrists have a foot in both the psychiatry and geriatric medical camps, but most of them have preferred to stay within psychiatry. This is unfortunate because much of the psychiatric 'action' among elderly people is in the district general hospital. The presentation of illness in old people often has a psychiatric flavour, leading to some doubt about where the patient should be referred. With dementia syndromes, help is often sought from a geriatrician or physician because of a concurrent physical illness, yet the management of the dementia syndrome is often of higher priority and importance than the physical illness, and requires the skills and resources of old age psychiatry.

Collaboration need not involve fully integrated services. It may be simply informal and episodic as the need arises, or may be done by holding joint ward rounds regularly. It is essential that there is a relationship of some sort between geriatric medicine and old age psychiatry to avoid the buck passing that can occur with patients suffering a mixture of physical and psychiatric problems.

Old age psychiatry is a very young specialty which is developing rapidly. Already the emphasis in training is for old age psychiatrists to have some senior level geriatric medical experience. Equally, all geriatricians should have some training in psychiatry. These developments should bring the two specialties closer together, and with increased resource limitations should encourage sharing of facilities like day hospitals, outpatient clinics, secretarial and other staff. Greater collaboration can only benefit patients.

MISCONCEPTIONS

There is still much confusion in the minds of both professional staff and the general public about the role of health care of elderly people. The most popular misconception is that the service exists only for the provision of long-stay beds for the very frail. In the past, geriatricians did indeed have control of very large numbers of long-stay beds, often in hospitals several miles from the main district hospital. Many of these hospitals have now shut, and the pool of long-stay beds is shrinking year by year. Modern health care for elderly people aims to provide a wide range of services (Table 39.1)

Table 39.1 Services provided by a Department of Health Care of Elderly People

Hospital inpatients
  Acute treatment
  Rehabilitation
  Shared management with Old Age Psychiatry
  Shared management with Orthopaedics
  Shared management with General Medicine
  Long-stay hospital patients

Hospital outpatients
  General clinics
  Shared clinics: diabetes, Parkinson's disease
  Memory clinic
  Continence clinic

Day hospital
  Medical/rehabilitation
  Psychiatric

Liaison with community services
  Home visits
  Liaison nursing
  Part 3 home visits
  Clinics in general practice

Training
  Trainees in general practice
  Nursing/medical
  Care staff in Part 3 homes
  Social work trainees

The range of tasks is daunting and not all are done with equal competence or enthusiasm. Preventive health care is seldom part of the service on offer, and increasingly it is recognized that prevention in old age is of value. The relationships with the private sector are not well developed in most parts of the UK. This large sector of care for very frail people is largely ignored by most departments of health care of elderly people. The challenge of increasing the number of very frail elderly people managed in the community has also yet to be faced by most departments. It is unrealistic to imagine that shifting the place of care of patients from hospital long-stay to the private sector or into patients' own homes will alter their need for the attentions of specialists.

Key points

- Elderly patients require a generalist to ensure that multiple pathology does not lead to multiple referrals, opinions and dilution of responsibility.
- The primary health care team provides a comprehensive approach, but many general practitioners require more training in health care of elderly people.
- Liaison between primary and hospital services is

vital, with easy communication and clear lines of referral.

- Sharing of work between general (internal) and geriatric medicine has evolved in three main ways: age-related (e.g. 75+ cut-off); integrated (i.e. no separate admission system); and needs-related (GP decides where to refer). There is no 'best' way of sharing the work; each method has advantages and disadvantages.
- Links with old age psychiatry services are crucial for patients with a mixed medical/psychiatric presentation.
- Health Care of Elderly People services are wide ranging and aim to be innovative and comprehensive to meet the challenges of an increasingly frail and dependent population.

FURTHER READING

Arie T (ed.). *Health Care of the Elderly*. Croom Helm, London, 1980.

Grimley Evans J. Aging and rationing. *Br Med J* 1991; **303**: 869–870.

Royal College of Physicians. *Ensuring Equity and Quality of Care for Elderly People. The Interface Between Geriatric Medicine and General (internal) Medicine.* Royal College of Physicians, London, 1994.

40 CARE IN THE COMMUNITY

- Background
- The NHS and Community Care Act 1990
- Care management
- Paying for care

BACKGROUND

The history of medical and social care of elderly people evolved from religious settings through the Poor Law system to workhouses and institutions. The 1950s was the period of recognition that people could become 'institutionalized' and the beginning of the move towards care of people in a community setting. The message was strongly reinforced by Peter Townsend's book *The Last Refuge,* published in 1962. He exposed the fact that many residents in institutions (local authority, private and voluntary residential homes) did not need care but were there because of homelessness, poverty and social isolation. A few years later began the first of many scandals within large institutions (Ely Hospital, Cardiff) resulting in a series of Government White Papers (Government proposals to change law) aiming to reform the care of the mentally ill and initiating the concept of closure of the huge hospitals.

The 1970s saw reform within local authorities. The Seebohm Report recommended that the separate and specialist services should come together as social service departments with generic staff able to deal with a

range of problems. At this time child care issues came to the fore, resulting in mandatory legislation to enforce provision of help to children from social services, a right few others have.

In the 1980s there was a marked shift in government emphasis concerning the funding of long-term care for elderly people. Previously only those with private means could seek accommodation outside that provided by the local authority (Part 3 homes — means tested) or NHS long-stay/continuing care bed (free). The then Department of Health and Social Security agreed to finance care in private and voluntary residential and nursing home *with no assessment of need.* Initially local limits were set and later national ones. This coincided with government-led closure of hospital long-stay/continuing care beds as well as the closure of local authority Part 3 homes. By the mid 1980s it became evident that the cost of this exercise of shifting the place of care from the statutory sector to the private sector was enormous, amounting to hundreds of millions of pounds and £2 billion by 1993.

The 1986 Audit Commission report identified one major failing in the institutional payment scheme. It encouraged institutional care at the exclusion of professional assessment and care at home with effective services. This report led the government to commission Sir Roy Griffiths to produce his report, *Community Care: Agenda for Action 1988* (the Griffiths Report). The main recommendations concerning organization and funding of community care services involved a shift of resources (then being spent by social security to pay for residential and nursing home care) to the local authority. This money should then be used to enable people to stay in their homes with effective services as long as possible, delaying or avoiding the need for residential, nursing or hospital care for many. Other changes included 'ring-fencing' this budget and changing the philosophy of local authorities away from being the sole *providers* of various services to being *purchasers* of services for their clients. To provide comprehensive care in the community local authorities would need to develop strategies with health and housing authorities, assess need, determine priority as well as encourage people to pay for the services they receive.

At the same time as Griffiths was recommending an organizational approach, Gillian Wagner produced a report concerning quality issues around residential care: *Residential Care: A Positive Choice* (the Wagner Report). Included in the report are 'five Cs', five themes that are the elements of good practice (Table 40.1).

Table 40.1 The 'five Cs': elements of good practice

Caring
Caring is personal, with residents feeling valued, safe and secure

Choice
The residents' right to exercise choice over their daily life is maintained

Continuity
Residents are given consistency of care from staff and can maintain past links

Change
Residents have the opportunity to continue to develop as individuals and staff are able to respond to changing care needs

Common values
Practice is based on a shared philosophy and values

The government's response to these two reports was *Caring for People 1989*. Only some of the Griffiths and Wagner reports recommendations were included and a new concept, that of 'targeting' people with the most care needs, was added. The report introduced six key objectives as listed in Table 40.2.

Table 40.2 Six key objectives introduced by the government report *Caring for People 1989*

1. 'To provide the development of domiciliary, day and respite services to enable people to live in their own homes wherever feasible and sensible.'
2. 'To ensure that service providers make practical support for carers a high priority.'
3. 'To make proper assessments for need and good case management the cornerstone of high quality care. Packages for care should then be designed in line with individual needs and preferences.'
4. 'To promote the development of a flourishing independent sector alongside good quality public services.'
5. 'To clarify the responsibilities of agencies and so make it easier to hold them in account for their performance.'
6. 'To secure better value for taxpayers' money by introducing a new funding structure for social care.'

THE NHS AND COMMUNITY CARE ACT 1990

Many of the changes required amendments to existing law and these proposals came at the same time as the NHS reforms. The changes were therefore phased in between 1991 and 1993. They included the transfer of responsibility for placing and funding a person in a nursing home to the local authority (the health authority must approve the placement). Other changes involved the setting up of complaints procedures, purchasing and contracting for services and making local authorities responsible for registration of private and voluntary residential homes and for the inspection of all residential homes in their area (via inspection units). Although local authorities purchase places for clients in nursing homes these are registered and inspected by representatives of the District Health Authority.

CARE MANAGEMENT

People who need community care services (be they at home already or in hospital awaiting discharge) must have an assessment of need performed and indeed the NHS and Community Care Act made this a duty for local authorities. This assessment is carried out by a social worker (employed by the local authority though may be based in a hospital team). There are different levels of assessment (from simple to complex). This process is part of care management leading to the development of a care plan containing 'a package of care'.

The budget holder or purchaser of some of the components for the care plan is the care manager. This person will be involved in all but the most simple cases. They will supervise the interagency working (health and housing) to ensure the most effective care package and will ultimately decide if the care plan is economically viable (i.e. the budgets are limited).

The assessment process requires detailed information about the client, their medical and social needs as a baseline, the involvement of carers and their 'need' perspective as well as a knowledge of what is available. To this must be added an awareness of financial entitlements, race and culture sensitivity and a view on risk, i.e. self-determination and independence versus responsibility to carers and neighbours, and the ability of the client to make informed decisions. Complex cases may require a case conference to be held to fully air the views of all groups potentially involved, including client (often advocate), carer, GP, district nurse, home care, housing, members of the hospital team. This process can be time-consuming, involving not only the assessment process (often via case conference) but also then the implementation phase for a package of care.

This can result in a considerable delay, especially if the elderly person is in hospital. Resources are finite and complicated care packages are expensive, resulting in the funding dilemma between costly packages of care to keep an individual at home and the possibly cheaper institutional alternative. Targeting on the most in need runs the risk of marginalizing and neglecting those with some need (who will eventually develop more needs if ignored).

One way to try to avoid this is the establishment of monitoring and review processes. These should highlight gaps in service, poor or ineffective service provision, inappropriate services or placement of clients, etc. The complaints and inspection procedures should also provide feedback and the whole process lends itself to an audit format concentrating an outcome measures.

Care in the community has been an ideal for many decades — a goal of helping people with care needs to live in a setting of their choice be it at home or elsewhere. Legislative changes have initiated that process.

PAYING FOR CARE

NHS long-stay/continuing care remains free whereas nursing home and residential home care is based on the ability to pay. People with private means can purchase whatever care they choose. Clients with an assessed need for residential or nursing home care have their income and savings assessed (including any capital assets, e.g. house). If a person has more than £8000 they pay the full cost; under this amount the person is means-tested and a contribution — the 'care element' — obtained. Some people will qualify on financial grounds for a residential allowance (paid as part of income support via social security) if they are placed in the independent sector and this will be included in the assessment of income, e.g. state and occupational pensions. A small sum for personal expenses remains for the client.

Clients choosing a home with fees higher than the local authority are willing to pay can only do so if they, their relatives, a charity or others pay the 'top-up'. The local authority has no responsibility to meet the 'top-up' and if the element of funding fails, the client will have to move to cheaper accommodation. Local arrangements with the local authority social service department are needed when one partner needs care leaving the other at home, payment being deferred.

Initially the government indicated that no person could be forced to accept nursing home care if they refused to pay for it. This was not sustainable and this potentially 'grey' area has only been partially resolved. Health and local authorities have agreed joint guidelines and indicators of need for NHS continuing care versus nursing home care. The government has also intervened with guidance indicating that long-term NHS care is for complex medical and nursing care patients whose needs cannot be met elsewhere. This is an area that will inevitably lead to repeated challenges.

Care in one's own home continues as pre-April 1993 with each local authority setting their own charges for services. This includes assessment of ability to pay and charges must be 'reasonable'.

Key points

- Care in the community is still an aim not a reality.
- The Audit Commission Report, the Griffiths Report and the Wagner Report helped shape the 1990 NHS and Community Care Act.
- Funding responsibility for all institutional care transferred to local authorities.
- Care management involves care managers, care plans and packages of care.
- Payment for all care needs is means-tested except NHS long-stay/continuing care.

FURTHER READING

Griffiths Report. *Community Care: Agenda for Action.* A report to the Secretary of State for Social Services. HMSO, London, 1989.

Meredith B. *The Community Care Handbook: The New System Explained.* Age Concern, London, 1993.

Wagner Report. *Residential Care: A Positive Choice.* Report of the Independent Review of Residential Care, chaired by Gillian Wagner. HMSO, London, 1988.

41 THE DAY HOSPITAL

- Medical day hospitals
- Psychiatric day hospitals
- Multidisciplinary teams

Borrowing the concept from Russia, UK psychiatrists developed day hospitals as places where treatment and management could continue while the patient lived at home. This successful idea spread to the care of elderly people at the inception of the NHS and now day hospitals form part of the spectrum of care options for most departments of health care of elderly people. The term 'day hospital' is often confused with 'day centre' (a social service resource providing meals, diversional therapy and companionship). A day hospital is an NHS unit which is usually part of a Department of Health Care of Elderly People and either a medical or psychiatric facility. A few day hospitals intentionally mix their clientele and hence the expertise of their staff. Day hospitals should be on the district general hospital site.

MEDICAL DAY HOSPITALS

Traditionally the aim is to provide an assessment unit where medical and rehabilitation treatments can be performed whilst keeping the patient living in the community (at home or Part 3 accommodation). This is achieved by providing:

1. concentration on rehabilitation but especially the maintenance of skills needed in daily living;
2. medical plus multidisciplinary team assessment, investigations and team follow-up of the 'problem list';
3. regular (short term) review of problems, monitoring of medical, therapy and social needs;
4. advice based on knowledge base of 'networks' and often involving home visits and liaison with community teams; and
5. support for the carer.

Referrals tend to reflect the rehabilitative nature of most day hospitals, and mobility problems (e.g. falls, stroke, Parkinson's disease and arthritis) form a large subsection of attenders. Problems such as urinary incontinence, weight loss, 'inability to cope', often account for another group. One-problem cases, by virtue of the multidisciplinary nature of the set-up, are in the minority yet when more time is needed than can be given in the outpatients clinic, the day hospital can be invaluable (e.g. intermittent blood transfusions, one-off procedures). Patients who have 'failed' or difficult discharges previously or those with anticipated peri-discharge problems often form another group of attenders.

PSYCHIATRIC DAY HOSPITALS

The 'provision' list is basically the same as for medical day hospitals plus the added emphasis on the psychiatric state of the patient. Some psychiatric day hospitals incorporate memory clinics in the range of assessment features offered. Memory clinics investigate people presenting with the symptom of memory impairment and thus help in the early detection of possible causes including dementia. Some clinics accept self-referrals, but most are via health care workers, especially GPs. The standard core of professional expertise within a memory clinic consists of a clinical psychologist, a physician and a psychiatrist. These people usually assess independently, collating their data to a cumulative profile (nursing input is helpful and social work involvement extremely valuable). The psychologist assesses any memory loss via testing instruments (e.g. Kendrick battery) and now computer-assisted tests. The physician excludes treatable causes of memory loss (e.g. hypothyroidism) and the psychiatrist assesses mental state (e.g. affective disorders).

Some psychiatric day hospitals further subdivide into those that deal with affective disorders (e.g. depression) and those that deal with mainly organic problems (e.g. dementia). As a generalization people attending psychiatric day hospitals tend to be mobile and the team geared to the more physically fit and ambulant person. Medical day hospital patients tend to be more frail and are often immobile. The two populations overlap, however, causing conflict when rigid definitions concerning attendance criteria have to be adhered to.

'Social' care is rarely a stated aim within day hospital attendance criteria yet most day hospitals have a small group of long-term attenders who cannot be discharged and who are too frail or difficult for a day centre. This social care role relieves carers and may keep the person temporarily out of institutions. This long-term care is not cheap and if a day hospital accumulates many such patients the multidisciplinary team can lose morale and also be unable to accept new referrals due to lack of space.

MULTIDISCIPLINARY TEAMS

Just as the multidisciplinary team is essential to effective management and discharge in a ward setting, the same is true in the day hospital. Most day hospitals have a manager or organizer who is often a nurse or occupational therapist by training. The range of 'core' expertise in most medical day hospitals includes medical (usually junior), nursing, occupational therapy, social work and physiotherapy. A standard routine (dependent on referral problem) involves a 'medical' clerking with nursing, occupational therapy and physio assessment. There are usually weekly meetings to review and agree the 'problem' list and to consider referral to other agencies usually serving a day hospital (e.g. dietician, speech therapy, chiropody, dentist, continence adviser, etc.). Attendance rates are decided and treatment plans organized with weekly meetings assessing progress until discharge can be contemplated.

Recently, however, day hospitals have come under more critical scrutiny, not only with regard to their role but also to their cost-effectiveness. In many areas their role has become rigid and they have not developed as the client/patient needs have altered. There has been a downward shift in dependency with very frail people living at home or in Part 3 accommodation (displacing the less frail type of client found there 10 years ago). Most attenders need transport which unless it is 'dedicated' (the day hospital having its own ambulance) has proved difficult. Patients often arrive late, leave early and spend many hours 'touring' their local district. Dedicated ambulances with escorts are an essential element to a successful day hospital.

The role of carers may not be fully appreciated and their needs assessed. Day hospitals should develop carer support groups and possibly run a 'rolling' series of talks aimed at carers and other non-professional groups to help them understand ageing, disability and the common diseases. Day hospitals need to 'communicate' more effectively. This can be directed towards the patient and carer via explanatory booklets and a 'diary' (a communication notebook kept by the patient in which day hospital staff note treatments performed and changes in medication and also into which patient and carer write when the need arises at home). All day hospital staff need to assess and monitor their effective contact with patients; surveys indicate communication between staff and patients to be poor and also reveal a lamentable lack of actual contact time with patients in all disciplines.

Day hospitals will not survive the economic straitjacket unless they can demonstrate that they have a cost-effective niche in the delivery of health care. This means that every day hospital has to evaluate its method of working, its acceptance criteria, cost of treatment and transport, throughput of patients, etc. Day hospitals must adapt to changing circumstances, perhaps acting as education and resource centres (the base for continence advisers, chiropody, dental and memory clinics), and rapid assessment for community care and general practice patients. Close cooperation with psychiatry and other specialties may enable a premises to be used more effectively. For example, there could be combined days for the elderly mentally ill (EMI) plus EMI with medical problems, joint clinics with neurology (Parkinson's disease and stroke) and orthopaedics. Increasingly the NHS will move away from the 9–5 day care/outpatient model. The US concept of 'polyclinics' (numerous specialties cooperating and allowing multiple assessments quickly and efficiently in one geographical area) is gaining support. The concept of day hospitals being open in the evening/weekends with varied use will develop. Liaison with social services is another area for study — there are already joint premises with day hospital, day centre and luncheon club under the same roof but often organized and run separately.

Day hospitals for the elderly are a unique and important facet in health care. Although economic factors will play their part, sufficient attention will have to be paid to the patient and client requirements and satisfaction levels compared with the alternatives. Hospital-at-home schemes are not always appropriate and need closer economic appraisal. Care in hospital is expensive and not 'user friendly', most people wanting to be at home as soon as is comfortable and safe. Day hospitals can bridge the gap between what is acceptable to the patient (staying at home or getting home sooner) yet fulfilling the professional needs of treatment and maintenance programmes. Transport, client mix, function, opening hours and staff levels and mix are all comparatively flexible parameters allowing day hospitals to adapt and flourish.

Key points

- A day hospital is an NHS resource (day centres are run by social services).
- Day hospitals provide multidisciplinary assessment.
- There is a concentration on rehabilitation and the skills needed in daily living.
- Psychiatric day hospitals may be organic (dementia), functional (depression) or both and may incorporate a memory clinic.
- Long-term attenders are a reality but every endeavour should be made to keep the numbers low.
- Dedicated ambulances are an essential element of successful working.
- Carer groups are an important aspect.

FURTHER READING

Brocklehurst JC, Tucker JS. *Progress in Geriatric Day Care*. King Edward's Hospital Fund for London, London, 1980.

Maczka K. *Occupational Therapists' Reference Book of the Bethnal Green Day Hospital*. British Association of Occupational Therapists, London, 1988.

Royal College of Physicians Report. *Day Hospitals*. Royal College of Physicians, London, 1994.

42 SEVERE CHRONIC DISABILITY

- Services for disabled people
- A typical day
- The carers: formal and informal
- Respite care or recurring admission?
- Who needs to be in a long-stay hospital or nursing home?
- Making the best of institutional care

Medicine seems to teach us that *cure* is the only outcome worth considering. Patients who are not cured are failures and highlight the doctor's impotence to solve their problems. This is simplistic, but does explain some of the attitudes surrounding patients with severe chronic diseases. In some way, they are not 'proper' patients because they do not get better; their problems are redefined as 'social' to ensure that doctors do not have to get involved. Often such patients are passed on to geriatric services because they can 'no longer be helped'.

Even in a rehabilitation unit, patients who do not do well are considered to be 'failures'. They fail to conform to the expectations of professionals and can suffer because of this. Less interest is taken in their futures, and little thought given to how they, and those around them, will cope.

SERVICES FOR DISABLED PEOPLE

Organizing services requires careful assessment. The first step is almost always a team assessment of disease processes, functional ability, continence, cognition and personality, mobility and social background. Once a complete picture of the relative strengths and weakness of the person has been put together it is essential to decide with the person and family what will be needed.

Sometimes medical treatment will continue to be needed for deteriorating chronic diseases such as heart failure, arthritis or Parkinson's disease. Usually rehabilitation will be needed, either to achieve a specific goal or to maintain a level of ability. Social work is vital, but often a very limited resource. The counselling tasks are as important as providing information on welfare benefits and home care services but are time-consuming. Access to these services is extremely limited in institutions, particularly in the private sector, and almost as poor for those people living at home.

A TYPICAL DAY

The best approach to thinking and acting for people with disability is to consider their typical day — the full 24 hours. Start with getting up in the morning, and try to relate what you would do with what the person might want to do, and can do. For each disability it is necessary to think of some way around the disability, thus creating ability. This is usually done by getting a relative or friend to stand in for the person. However, with more thought and creativity, and advances in technology, disabled people can be given more autonomy, and their dependence on other people reduced — if that is what they and those around them want (Table 42.1).

The key to producing a viable plan for disabled people is to involve them and their relatives in deciding what is wanted. For example, some people may simply want to spend the whole morning in bed, only getting out to go to the lavatory. They may wish to conserve their energy for later in the day, or may simply see little point in being up for no obvious reason — however much it accords with a professional view of how the morning should be spent. Some people may prefer to be incontinent of faeces, using an incontinence pad, rather than go through the business of two transfers, a cold lavatory, and an undignified wipe of the bottom by a close relative. The secret is to ask the person, and not impose artificial standards.

Table 42.1 The disabled person's morning

	Task	Substitutes
Waking up	Orientation: time	Alarm clock radio
	Alert others	Radio on
	Hot drink	Teasmade/thermos, may need straw
Getting out of bed	Assisted transfer to wheelchair	Done by spouse + mobile hoist
		May need nurse if spouse unwell
Going to lavatory	Assisted transfer to lavatory	Done by spouse
		Toilet raise + rails, one-handed paper dispenser, one-handed suppository applicator
Shower	All over wash	Modified shower room, with seat, soap on a rope
		Towel dressing gown + help from spouse
Breakfast	Making breakfast	Assist spouse using modified bread board, electric toaster and tea dispenser
	Eating	Able to manage independently
Daily news	Read newspaper/switch radio/ TV channels	Spouse reads items out loud/use hand-held channel changer
Arrival of friends	Open front door, open curtains, move to living room	Remote control door lock + video camera
		Environmental control electronics: curtains, power points, appliances
		Self-propelled wheelchair

Equipment and adaptations

A major difficulty in deciding what would be useful is the limited opportunity for 'road-testing' expensive pieces of equipment. The Disabled Living Foundation now has showrooms where equipment can be seen and tested, and local authority occupational therapy departments are setting up Aids and Appliances Centres. These may facilitate choice and loans of equipment until the person knows whether the item really suits.

Given the individual nature of disability and handicap it is very difficult to give a formula plan of action that will suit every patient. There are so many different aids and appliances that may help. Keeping up to date with changes is the task of occupational therapists, and their help should always be sought when considering equipment.

Lifting

These tasks are frequently too much for a frail carer. In some cases, a small hoist at home will make the difference between success and failure of home care. The range of hoists is large, and style of slings, their size and manoeuvrability also vary. Sometimes a hoist is not the answer, but advice about lifting, a transfer board or a higher chair may be all that is needed.

Mobility aids

Assessment by a physiotherapist and occupational therapist working together is the best means of ensuring the patient gets a good deal out of mobility aids.

Wheelchairs are often provided but not used as they are not a complete solution to the problem of immobility.

The first decision is about who will be providing the effort — patient or carer. If the chair is exclusively for outings with the rest of the family, a collapsible assisted wheelchair is best. If the patient is going to propel him- or herself, then the questions of who will assist with transfer into the chair, will it fit through doorways, and does the patient have sufficient reserves of stamina must be answered. Inspection of wheelchairs should be systematic: brakes, tyre inflation, foot plates working, seat padding should all be examined.

Walking frames are robust and need little maintenance, but handles do crack and the collapsing type may prove unstable for some patients. Walking sticks can transform a patient with osteoarthritis of the hip, and boost confidence. The length is important: it is best measured by inverting the stick and placing it alongside the patient's wrist with the arm straight down. The correct length should correspond to the crease of the wrist joint and can be marked on the end of the stick should it need to be cut down. 'Quad' sticks (those with four legs at the base) used to be popular for patients who had suffered strokes but tend to encourage a poor walking pattern and are not often used now.

Battery-operated wheelchairs and tricycles are expensive and often bought with little practical assessment. This is a pity since they are of only limited use and careful assessment will demonstrate who will benefit. Stair lifts too are expensive to fit and may turn out to be inappropriate for many patients.

THE CARERS: FORMAL AND INFORMAL

A major part of the care plan for people with complex severe disability is attention to the needs of the carers. Carers include all of those people, both professional and family, who help the disabled person. Professional carers gain support and confidence in the tasks they do through their training and experience. They often work in groups which provide extra psychological and practical support when work gets tough.

For informal carers — wives, husbands, children, friends and neighbours — the set-up is very different. There is little recognized training for caring, no support and no extra help when things get difficult. Many carers are elderly themselves and have their own health problems and yet they are often expected to do a job of work that few health professionals would consider feasible. Recently national and local carers' networks have been set up to increase the attention given to the problems of carers, and to increase the number of support and training schemes available.

It is vital to recognize the essential resource of informal carers. Without them the health and social services would collapse, but as a society we place so little value on their role that we do not pay them and give scant attention to their views.

In general, carers need training to carry out the tasks of assisting disabled people. The best training is one-to-one with a therapist and carried out in the home. This gives the carer the confidence to ask about practical problems: How do I get him on to the toilet here? How do I get him into this bed? The ideal situation of the hospital is so far removed from most people's homes that it only gives a limited view of what the person will be able to do at home.

RESPITE CARE OR RECURRING ADMISSION?

Carers need a break from caring, and disabled people may need breaks from their carers, particularly for periods of 'top-up' rehabilitation and nursing care. Flexible 'respite' is frequently asked for but unfortunately is often not available. Respite may be given by admission to hospital or a Part 3 old people's home (depending on physical and mental condition of the person) for a week or two, by a regular cycle of admissions (e.g. two weeks in and six weeks out), or by occasional nights spent as an inpatient, or by a night- or day-time sitter who will cover for the carer.

The nature of 'respite' care needs better definition. In some cases it is simply to give carers a respite from the burden of caring. However, it is often better to think of it as a recurring admission to a rehabilitation environment where the patient may benefit from team assessment and a short course of treatment aimed at maintenance of function. This may be a more acceptable reason for admission for many carers who may find it difficult to accept their own needs for support and respite.

WHO NEEDS TO BE IN A LONG-STAY HOSPITAL OR NURSING HOME?

The answer varies depending on where you live. In some parts of the world (e.g. UK, New Zealand) where there are financial incentives to use private and public sector care for disabled elderly people, large numbers find themselves in institutions. In general, most disabled people want to live in their own homes and lead as normal a life as possible. The aim therefore should be to promote care within the person's home.

Even amongst the most severely disabled elderly people, a fair proportion (30 per cent) can be looked after at home. The reasons why many of them are in institutions are shown in Table 42.2.

Table 42.2 Reasons for institutional care

Inadequate pre-admission assessment
Lack of a carer
Unsuitable housing
Type of disability (e.g. faecal smearing or screaming)
Poor community services
Wishes of the person
Financial incentives (state subsidies)

Among those unfortunate people with moderate to severe dementia syndromes it is worth noting that no amount of 'care in the community' can avoid the need for institutional care for a proportion. Such people often need total supervision to avoid catastrophes or neglect. At present we tolerate a large degree of neglect and deal with crises as they arise, which does not constitute good quality care.

As the level of disability of a person increases, their care needs will increase. It is likely that at some point it becomes cheaper to look after a person in an institution rather than at home. This point is usually reached when the person needs help more often than every 4–6 hours, or requires help during the night, and has no immediate informal, *free* carer. The needs of younger chronically disabled people are increasingly often met by setting up group living homes, with resident care staff. For elderly people we are a long way from offering this sort of choice.

MAKING THE BEST OF INSTITUTIONAL CARE

It is possible to make an institution more homely, and this is best done by removing as many of those aspects of hospitals and nursing homes that are designed to suit staff and 'the system'. The first question to ask about any aspect of the care given to patients is 'In whose interests is this done?' For example, bathing routines: Is the preference for a bath or shower taken into account? Does the frequency of bathing match the person's usual practice? Is privacy possible? The same questions should be asked of all aspects of the resident's day. If there is any doubt, it usually means that patterns of care are done to suit staff rather than residents. One of the best examples of what can be done with long-stay wards is provided by the Bolingbrooke Hospital in south west London, which owes much to the enthusiasm of Professor Peter Millard.

Individualism

A further approach is to try to imagine what it would be like to live in the institution yourself. What things would irritate you? What could you live with? What would you change? Perhaps the most important aspect of care is the extent to which individualism is accepted and encouraged in an institution. Respect for individuals does not just happen, it has to be worked at. Simply seeing a frail, white-haired woman as an individual can be difficult. She looks just the same as the other 20 women on the ward. The key is to focus on the person's life history, to know what they looked like in their prime, to ensure that the person's own clothes are used, that mementoes and photos are on display.

Autonomy

Autonomy is also vital. It is easy to confuse the two concepts of autonomy and dependency, assuming that dependent people are incapable of exerting autonomy (or choice) over events. Dependency is a relationship between a person, another person(s), and an environment. Obviously many people without disability are dependent to some extent on others. The dependency relationship should not lead to removal of choice. In hospitals, it has become more and more difficult to encourage autonomy amongst the ever frailer residents, most of whom have some degree of cognitive impairment. In old people's homes and in sheltered accommodation it is easier as people are in greater day-to-day control of their lives and are usually less intellectually impaired.

Routines

Fixed routines are the hallmark of institutional practice and should be avoided where they contribute nothing to residents' well-being. Waking-up times and bed times should be decided by individual preference and not routine, whereas mealtimes give shape to the day, should be pleasurable, and are an opportunity for social engagement. Some variation in the residents' day is valuable, giving the idea of something to look forward to, something to enjoy and live for.

A ward in a hospital may be 28 beds, and a home may have 50 residents. This does not mean that every activity in the institution has to be done in these large groups. Smaller groupings can be more informal and more spontaneous, and certainly allow care staff to get to know residents better.

Privacy

Privacy in an institution can be a rare commodity. Nothing is private, not even a bath or bowel action. It is worth considering how privacy can be maintained in institutions. More single rooms, fewer shared bathrooms and lavatories would all help. Greater use of personal stereos and televisions might help reduce the noise pollution in many institutions, which can be difficult for some residents to endure. Perhaps an overprotective attitude on the part of staff leads to a desire to reduce risk of falling, or of dying, without someone knowing and seeing. In practice the use of name plates and bells on residents' doors, staff who encourage residents to exert their choices and preferences, and acceptance of a degree of risk go some way to improving privacy.

Relatives and friends

Involvement of relatives and friends is essential to running a happy institution. Relatives are anxious to ensure that standards are high, but may be viewed as trouble-makers by busy, pressured staff. Relatives are a major resource in an institution, and are the residents' only link with the outside world. Their comments should be taken seriously, complaints acted upon, and their involvement in the day-to-day care of residents encouraged. It is important that relatives get to do some of the nice things and the nasty things; taking granny out for a smoke in the garden is enjoyable for everyone, but taking her to the lavatory or cutting her finger nails should not be viewed as a strictly nursing task.

Relatives should be encouraged to view the institution as a home from home, where they can make choices themselves, and have a degree of control over what happens.

Key points

- Chronically disabled people require a diary of their day, establishing what has to be done and by whom.
- People should be allowed to 'road test' expensive equipment (such as hoists, battery wheelchairs) prior to deciding whether to make an order.
- Carers require much greater consideration for all the free care provided. Their needs are for training and for respite from caring.
- Long-term institutional care is often used by people who do not require it. Reasons include financial incentives through state subsidies, inadequate pre-admission assessment, and lack of a carer.
- Avoiding the worst aspects of institutional care requires the question 'in whose interests is this done?' to be asked of all practices (e.g. mealtimes, bathing regimens, bedroom allocation).
- Autonomy should not be confused with dependency. Dependent people should be able to exert their own autonomy (choice). Needs for privacy do not disappear in institutions.
- Relatives and friends should be actively engaged in the running of the institution.

FURTHER READING

Denham M (ed.). *Care of the Long-Stay Elderly Patient*, 2nd edn. Chapman & Hall, London, 1990.

Mulley G. *Everyday Aids and Appliances*. BMJ Publications, London, 1989.

Patrick DL, Peach H. *Disablement in the Community*. Oxford Medical Publications, Oxford, 1989.

Royal College of Physicians Report. *High Quality Long-term Care for Elderly People: Guidelines and Audit Measures*. Royal College of Physicians, London, 1992.

43 PREVENTION IN OLD AGE

- Primary prevention
- 75+ health checks
- Screening
- Case finding and surveillance
- Tertiary prevention

'Prevention is better than cure' is a well-established dogma. Among elderly people, the opportunities for prevention may seem small compared with those for children and younger adults. However, survival has increased so much in the last century that the majority of people who reach retirement can expect to live another 15–20 years. This is a long time, and the prevention of diseases during this time is becoming much more relevant. Also the increased levels of disease and disability amongst the very old suggest that ways of preventing problems must be looked for and implemented. Table 43.1 summarizes the three-pronged approach discussed in this chapter.

Table 43.1 Classification of prevention

Primary
The prevention of disease occurrence (e.g. immunization)

Secondary
The early detection of disease at a presymptomatic stage (e.g. screening for cancers)

Tertiary
Prevention of complications of established disease (e.g. contractures after stroke)

PRIMARY PREVENTION

There are many diseases that are either common among elderly people or can be easily prevented. The modern health promotion movement has emphasized the things that people can do for themselves to prevent ill-health by lifestyle modification. Elderly people are as keen as younger adults to achieve greater control over their destiny, and wish to be involved in anti-smoking, exercise and dietary changes. Unfortunately, many health professionals are rather negative in their attitudes, which leads to health promotion for elderly people being seen as a low priority.

Immunization

We tend to think of infectious disease as affecting only babies and children and are used to ensuring that they get their 'jabs'. However, rare diseases like tetanus now only occur to any extent amongst elderly people, and others such as influenza and pneumoccal pneumonia only cause serious levels of mortality among the very old. Therefore there are good reasons to ensure that elderly people get their jabs as well.

Exercise

The panacea for all the ills of old age is now exercise. The evidence that exercise is of benefit to elderly people is incomplete, and would not satisfy every scientist. Doubts remain over how much exercise to recommend, what type of exercise, what risks might be involved, and the precise benefits that might be expected. Well-designed experimental trials will be needed to give answers to these questions.

However, the health professional has to decide what to do now, not when all the evidence has been collected and sifted. There are beneficial effects on well-being and physical fitness in simply setting up opportunities for elderly people to join in some sort of regular activity. Even the very frail elderly have been shown to gain useful improvements in muscle strength from a short course of exercise. But exercise needs to be continued for the benefits to be maintained. Old people decondition just as fast as young people.

Many health centres and local authorities now have active programmes to encourage the 50+ population to take regular exercise. Among younger adults the aim is to get people to exercise at least three times a week for at least 20 minutes, doing something that makes them sweaty or out of breath. For older people, this intensity of exercise may not be feasible, and lower levels, such as brisk walking, may be better.

Stress management

Elderly people suffer from remarkable stresses: bereavement, poverty, disability for example. Not surprisingly, when asked about their needs for prevention, stress management and relaxation are firm favourites. Successful group activities may involve a period of exercise followed by quiet relaxation achieved through breathing exercises, lying quietly, and listening to music. It is important to discuss the causes of stress and discover how people try to help themselves with difficulties. This can be a great source of group bonding.

General measures

To enjoy the benefits of exercise and to attend groups, many elderly people will need chiropody, help with arthritis and other sources of pain, and reliable transport. It is necessary to examine the nuts and bolts of preventive activities to ensure that it is feasible for elderly people to take an active part.

The location of activities is also important. No one likes to be surrounded by other similar people all the time. The geriatric ghettos of our day centres and senior citizens' clubs are unlikely to suit everyone. A health centre is an excellent base because it provides prevention for the whole population, not just the elderly. In other areas of health promotion, one-to-one contact with a health professional is one of the most effective means of achieving changes in behaviour and lifestyle. Opportunities for elderly people to discuss their health with primary health team staff must be developed in addition to group activities.

75+ HEALTH CHECKS

In the UK, general practitioners now have the responsibility for assessing all their over-75-year-old patients once a year. This policy has been criticized because there is doubt about whether the time and energy invested will be rewarded by better health. However, the health checks do provide a good opportunity for health promotion, although this is not required under the terms of the contract.

Specifically, the health check requires that the problems listed in Table 43.2 will be looked for annually. Identification of such problems is best viewed as tertiary prevention rather than primary prevention (see below).

Table 43.2 Problems assessed during annual health checks

Visual and hearing impairments
Immobility
Mental condition (depression and dementia)
Physical condition (incontinence)
Use of medications

SCREENING

Screening is the detection of disease at an early, pre-symptomatic stage before the patient would normally seek medical help. The best examples of screening are looking for high blood pressure, cancer of the breast and the cervix. There is good evidence to support screening for all three of these diseases, certainly up to the age of 75 years. However, policy does not accord with scientific evidence in this area, and many doctors and nurses do not think it is worth including elderly people routinely in such screening.

In practice, the benefits are likely to be at least as great, if not greater, amongst elderly than among young people. Why should this be? Taking high blood pressure as an example, many trials have now shown that treatment will reduce the risk of suffering a stroke by up to 75 per cent. Young adults have such a low risk of having a stroke that even a very large reduction in risk will lead to only a handful of strokes prevented for many thousands of patients treated. Among older people, the risk of stroke increases dramatically, so the same scale of treatment effect will lead to around 20–30 strokes prevented for every thousand patients treated.

The same arguments apply to cancer of the cervix and breast. The UK policy is not to screen routinely women over 65, provided they have an adequate previous screening history (at least three previous negative smears, the most recent in the last 3 years). This policy is not supported by evidence but is the view of an expert committee. Mammography screening has only recently been introduced in the UK with an upper age limit of 65 years. The evidence suggests that older women will probably benefit to the same extent as younger women so again the policy is not informed by the scientific evidence and reflects ageist attitudes amongst policy makers. The best advice for women over 65 years is to request a cervical smear test every 5 years and mammography every 3 years, since the policy does not preclude patients seeking a test. By making regular demands of these services elderly women will ensure that they are not ignored and may begin to influence policy makers.

CASE FINDING AND SURVEILLANCE

Case finding and surveillance are terms often used to describe the opportunistic detection of disease or problems. For example, case finding for high blood pressure is done by measuring the blood pressure of everyone turning up at the surgery. Screening, by contrast, would aim to measure all those people who do not turn up at the surgery. The costs and ethical aspects of the two approaches are quite different. Case finding, because it fits into the routine of practice is relatively cheap and raises few ethical problems. Screening, because it has to seek out everyone, is more expensive,

and because the initiative is by the profession implies that the services are sufficiently good to deal with all the problems detected. For problems such as high blood pressure and cancer screening, a case finding approach is recommended.

TERTIARY PREVENTION

This is what many health professionals understand by 'screening' in old age. In fact it is detecting disease that is certainly symptomatic but largely unrecognized or unreported. Elderly people are much more likely to have covert problems — incontinence of urine, depression and early dementia, immobility, falls, visual and hearing impairments — that are usually attributed to the ageing process by both patients and health professionals.

Unrecognised or unreported problems should be uncovered by the annual 75+ health check. It is hoped that detection and treatment of these problems will lead to improvement in the patient's physical, mental and social well-being. The evidence that sending a nurse or health visitor to look for such problems leads to improvement in health and well-being is extremely hard to find. Several trials have been conducted and resulted in equivocal results, suggesting that screening may save lives, but at the expense of greater disability in survivors, may save hospital admissions (in the days when there were more hospital beds), and may improve patients' morale (Fig. 43.1).

There is little doubt that many patients welcome the attention and do wish to have an annual checkup. It is likely that such check-ups will reveal problems that require action, and it is less clear whether, as a society, we have the resources to meet such needs. In large part this will depend on the style of action wanted (or expected) by patients and offered by health professionals. Some evidence shows that elderly people are quite satisfied by their existing support systems, have tried several treatments for problems, and do not want any further action for their problems. This may of course be because past experience of health and social services has been so bad that expectations are very low.

It is likely that the new contract will lead to increased demands for hearing aids and ophthalmology clinic attendances, for referrals for social service home support, for investigation of incontinence. At present the skills of primary health care teams are not yet at a point where much of this work could be done within

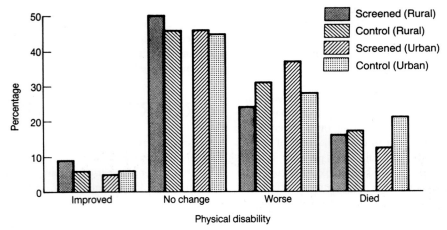

Figure 43.1 Results of a screening experiment in Wales, 1980/82 (Vetter, Jones and Victor, 1984)

the health centre. Indeed, the time and special facilities required to assess a confused, incontinent or depressed elderly patient make it unlikely that it will ever be a major part of primary health care work.

The most optimistic view of check-ups for old people is that they give an excellent opportunity to review social networks and identify pre-crisis states. Much of the health service work with elderly people occurs around a 'crisis' that has been going on for many months, and usually years, without any sort of support for hard-pressed carers.

The most useful approach will be to focus on those problems that patients want help with and are within the competence of the local services to solve. There is no reason why annual review of prescribing should not lead to fewer iatrogenic problems, why demented patients should not be referred to local support services and discussions on long-term care started and plans made, why increased numbers of frail dependent people should not be offered various types of respite care. The precise mix of what is possible will vary from area to area, depending on resources, and deficiencies will, of course, become much more apparent. Whether this will lead to increases in resources for elderly people is much more debatable, and will depend much more on younger elderly people exerting their political clout.

Key points

- Elderly people are much more interested in modifying their lifestyles to achieve better health than health professionals think.
- Primary prevention has much to offer old people: immunization (tetanus, influenza, pneumococcus); exercise; stress management.
- Case finding for common problems (i.e. high blood pressure, breast and cervix cancer) in younger adults should be extended to the adults aged 65–75 years. Above this age the evidence of benefit is not available, but up to 75 years the evidence suggest that the cost–benefit ratio is greater than at younger ages.
- The 75+ health checks require GPs to offer a home visit to every person over 75 years to assess vision and hearing, mobility, mental state, physical condition, continence and medications. It is hoped that this will lead to improvements in the physical, mental and social circumstances of old people. There is no evidence to support this notion.

FURTHER READING

Gray JAM. *Prevention in Old Age*. Churchill Livingstone, Edinburgh, 1985.

Vetter NJ, Jones DA, Victor CR. Effect of health visitors working with elderly patients in general practice: a randomised controlled trial. *Br Med J* 1984; **288**: 369–372.

44 SEEING PATIENTS AT HOME

- Advantages of domiciliary consultation
- Disadvantages of domiciliary consultation
- Home visit before discharge

A unique feature of the National Health Service is the practice of home visiting by hospital specialists in health care of elderly people. Within the system there are two types of home visit.

1. Domiciliary consultation: the consultant visits to give a second opinion requested by a general practitioner. A fee is paid.
2. Home assessment: the visit is suggested by the hospital specialist to assess the need for admission. No fee is paid.

In the former case the GP is expected to be present if possible and in the latter case the GP usually does not attend.

Soon after the start of the NHS when responsibility for the chronic sick was transferred to the hospital service the practice of hospital specialist visiting (often accompanied by a social worker) to assess urgency of admission was commenced. In the specialty of health care of elderly people this pre-admission assessment was often forced due to lack of resources, especially acute hospital beds. Such visiting continues to form the cornerstone of a few departments in the country. In most units such assessment visits have ceased although paid domiciliary consultations continue.

ADVANTAGES OF DOMICILIARY CONSULTATION

Second opinion at home

One advantage of the system is that the GP can request a second opinion in the patient's home. Sometimes social conditions make it difficult to specify which problems should be regarded as contributing to the need for admission. A domiciliary consultation from a consultant is often requested in these circumstances.

History-taking

There can be considerable advantages gained from seeing elderly people in their own homes. History-taking may be difficult due to deafness, poor memory, speech impairment or confusional states. At home it is usually possible to obtain a more accurate and comprehensive history from a relative or neighbour who may well not be present in the outpatient department or on admission. The true problems are often identified in this way.

Educational value

Joint visiting (when GP and hospital specialist meet at the patient's home) can often benefit both: the GP being informed of new and previously hospital-based therapies and the specialist having the totality of the patient's dilemma illuminated by the GP's unique longitudinal information. Many hospital specialists take medical students on the domiciliary consultation, adding to their insights into the complexities of health care in this group.

Alternatives to admission

After the visit advice can be given concerning the diagnosis, the likely chain of events and possible intervention using physical or drug remedies. A particular style of living may need to be adopted temporarily (e.g. one-room living with commode) and/or the use of social services may then prevent a hospital admission. Some districts have 'hospital at home' schemes or other forms of extra care provision to help keep a person in the community. Occasionally simple ideas may aid carers, such as advice on lifting, or the provision of continence aids.

Knowledge of home circumstances

This aspect of home visiting may be the most important aspect but its true value only appreciated later (following a subsequent admission when discharge plans need to be made). This insight by clinicians is unique. Note can be taken of accident hazards (difficult stairs, worn or loose carpeting, low furniture, uneven low beds or an outside lavatory). There may be signs of self-neglect or neglect of the home with inadequate heating, poor food store provision and the non-functioning of the bath and toilet. This information is of great value when planning an eventual discharge as these problems stay vividly in the mind when seen at home prior to admission. However, domiciliary visits have been known to be conducted through the letter box and the cause of immobility diagnosed through the kitchen window. Official identification is essential.

Consultation with relatives

Relatives or carers may be approaching exhaustion or already totally 'burnt out'. Some severely stressed relatives expect (even demand) that the visiting doctor take the patient away immediately even if the patient's condition does not warrant this. However, if help is needed it is essential that this is given as soon as possible and in some cases immediately (admission, day-hospital, etc.). This promptness helps later when discharge is contemplated and relatives/carers then know that they will be supported in their caregiving role. It is important that admission should be arranged before the situation becomes so critical that the relatives/carers feel that they cannot perform that role again. During the domiciliary visit time should be allocated to listen to the carer's point of view and then to outline the planned policy of treatment, rehabilitation and eventual discharge. In this way the carer realizes that admission to hospital will not be permanent.

Palliative care

Sometimes a visit reveals that a person is terminally ill and that death will be soon or inevitable. In these circumstances transfer to hospital may not be justified and a better course of action is to discuss the prognosis frankly with the relatives (and usually with the patient if the circumstances are appropriate) giving time to listen to the worries of all concerned. Then by liaising with the GP it is usually possible to arrange for extra home support (district/'Macmillan' nursing) by day and night.

Insight into social networks

Through domiciliary visiting one becomes aware of the unique nature of the individual and their social network. One comes to realize that there is no such thing as total independence, for each of us is dependent upon others. Rather one realizes that there is relative acceptance and tolerance. The medical diseases may be the same but the social networks are not and a plan of management that ignores this holistic approach is doomed to failure.

DISADVANTAGES OF DOMICILIARY CONSULTATION

Conflict

Rarely conflict may arise when there is a difference of opinion as to treatment options between GP, consultant and carer.

Delay in gaining treatment

Most visits should be carried out within about 24 hours of the request unless otherwise specified. If a change in treatment results or admission is needed the domiciliary consultation may lead to an extra delay. This can be lessened by the specialist and GP meeting on the visit (as is theoretically required) or by the use of the telephone once the assessment is over. However medical ill-health does not present classically in elderly people, and while a 'classic' urgent presentation may result in a quick admission, a slower 'gone off their legs' or 'failure to thrive' may be presented as a 'social problem' with inherent delays along the way. Also it should not be forgotten that in rural areas (and in heavily congested inner cities) considerable amounts of consultant time can be spent in the car travelling from hospital to home and back.

Lack of diagnostic facilities

Poor home circumstances can mean that the patient is not examined fully and an outpatient or day hospital appointment needs to be arranged so that a thorough clinical examination can be undertaken. In addition, apart from clinical acumen the investigations that are possible are obviously more limited than when the person is seen at the hospital. Some doctors consider that these clinical disadvantages are sufficient to make home visiting impracticable whilst others think the benefits far outweigh the disadvantages.

HOME VISIT BEFORE DISCHARGE

A home visit is also the term used when hospital-based therapists (occupational therapists, physiotherapists) accompany a patient home for a few hours to assess all of the discharge needs. Other professionals (e.g. social worker) may also be present as well as carers. This visit can assess the patient's stamina, physical and mental skills as well as the home circumstances (furniture, stairs, hazards, etc.). It is a good opportunity to meet relatives and neighbours who may strongly express their concerns. Tasks may be set and their completion reassure both therapists and carers. The patient may do very well on the visit and concerns be allayed. However, there may be further rehabilitation needs identified or structural alterations deemed necessary. The need for formal and informal carer input can be assessed and a discharge plan identified with agreement

that a certain level of input (from whatever source) can actually be achieved.

Home visits on the day of hospital discharge should be discouraged. Unexpected problems may arise and therapists and carers may be put under extra stress to prevent a readmission to hospital. In difficult circumstances a 'trial' at home is arranged with the appropriate professional calling in to the patient's home to check on progress. In ideal circumstances a post-discharge 'check' home visit can be used to allay fears and monitor the peri-discharge process.

Key points

- Domiciliary consultations are requested by the GP and are for the purpose of giving a second opinion on a patient's diagnosis and/or management. They are not used to assess the need or priority for admission to hospital.
- Advantages of domiciliary consultations are: ease of obtaining a second opinion; a more accurate and comprehensive history may be obtained; educational value; may be an alternative to hospital admission; knowledge of home circumstances may be valuable in management; relatives may be seen more easily and insights gained into social network.
- Disadvantages of domiciliary consultations are: conflicts may arise between doctors, patient and family; delay in treatment may occur; there is a lack of diagnostic equipment available.
- Home visits may be done prior to discharge from hospital by various members of the ward team. This allows better assessment of the patient's needs on discharge.

FURTHER READING

Arcand M, Williamson J. An evaluation of home visiting of patients by physicians in geriatric medicine. *Br Med J* 1981; **283**: 718–720.

Coupland AL, Todd GB. Pattern of domiciliary consultations in the Trent Region. *Br Med J* 1985; **290**: 1399–1402.

Dowie R. National trends in domiciliary consultations. *Br Med J* 1983; **286**: 819–822.

Littlejohns PC. Domiciliary consultations — who benefits? *J R Coll Gen Pract* 1986; **36**: 313–315.

Mulley G. Domiciliary visits. *Br Med J* 1988; **296**: 515.

Smith MV, Blythe JD. Domiciliary consultations. *Update Plus* 1971; **1**: 135–139, 149.

45 THE ELDERLY PATIENT IN ACCIDENT & EMERGENCY

- The problem
- The medical diagnosis
- The social set-up
- Appropriate referral
- Returning home
- Local authority Part 3 admission
- Admission to hospital

Elderly people form a disproportionately large part of the work of the A&E departments which have yet to come to terms with their needs. It is now accepted that children should be seen in a separate part of the A&E department, that special training and consideration of both child and parents are needed to ensure high standards of practice. The same could be said of elderly people, but it will take much effort to persuade A&E departments of the wisdom of treating elderly patients as a priority.

THE PROBLEM

The problem is all too familiar: an elderly woman arrives by ambulance in a confused state, with a daughter who is upset having found her mother on the floor at the bottom of the stairs. The patient does not seem too bad, and nothing medical seems to be wrong. The daughter then tells the casualty officer that it is obvious that her mother cannot go back home tonight.

In these circumstances, the casualty officer is forced into a role of gatekeeper to a scarce resource — a hospital bed for an elderly, confused woman. A confrontation seems likely, which makes the casualty officer annoyed, so he appears aggressive. There are no geriatric beds, the last one was filled hours ago, and the medical take-in team do not like 'confused grannies'. The patient lives alone, and was not coping too well anyway according to the daughter. Things really came to a head when the next door neighbour was taken ill and went into hospital the previous week.

The problem is the usual undifferentiated mix of medical problems, social support mechanisms, and immediate placement — or disposal from A&E. Unfortunately, it is very easy to muddle these different aspects of the case, and thus fail to come to the correct solutions. The crucial first step is to tackle each dimension of the problem separately, before making a judgement. This does of course take time, and requires just the same patience and tact as dealing with a two-year-old who may or may not be seriously ill.

THE MEDICAL DIAGNOSIS

Elderly patients present non-specifically (just like children), and multiple pathology is frequent. It is usually necessary to rule out various common diseases systematically (Table 45.1).

Table 45.1 Questions the house officer should ask before sending an elderly patient home from A&E

History
  Is the patient normally well?
  Is the patient on any medication?
  Is the patient normally rational?

Examination

General
  Is the patient confused?
  Is the patient pyrexial or cold?
  Is there a tachycardia?
  Is the patient dehydrated?

Chest
  Is there evidence of respiratory distress (count the rate)?
  Is there evidence of pneumonia?

Heart
  Is there evidence of heart failure?
  Is there postural hypotension?
  Has the patient had a silent heart attack?

Neuro/locomotor
  Does the patient have evidence of a stroke?
  Can the patient walk?
  Could the patient have a hip fracture?

Miscellaneous
  Could it be a urinary tract infection?
  Could it be an overdose?
  Is there blood on rectal examination?

Investigations

Urea & electrolytes:	Electrolyte disturbance?
Chest X-ray:	Signs of pneumonia or heart failure?
Urine/MSU:	Blood and/or pus cells?
ECG:	Acute infarct or dysrhythmia?
Blood sugar:	Diabetic or hypoglycaemia?

All this may seem 'over the top' to the busy casualty officer with plenty of 'real' patients to see. However, it is extremely rare for such a medical diagnostic approach to be negative, and even rarer for presentation at A&E to be precipitated for purely 'social' reasons. If a social crisis does appear to be the prime cause of attendance, it is always worth asking whether it was precipitated by an acute medical problem. Often that problem will turn out to be confusion.

Assessing the confused elderly patient is not easy without some history. The crucial point to decide is whether the confusion is of recent and acute onset, or whether the patient has been gradually deteriorating for a period of many months or years. The patient will never be able to tell this piece of information to the doctor, so some other witness must be found. This may involve telephoning relatives, neighbours, the community psychiatric service, social services, or the family doctor.

It is simply negligent to state that due to confusion no history or examination could be done. It is also surprising how information can be obtained if it is asked for — even old hospital records can be found and may contain much-needed clues to the present problem.

A side-effect of fully investigating elderly people in A&E is that it takes time. A&E trolleys are hard with mattresses that are far too thin to protect elderly patients' skin. Pressure sores frequently have their origin in the A&E department, but are too often blamed on the receiving admissions ward. Pressure sore prevention measures are as much the responsibility of A&E staff as any other hospital department, and appropriate mattresses should be used for immobile elderly patients.

THE SOCIAL SET-UP

Elderly people live within social networks, just like anyone else. Sometimes these networks are very supportive, sometimes they are as frail as the elderly patient. It is necessary to make enquiries about social networks, to work out who are the key people in this particular patient's life, the services received, the type of home lived in. This background information is essential in making a decision about referral. If the patient is to go home, the A&E department has a responsibility for knowing what 'home' means (e.g. outside lavatory, no central heating, and no home care services).

Often, local social service departments run 'good neighbour' schemes, or frail elderly schemes to help with the acute support of patients who do not require hospital admission but are unable to look after themselves for relatively short periods of time. It is only by contacting local social services that such information can be obtained. Contact should be made regardless of the expected outcome (i.e. going home or admission). In the latter case services may have to be cancelled, and considerable anxiety (and broken down doors) can be avoided by telling a home help that the person is in hospital. The task may of course be delegated to a social work assistant attached to the A&E department.

Communication with the family doctor is also of vital importance. The family doctor may have information about diagnoses, medication, and if the patient is going home, must be informed so that the patient can be reviewed the following day. Formal methods of communication between A&E and family doctors are frequently poor, and should not be relied on for frail elderly patients. The responsibility rests with the casualty officer to contact family doctors by phone at the end of the shift.

APPROPRIATE REFERRAL

Having made a proper medical assessment, it is usually clear what the next steps must be. Admission to an acute medical ward is not always necessary, although this is often seen as the easiest way out of a confrontation, and avoids the need for collecting so much information. It is often not in the patient's interests to be admitted to hospital unless essential. Typically, a request is made to admit an elderly patient with a toxic confusional state. In practice the diagnosis frequently turns out to be a dementia syndrome that is obvious after the first telephone call has been made to a relative.

RETURNING HOME

It is often necessary to discuss return home with friends and relatives, who may feel that they have 'done their duty', and that they no longer wish to provide care and support for this frail elderly person. Such feelings are understandable and need to be talked through. Often a compromise can be reached enabling the elderly patient to return to their own home, while a more durable plan is built up with the help of the appropriate hospital and community services. Indeed if the problem has been precipitated by an acute illness, it is likely that things will return to normal within a few days. Such negotiation is not normally part of the training of casualty officers, and is probably best done by specialists in health care of elderly people.

LOCAL AUTHORITY PART 3 ADMISSION

All social service departments have an on-call duty officer around the clock, and emergency places are available in Part 3 old people's homes. These are intended for genuine social emergencies (e.g. the death, or admission to hospital, of a carer). The patient has to be reasonably well: mobile, continent, and needing only minimal help in activities of daily living. Increasingly, local authorities are reducing their stock of Part 3 homes and this sort of admission will be more difficult to organize in some parts of the country. It is probable that the voluntary sector and acute hospitals will fill the gap by means of night sitters and temporary admission respectively.

ADMISSION TO HOSPITAL

If the medical problem is surgical or orthopaedic this does not usually present any difficulties. With medical problems there can be confusion over referral to geriatricians or physicians. Most hospitals now have an acute medical take-in policy which aims to clarify relationships between the two specialties (see Chapter 39). Policies are either integrated with general medicine or age-related (e.g. over 75 years). It is important to know which system operates in the district, so that time is not wasted contacting the wrong service. However a degree of patience is needed, because whatever the policy, beds are never empty when they are needed, and it will always take at least one more phone call than expected to discharge an elderly patient from A&E. Casualty officers who have done a sensible job of making a diagnosis, of finding out about the social set-up, and working out an appropriate plan should have little need to play 'pass the parcel' with their elderly patients. It should be obvious where they need to go.

A further trap for the unwary is catchment areas. Most geriatric and psychiatric services admit only those people living in the district, and do not take admissions from out of the district. This is largely because of resource constraints, rather than bloody-mindedness!

Key points

- An elderly patient presenting to A&E requires a thorough assessment. Corners cannot be cut, and obtaining background history is essential.
- Casualty officers should have a standard framework for their enquiries to aid ruling in or out common problems such as infection, stroke and heart failure.
- Social services do provide help for genuine social emergencies, but are not a dumping ground for people with undifferentiated problems.
- A&E departments should be aware of the geriatric and general medicine admission policies, and local catchment areas. Provided the patient has been

properly evaluated, discharge from A&E is seldom a problem.

- Old people are vulnerable to developing pressure sores while waiting in A&E. All beds and trolleys for immobile old people should have adequate pressure-relieving devices.

FURTHER READING

Dove AF, Dave SH. Elderly patients in the Accident Department and their problems. *Br Med J* 1986; **292**: 807–809.

46 DISCHARGE FROM HOSPITAL

- Discharge planning
- Care plans
- Informing the general practitioner
- The first 48 hours
- Checklist

During a patient's stay in hospital the aim is to get them well enough to leave and return home. If at the end of their treatment the discharge is unplanned, the effect is to undo all that has been achieved and possibly cause a traumatic period at home or a readmission. This can severely undermine a patient's confidence in their ability to manage ever again.

DISCHARGE PLANNING

This begins on the day of admission and is based on a full physical, mental and social assessment. It is very important to ascertain the patient's pre-admission lifestyle, i.e. prior to the acute illness. This information may need to be obtained from many sources, especially when dealing with a confused patient. In the course of the total assessment answers should be obtained to the questions listed in Table 46.1.

Careful interviewing technique is essential to avoid such devastating comments to carers such as 'your mother must never be left alone again'. Such thoughtless remarks can ruin lives.

Table 46.1 Questions to be asked early in discharge planning

What is the type and position of accommodation?
Is it owner-occupied or rented accommodation?
How many floors and stairs are there?
What is the position of bathroom and toilets?
Does the person live alone, with family or with others?
What is the frequency of visits or trips out?
What about shopping, clubs, church, social activities?
What is the frequency of visitors?
Is there any support from relatives or neighbours?
Are visits from social services or health services arranged?
What is the family/carer's perception of the client's well-being?
What is the client's perception of well-being?
What does the client want on their return home?

Set realistic goals

A picture of a patient's lifestyle prior to admission is formed taking into account their present physical and mental state, and rehabilitation targets can be set. These must be realistic, i.e. a patient who has not walked for 5 years but managed at home is unlikely to walk again simply because of an admission to hospital. Discharge planning requires teamwork but central to this theme is that the patient understands and agrees to what everyone is trying to achieve.

Home assessment

It may be necessary for the occupational therapist or physiotherapist to undertake a home visit prior to discharge. Only then will the team know what difficulties the patient still has (if any) and what extra help will be necessary. The visit must be explained and agreed with the patient and often the carers, who in certain circumstances find this a threatening situation (e.g. the potential discharge of a patient whose carers consider should be 'in care'). All aspects of daily living can be assessed as well as orientation within the home surroundings. It should be remembered that some aids and adaptations may take many weeks to organize and a priority list should be made (i.e. essential, advisable, non-urgent, etc.). Adjustments should be made only with the patient's agreement (i.e. they see that the change is helpful). During the visit the opportunity can be taken to talk to neighbours. It may be possible to find out what help, if any, they are prepared to give but it is important that unreasonable demands are not placed upon them and that they should know where to turn to for help.

Following the visit it may be necessary for the team to meet with the patient and family/carers and decide on what needs to be organized, especially the role of new or extra help. The social worker usually plays a key role in discharge planning (with the ward nursing staff) and is often the patient's advocate, aware of their attitudes to the discharge and the future.

Timing and coordination

A crucial decision is the day of discharge. It is irresponsible to discharge an elderly person living alone and dependent on services home on a Friday. A Monday discharge means that they have the benefit of five days of help and support prior to the weekend. On the other hand a weekend discharge is often best when the person is returning home to relatives/carers/neighbours who otherwise work and who provide a lot of input. Patients and relatives should have the telephone numbers and addresses (and even the names) of the support staff who are going to visit them at home (e.g. district nurses, bath assistants, home help, meals on wheels organizer). If there is then a problem the relevant person/organization can be contacted directly with minimal delay. Many services now insist on assessment visits so that the services themselves decide with the client what they

need and how it will be provided. This may mean some degree of uncertainty prior to discharge as patient and carer can only be told that a service has been applied for. Some services are under severe strain in certain areas (e.g. bathing attendants, weekend meals on wheels, evening/twilight nursing) and the hospital staff should not imply to patient or carer that a service is automatic. It is far better to let the service manager discuss the situation with the client/carer and if it is a vital service necessary for discharge one should endeavour to arrange a meeting of the relevant parties on the ward. Early referral to any service is essential. In difficult circumstances a case conference may prove necessary.

Prior to discharge any drug regime should be made as simple as possible and doctors, nurses and pharmacist should ensure that either the patient is safely self-medicating or that suitable alternatives are made (carer, district nurse, etc.). All patients should be issued with a drug card stating the drugs being taken, the dose and reason for prescribing (colour and shape can be useful). Any changes in medication must be noted on the card by the patient's GP.

CARE PLANS

The implementation of the Care in the Community legislation in April 1993 resulted in the use of care plans. The hospital social worker dealing with a particular patient must prepare a care plan for their discharge from hospital should any services be required. The care plan is a detailed assessment of the patient's social needs including some medical details (usually obtained from the ward doctor). The plan is usually either simple (day care services) or complex (frequent multiagency input or residential care request). In theory the patient cannot be discharged until the care manager (social services), who is the fundholder, agrees to finance (i.e. pay for) the care plan package. Each discharge therefore involves a multipage form being faxed (or posted) after the multidisciplinary ward meetings and agreement sought. In 'complex' cases care managers usually insist on a care conference with themselves or a deputy present.

INFORMING THE GENERAL PRACTITIONER

Close cooperation and communication between the hospital doctors and the patient's GP are essential.

Ideally the GP takes part in discussions prior to discharge (especially in difficult cases). Failing this the GP should be contacted on the day before discharge by telephone informing them of the diagnosis, treatment and medication as well as the support service arrangements and follow-up. This information should also be sent out by post in a short letter unless the discharge summary (a brief document containing only essential information) is sent within 24 hours of discharge (Fig. 46.1). Outpatient or day hospital attendance arrangements should be made in advance and the patient, carer and GP informed.

THE FIRST 48 HOURS

This is the crucial period for many elderly people discharged from hospital. Some units have discharge teams (social workers or health visitors) who monitor the person's progress and report back. They are also available for any crises that may occur. 'Social' crises invariably arise due to an underlying medical issue and the GP with the information from the recent admission will be able to decide what action needs to be taken. Occasionally problems arise due to carer 'breakdown'.

DISCHARGE SUMMARY

Name:
Address:

DoB:
Hosp number:

Consultant:
Admitted:
Discharged:
Ward:
Discharge address:

GP:
Address:

Dictated:
Typed:

PROBLEMS   ACTION

PRESENTATION

DRUGS
Admission   Discharge   Allergies

Drug card(s)

DOMICILE   CARER

FUNCTION
Previous   Discharge   Mental
                                       Test

SUPPORT SERVICES
Previous   Discharge:
Service   Frequency   Service   Frequency

FUTURE PLANS
Follow up   Points for follow-up

Long-term plans

INFORMATION GIVEN

SHO name: Bleep number: Signed ....

Figure 46.1 Discharge summary

These can be minimized by adequate pre-discharge planning and counselling. Pre-discharge arrangements should ensure that services are organized. In the event of problems the patient/carer must know where to obtain the relevant and specific explanation. Unavoidable readmissions do occur, often due to new illness episodes, unrecognized illness 'brewing' during discharge planning or unexpected accidents (falls etc.). These should become learning exercises and form a specific part of a unit's auditing process. Avoidable readmissions are time-consuming, wasteful of resources and an unpleasant upheaval for the person concerned.

CHECKLIST

Attention must be paid to the 'small' but essential items; food at home, keys, home security (during admission and post-discharge), adequate heating, aids fitted/delivered, spectacles/hearing aids/teeth return home with the patient, transport booked (the correct type) and follow-up arrangements made.

It is important to find out if the patient wants to return home. Many patients have anxieties but in spite of these they wish to be at home. For a few, however, going home is an appalling prospect. They consider it lonely, often frightening and either wish to stay in hospital or move to what they consider to be more suitable accommodation. The patient may not volunteer this but then perform unexpectedly badly on a pre-discharge visit. The patient should be counselled and as many anxieties as possible worked through. Except in the most difficult cases, however, the person usually has to return home while alternative arrangements are being made. For a few their anxieties are so great that despite performing well on the ward the discharge fails dismally and readmission is necessary.

Table 46.2 gives a checklist of questions to answer prior to discharge.

Given the motivation to stay at home, careful planning and a modicum of luck the return home of the majority of patients will be a safe and happy event.

Table 46.2 Questions to be answered prior to discharge

Is the person really medically fit enough?
Do they want to go home?
Is the discharge date and timing suitable for the carers and services?
Have the points noted in the home visit been answered?
Have the ambulance (correct type) and services been ordered? (Usually 48 hours' notice required)
Is the drug regime the simplest possible?
Does the patient have a drug card?
Have the patient, carer and GP been told?
Has the follow-up (and its transport) been arranged?
Before the person leaves the ward do they have all their belongings, especially teeth, spectacles, hearing aids, keys, money, as well as medication?
Has the care plan been outlined and agreed by the care manager?

Key points

- Discharge planning begins on admission with a full assessment.
- Realistic goals help patient morale.
- A home visit/assessment is necessary for many elderly patients, especially if there are team or carer doubts concerning the patient's ability.
- Day of discharge is important: early in the week is best for patients being supported by services, whereas a weekend may be more convenient for carers.
- Give the client and carers the names and telephone numbers of the services that have been booked.
- Liaise with the GP *prior* to discharge in difficult cases.
- Review and audit readmissions; they provide good learning exercises.
- Develop a discharge checklist.
- For most patients a care plan must be implemented and the financial responsibility agreed.

FURTHER READING

Gay P, Pitkeathley J. *When I Went Home: A Study of Patients Discharged from Hospital.* King Edward's Hospital Fund for London/Pitman Medical, London, 1979.

Simpson PJE, Levitt R. *Going Home: A Guide for Helping the Patient on Leaving Hospital.* Churchill Livingstone, Edinburgh, 1981.

47 THE ROLES OF THE TEAM MEMBERS

- Carers
- Chaplains
- Chiropodists and podiatrists
- Clinical nurse specialists
- Clinical psychologists
- Community psychiatric nurses
- Continence advisers
- Dentists
- Dieticians
- Doctors
- Health visitors
- Hearing therapists
- Hospital management
- Nurses
- Occupational therapists
- Pharmacists
- Physiotherapists
- Placement officers
- Social workers
- Speech therapists

CARERS

The holistic approach to patient care must involve the main carer in decision-making processes. Patient autonomy and independence must be respected but health care professionals must listen to the wishes and needs of carers and together (patient, professional and carer) achieve realistic aims. The carers are an important source of detailed information during the hospital admission, especially in the mentally impaired client. They are essential elements in the pre-discharge discussion process and when it comes to talking about future patterns of care. The concepts of duty and burden can be difficult to disentangle from care, and carers often take their cue from professionals and hence enter into a long-term commitment. These decisions may affect their own family, job and indeed health and hence advice should never be offered lightly in terms of 'your mother shouldn't be left alone', for example. Stress and caring is another difficult area. Many carers do not wish to be placed in that position or through physical or mental problems should not be expected to fulfil the task. It is accepted that looking after a frail or demanding person can affect one's physical and psychological well-being. Lack of sleep affects everyone. The role of 'stress', however, in subsequent problems such as ill-health or as a cause of abuse of the older person is far from clear. The role of respite care in reducing stress is also not clear-cut, though in all of these situations one should err on the side of providing as much help as possible to both carer and client.

Carers, as far as is ethically possible, need to be kept fully informed as to a person's disease state, progress and prognosis. Most patients want their carer to be as involved as they are though exceptions do occur and the cue for information-giving must come from the patient. Disease states need to be explained fully, especially in 'chronic' conditions such as Parkinson's disease and Alzheimer's disease. Health care professionals need to have pamphlets or books at hand to recommend for further reading as very little information is retained in the formal setting of doctor/patient/carer interview or meeting.

Where possible the patient and carer should be offered the referral to voluntary organizations specializing in the field concerned, e.g. Parkinson's Disease Society, Alzheimer's Disease Society, etc. These groups act as further information sources, research bases and as carer/patient support systems. They can offer very useful and practical advice on the particular difficulties of caring from someone with a certain condition. In addition there is the Carers National Association, an advisory group dealing and helping with all aspects of the carer's role.

Caring is not a new phenomenon but it is occurring under new circumstances for many people. In past generations the extended family assimilated grandparents, older aunts, uncles or cousins with disabilities because usually they lived under one roof and there were few alternatives to 'caring'. People were no better at the role in days gone by, the same stresses, frustration and problems were present.

Now, however, most children move away from home and have considerable periods of freedom away from such commitments (often until late middle life). Alternatives are available but 'society' still looks (as does the recipient) to family — especially daughters — to fulfil the caring role when it is required. Altering work and home schedules after such long periods of time is undoubtedly very hard. It must be remembered that for the first time in history, four generation families are commonplace with the oldest being cared for by their adult children who are themselves over retirement age.

The amazing thing is that so many people continue to do it, whether out of love, caring or a sense of duty. At any one time there are approximately six million people caring for others in the UK — a truly impressive statistic.

CHAPLAINS

In many hospitals the chaplains (either hospital-based or from the local church) provide a multifaceted service. Their visits may be regular or occasional. They provide the hospital religious services for staff, patients and visitors but also offer the individual patient spiritual help. This may be supportive or in the form of counselling or be at a time of crisis (i.e. severe illness, impending death).

As the community becomes more multicultural so do the religious needs of patients. Religious guidance for many faiths may be needed on a single ward, not only to serve the patients but also to advise the staff on the special needs and practices essential to that religion. The chaplain may assume the role of visitor, friend or advocate and where a close relationship exists they should be part of the team process. The role also extends into teaching so that medical, nursing and other students are exposed to the holistic approach involved in the best care of patients.

CHIROPODISTS AND PODIATRISTS

Despite the concern over mobility in elderly people, interest in their feet tends to be aroused only at a very late stage. Elderly patients may be unable to see their feet or reach them. They may have accepted painful feet as an ageing process or indeed sensation in the feet may be impaired or even absent.

The chiropodist is not trained simply to trim nails and cut and attend corns (which can themselves render a patient housebound and immobile, but are usually treated by a foot care assistant) but to diagnose and treat congenital and acquired foot problems. Podiatrists are chiropodists who have undergone further postgraduate training to equip them to perform operations on the feet. They may range from the minor to the correction of toe deformities performed under local anaesthetic using fully sterile techniques. The operations are usually performed as day cases and podiatrists often have joint assessment clinics with orthopaedic surgeons to assess and select suitable patients. Chiropodists recognize and treat the pedal manifestation of systemic diseases; for example, the patient who presents with plantar perforating ulcers as a result of diabetic peripheral neuropathy or the ischaemic changes seen in peripheral vascular disease, confirmed using clinical examination and Doppler studies. Diabetics, however, have a special need for regular chiropody.

The NHS chiropody service is available free to the following categories of patient:

1. men aged 65 and over;
2. women aged 60 and over;
3. expectant mothers;
4. mothers with children under one year old;
5. children under school-leaving age;
6. physically handicapped persons;
7. diabetic/medically at-risk persons on referral from a consultant.

Treatment and advice can be obtained from health centres, hospital outpatient clinics, day hospitals and day centres (if mobile). If the patient is housebound a domiciliary visit can be made. Transport should be available to take a person to a community clinic or hospital.

In many parts of the country the number of chiropodists is totally inadequate, resulting in long waiting lists and practically no domiciliary service. Private clinics are increasing as the NHS service collapses. There is an urgent need to train more foot care assistants.

CLINICAL NURSE SPECIALISTS

Clinical nurse specialists are nurses with postgraduate training in a specific field. The areas of expertise covered include tissue viability, stoma care, nutrition and palliative care. They are not only responsible for practical advice to clinicians, nurses and others but develop treatment protocols, care guidelines, standard setting, education courses, etc. They are often part of larger teams, such as nutrition teams or wound healing teams. In view of their comparatively small numbers many develop the concept of key 'link' nurses in ward areas to act as a more local focus to devolve the expertise.

CLINICAL PSYCHOLOGISTS

The clinical psychologist is concerned with the application of psychology to clinical problems.

Advice
Assessment and diagnosis

There is evidence that psychometric evaluation is able to contribute to the differential diagnosis of functional and organic conditions in the elderly. It can help in the difficult discrimination between dementia and depressive pseudodementia. In addition, careful objective assessment can be helpful in the identification of cognitive and functional deficits and advising staff on rehabilitative procedures. Baselines can be established to guide staff in assessing rate of change and areas of improvement or deterioration.

Treatment and management

Treatments for the confused elderly are directed towards helping the individual to remain at home or in the community, and/or easing problems that create special difficulty within the home or institution. These may include treatments for specific behavioural problems which can prevent the elderly person from coping at home (e.g. incontinence, faecal smearing, wandering, importuning, noisy or aggressive behaviour).

Psychologists may be involved in working individually with patients (e.g. treating fears or phobias which may be incapacitating, and in employing psychological approaches to the treatment of depression. They may also be able to help with other problem behaviours which may be causing stress within the family. Such interventions are primarily concerned with counselling of and in some cases training of relatives and care staff.

Recent developments
Cognitive change and age

Developmental psychology has produced a broader knowledge concerning the effects of ageing and there is now increased insight into the complexities of cognitive change in the ageing brain. There is no evidence of a simple progressive intellectual deterioration with increasing age. Some of the behaviour changes reported in the elderly which have been attributed to intrinsic causes probably relate to environmental variables. Even in dementia where impairment of learning and memory function is established, the residual adaptive capability is being explored as are programmes which minimize the detrimental effects of learning deficits. In some dementing illnesses certain research conditions can produce near normal levels of retention of previously learned material. The exact nature of the memory deficit is still a controversial issue. Clinical psychologists are interested in the practical implications, such as the management of the memory-impaired person, devising memory aids, etc.

Environmental factors

Knowledge of the impact of physical, environmental and social influences on behaviour, particularly in institutions, is also expanding. A wide range of environmental factors are involved including the role of the individualized environment, privacy, 'territorial' behaviour in maintaining a sense of personal identity, the effects of imposed 'social' space and the effects of staff attitudes. The effects of the physical environment are also becoming better understood. A reduction in light level may produce disorientation and falls, certain colour contrasts can produce misperception of depth — hence psychological interventions may involve environmental modification.

Institutional care

Despite some advances in institutional care, publications and official reports still indicate that the environment of old people in institutions is unstimulating, non-therapeutic and creative of high dependence in residents and low job satisfaction in staff. Greater involvement by psychologists has been requested in helping to develop a therapeutic milieu in wards and day hospitals and to develop programmes to help elderly people adjust to any failing functions. Evidence is accumulating to indicate that some deterioration is related to these environmental variables. Improvement may be seen following the use of:

1. *Stimulation and activity approaches.* The improved effects do not seem to continue after the outside stimulation has ceased.
2. *Reality orientation techniques.* This aims to reduce disorientation and maintain a sense of personal identity in a confused person by continually presenting him or her with information about their current reality, the day, date, time, name, place, etc. Several studies show improvement in intellectual, social and word behaviour with these techniques.

3. *Milieu approaches.* These aim to counteract social deterioration by attempting to provide patients with normal social roles (e.g. encouraging an elderly person to take as much responsibility for their care and management as possible including the making of decisions concerning group living in old people's homes). There are clinical reports of increased social cohesion and better self-care, increased responsiveness and reduced levels of incontinence using this approach (dependent to some extent on changes in attitude of care staff).
4. *Behaviour therapy.* This is based on a careful analysis of the interaction between patient and his or her past and present environment to throw light on the process leading to disturbed behaviour. It can be used to try to improve various functional deficits including problems in self-care (toileting, dressing, eating habits), social interaction and disturbed behaviour which are often accepted as part of a chronic confusional state.

COMMUNITY PSYCHIATRIC NURSES

Community psychiatric nurses are qualified in psychiatric nursing and in addition often have general nursing training. They can work out of hospitals or be attached to community health centres. They assess, monitor and treat all aspects of psychiatric illness in elderly people, liaising with consultant psychiatrists. They have roles in education (client and carer) and in supporting both groups in the community. They tend to specialize in some areas such as the management and treatment of depressive disorders and the organic illnesses such as dementia. Some are involved in crisis intervention teams.

With an increasing number of mentally ill elderly patients requiring assessment and long-term support, the role of the community psychiatric nurse is one of great importance. By building up and liaising with the supportive social networks and generating trust with both patients and carers, they are often able to maintain very mentally impaired people in the community.

CONTINENCE ADVISERS

Continence advisers are trained nurses with a special interest in the problems of both urinary and faecal incontinence in both sexes. They may be based either in hospital or in the community and can help in diagnosis and management. They work closely with other specialists, e.g. urodynamics department, gynaecology, etc., but usually initiate some investigations and refer on if necessary. Some advisers work out of specialist urodynamic units and hence are involved in conducting the more detailed investigations. They are experts in the management of incontinence and are able to give specific advice concerning all the continence aids available, their use by client or carer. Most will perform home visits for the very disabled and have knowledge of the services available in a community (laundry service, delivery of pads, etc.). In hospitals their help can be invaluable for the 'difficult' patient and in an education and teaching role. They need to be consulted early and certainly before discharge is contemplated. They are also a source of information on equipment such as the latest catheters, their different uses, cost and drawbacks. Their expertise is available to institutions such as Part 3 homes.

DENTISTS

Many elderly people have poor dental health and are handicapped by their dental condition. One sociodental investigation of elderly people living at home revealed that:

1. 74 per cent were edentulous and many were wearing unsatisfactory dentures;
2. 59 per cent had lesions of the oral mucosa (mainly related to dentures);
3. 32 per cent complained of oral pain;
4. 30 per cent had difficulty in chewing their food; and
5. 13 per cent felt embarrassed by their appearance with dentures dropping during social contact.

Most dental treatment is carried out by general dental practitioners. Although people over 65 years of age take up a very small percentage of NHS courses of treatment they pay a comparatively large percentage of all the charges because their treatment often involves expensive items such as dentures. Most elderly people have very low expectations of their dental health and are not particularly demanding. This situation will change in the future as more people retain their natural teeth into old age and higher levels of care will be required.

Old people often face serious dental problems if they become ill. Poorly fitting dentures previously skilfully controlled may suddenly become unwearable. For the increasing number of dentate elderly people with heavily restored mouths a high level of oral hygiene is required. If this is difficult to achieve because of severe illness, recurrent caries and progressive periodontal disease may necessitate removal of the teeth, leaving the patient edentulous with no previous denture-wearing experience.

In hospital a hospital dentist may be available. Alternatively the FHSA (Family Health Services Authority) can provide a list of dentists who may be able to help. Similarly, if a person is housebound a dentist prepared to do domiciliary treatment may be contacted via the FHSA.

The Community Dental Service can treat handicapped adults if they cannot arrange treatment from other sources.

Treatment

Initially an assessment is made and emergency treatment to relieve pain carried out. It is then necessary to make a long-term treatment plan which may include:

1. prevention of further dental disease by
   (a) scaling and polishing natural teeth,
   (b) cleaning dentures,
   (c) advice on oral hygiene and diet;
2. treatment by
   (a) restoration of teeth,
   (b) provision of training appliances or new dentures.

New techniques such as palatal training devices (for use in dysphagic patients after stroke), postgraduate dental advice from dentists specifically trained to deal with the elderly (e.g. an MSc in Gerodontics is offered by the London Hospital Medical College) and the very disabled (e.g. Parkinson's disease) may be available in some areas.

It is strongly recommended that all dentures are marked. The loss of a denture can be extremely distressing and it is often impossible to produce satisfactory replacements. This is particularly important for patients in continuing care settings.

DIETICIANS

Formal studies have revealed what has always been suspected — there is a lot of malnutrition amongst elderly people. A high degree of suspicion is needed for diagnosis since most sufferers will have a subclinical picture. Florid scurvy is rare but does still exist. The role of the dietician working with the elderly includes:

1. giving advice on nutrition in health and disease;
2. educating all people who work with elderly people understand the need for a special knowledge concerning the importance of nutrition;
3. the nutritional assessment and treatment of referred patients; and
4. being a fully involved member of the multidisciplinary team.

Elderly patients requiring nutritional advice both in hospital and in the community will be seen by the dietician usually following receipt of a referral form from the hospital doctor or general practitioner.

A person may be at risk of malnutrition if he or she fulfils three or more of the conditions listed in Table 47.1.

One area of particular interest for the dietician is the swallowing-impaired patient (most commonly post-stroke). The dietician is involved from the outset with many other specialists (e.g. speech therapy) in assessing the swallow reflex and nutritional states and advising on the best regime. Foods with varying consistency may need to be provided or if nasogastric feeding is implemented (short or long term) the dietician advises on the total body requirements.

It must not be assumed that people living within institutions will be well nourished. In one study 30 per cent of long-stay patients in hospital were at risk of scurvy. Others who did not go out in the sun were at risk of osteomalacia.

DOCTORS

Life is short and the art long; the occasion fleeting; the experience fallacious and the judgement difficult. The physician must not only be prepared to do what is right himself but also to make the perfect patient, the attendants and externals cooperate. *Hippocrates–Aphorism 1*

Hospital doctors work in a hierarchical structure whereby ultimate responsibility for medical treatment resides with the consultant. Consultants expect the junior doctors to show that they have done their work to the best of their ability. They are expected to demonstrate that they have taken a first class medical and social history (often needing details from relatives, carers and others), thoroughly examined the patient,

Table 47.1 Risk factors for malnutrition

Social
  Isolation — living alone
  Recent bereavement
  Few or no outside interests

Mental disturbance
  Acute confusional states
  Dementia syndromes
  Depression

Physical disability
  Immobile or housebound
  Arthritis
  Blind or partially sighted

Effects of drugs
  Causing nausea — chemotherapy, digoxin, antituberculous drugs, antibiotics
  Metabolic effects — anticonvulsants, aspirin/anti-arthritic drugs, diuretics, anti-Parkinsonian drugs (L-dopa)

Ignorance of nutrition
  Widowers
  Those eating only one meal per day
  Pre-existing poor dietary habits
  Obsessive ideas about food
  Restricted variety of diet

Impaired appetite
  Following illness
  Due to other factors, e.g. social, mental, drugs

Economics
  Pensioner alone
  Other high expenses, e.g. heating
  Poor knowledge leading to poor choice and unwise use of available money

Increased nutritional requirements
  Bed-rest
  Pressure sores/chronic wounds
  Pyrexia (esp. long term)
  Post-trauma, e.g. fall/fracture
  Pre- and postoperatively

Poor dentition
  No teeth
  Ill-fitting dentures
  Decayed teeth
  Poor gum condition

Regular use/abuse of laxatives

High alcohol intake
  Replacing meals
  No money for food
  Impaired vitamin metabolism

Recent discharge from hospital

Institutionalization

written legible complete notes and requested the correct investigations. Junior staff are not expected to know everything, nor get everything right but they are expected to demonstrate first that they have tried and secondly that they are aware of their limitations.

Doctors who do not give of their best let themselves, their patients and their colleagues down. Excuses for failure to write notes, obtain X-rays, etc. are unlikely to be accepted — remember that the consultant was once a junior too.

The biggest failing at all levels is medical arrogance. The belief that one knows it all is surely tested by regular post mortems. Always remember that the other non-medical members of the team know much more about their subject than the junior doctor. A useful tip is always ask the question *why?* Identify the problems and try to group them together. Some doctors routinely use a problem list (e.g. problem-orientated medical records) or a disability profile to ensure that problems such as deafness and incontinence are not ignored. A biochemical profile is a useful addition to all notes. In acute wards a note should be written each day and on each occasion a procedure is carried out, drugs changed or a significant event has occurred (including summaries of conversations held with carers). In long-stay (continuing care) wards a progress note should be written weekly.

The house physician is the 'key worker' for the majority of patients in the ward. He or she should know everything that is happening to the patients and is responsible for ensuring that other staff, the patients and carers know as well. This is the art of communication, it entails patience, good telephone skills and a pleasant manner, often in the face of difficulty. The house physician is a collator of information. When talking to relatives junior doctors should collect relevant information but must be careful about making value judgements or hasty statements (e.g. 'she should not be left alone' or 'she can never go home'). Sitting in with the consultant at difficult interviews (angry or anxious relatives) can be invaluable experience in learning how to handle these situations. It is essential to record significant events in the notes; examples include not only changes in the medical condition but issues around medication, falls, conversations with relatives (especially if it involves a complaint) or changes in management (medical or social).

The house physician should prove a good link to the general practitioner in the primary health care team in the community. In all potentially difficult discharges (patient or relatives) the GP should be alerted prior to the discharge date. Similarly in cases where the GP should be forearmed with knowledge (recent diagnosis of carcinoma, unusual drugs, etc.) a telephone call is polite and valuable. Discharge letters and summaries should be prompt, short and relevant (see Chapter 46).

Requests for admission by GPs should not be questioned by junior doctors.

HEALTH VISITORS

Hospital-based personnel are often vague as to the precise qualifications of a health visitor. They are all fully trained nurses and midwives with several years' experience followed by a one- or two-year postgraduate diploma course at university or polytechnic. Health visitors are usually based in the community either in child health clinics or sometimes within general practitioner's premises. Comparatively few specialize in the health care needs of elderly people.

There are four main functions of health visiting:

1. prevention of mental, physical or emotional ill-health;
2. early detection of ill-health and surveillance of high-risk groups;
3. recognition and identification of need and mobilization of appropriate resources where necessary; and
4. provision of care: this includes support during times of stress, advice and guidance in case of illness and in the management of children.

In the community the first priority is to children under five with a view to counselling the whole family. The basic role changes little on joining the team involved in health care of elderly people in that expertise in working with the whole family remains a very important part of the work. This is coupled with support of and liaison with the professional team.

The health visitor provides a link between the contrasting worlds of home and hospital. This is accomplished by visits to the home before, during and after admission and attendance at ward rounds for the sharing of knowledge. The health visitor can provide information and opinions on the following.

1. Housing conditions — will the patient be able to cope with their immediate environment or will changes need to be made?
2. Relative support — assessing the level of support carers will be able to provide following discharge.
3. Neighbours' attitude — often provides clues to the patient's inability to cope with emergencies.

In an ideal world (or at least an ideal NHS) every suitable elderly patient would have the benefit of a health visitor's assessment whilst in hospital and care after discharge (even if only for a short period in most cases). The peri-discharge period is fraught with complex difficulties and the expertise of a health visitor liaising between hospital and community can make the difference between a 'soft' and a 'hard' landing (or no landing at all and a readmission).

HEARING THERAPISTS

Hearing therapy is a relatively new discipline, introduced to provide more continuous and comprehensive help than was possible by issuing hearing aids alone. The therapist tries to help individuals with an acquired hearing loss make the most of their residual hearing, by teaching them to use every available auditory and visual clue, thus making it possible for them to live in a world that relies on language for communication with less anxieties.

The hearing therapist is concerned with rehabilitating the hearing-impaired person via programmes which include:

1. auditory training — encouraging a person to listen again through a hearing aid where speech is frequently distorted;
2. lipreading — teaching a person to watch facial expressions and lipshapes to assist their understanding of speech;
3. help with a hearing aid — how to operate the controls and how to fit the earmould in the ear;
4. advice about environmental aids — television, telephone and doorbell etc.;
5. advice on how to cope with a hearing loss — counselling about the problems concerning home, work and social situations.

The disability of deafness

Society relies on the spoken word for exchanging ideas, commenting on events, expressing pleasure, relaying information and idle chatter, all of which add meaning to our lives. Failure to appreciate the spoken word can cause withdrawal from society (Beethoven being only one famous example). Most people perceive deafness as an inability to hear anything and assume that the only way to communicate with the deaf person is to shout. It is a widely held view that with a hearing aid a deaf person will comprehend all spoken language and if the hearing aid is not worn then the person is being uncooperative, antisocial or even aggressive. Due to their behaviour the deaf person may be shunned and ignored. It is easier for people with good hearing to talk to someone who understands them rather than take the time and effort to communicate with the deaf person. Deafness affects one in three elderly people and its onset can make a cheerful person become sullen, withdrawn, aggressive and overanxious.

Recognizing the patient with hearing loss

1. Visual clues — leaning forwards, cupping hand behind the ear.
2. Auditory clues — complaining about others mumbling, speaking loudly.
3. Social history — door not answered, TV too loud, not attending family gatherings.

Action

1. Examine ears for wax.
2. Refer to ENT, for medical assessment of hearing.
3. Refer to ENT technician if hearing aid malfunctioning.
4. Refer to hearing therapist.

Hearing aids

A person who wears a hearing aid successfully will feel more confident and less depressed and isolated. They will not receive clear speech automatically. A hearing aid amplifies all sounds equally, it does not correct impaired hearing but only amplifies sound. The controls on the hearing aid are difficult for many elderly people to adjust and the earmould is not easy to fit.

How to assist the hearing-impaired patient to communicate better

1. Attract the person's attention before you start to speak.
2. If possible exclude peripheral noise.
3. Speak slowly and clearly in a moderate voice.
4. Do not exaggerate lip movements.
5. Write down important facts.
6. Check if spectacles are worn.
7. Look at the patient when speaking with the light towards your face.
8. Sit at the same level as the patient.
9. Do not speak with your face covered.
10. Keep your hands still.
11. Check that the hearing aid is working.
12. Try an easi-com communicator.

HOSPITAL MANAGEMENT

In the late 1980s the first Griffiths Report on the Health Service recommended the introduction of a new management structure to improve communication, cut out delays in decision-making and introduce the concept of budgets (cost-effectiveness) within a health care setting. Each health district gained a District General Manager (DGM) with specific Unit General Managers (UGMs) accountable to them. A new tier of finance managers was also incorporated and with the addition of medical and nursing representatives district management teams evolved.

In April 1991 hospitals and their community services became the providers of health care whereas the District Health Authorities and GPs became the *purchasers*. At the same time some hospitals were encouraged to become trusts. Though still within the NHS and under the rules of purchaser/provider they were able to raise some capital independently (e.g. borrow money to fund new schemes) and have more autonomy in management decision-making, hence improving their competitiveness. At the same time GPs were encouraged to group together and become *fundholders* and act as purchasers of health care in parallel to the DHA.

Purchasing and providing has developed a sophisticated system of contracts by which health care is transacted at a business level. Contracts involve numbers of clients, costs (either individually or large groups) and issues around quality. This system has evolved into a series of contract meetings between purchaser and provider with each area of service (e.g. care of elderly people, ENT, etc.) having a separate allocation within a total contract review.

The overwhelming majority of provider care is now dealt with by trusts (either acute or community — an initial allowing of joint trusts has been abandoned). Purchasers have tended to amalgamate and form consortia, i.e. powerful contracting negotiators able to influence markedly how a trust provides its service. Crude tools include the possibility of withholding or redirecting contracts unless changes are made; more sophisticated ones use clinical audit using outcome measures to ensure higher standards of service for clients.

Purchasers need to ensure that providers meet not only contract specifications but government targets specific to the *Patients' Charter* and *Health of the Nation*. GP fundholding has been taken up only by a minority of practitioners but the government target is to get the majority involved.

Trusts are run on business lines with a chief executive and a management board usually consisting of executive directors, e.g. director of finance, estates, human resources, medical director. Non-executive directors are often chosen for their business and management expertise. Different models of management can be applied within a trust, acute trusts often using the clinical directorate model with each service area or department having a clinical manager with general and financial management support. In other models clinicians have a lead role (advice etc.), but the specific unit is run by a manager. The role of clinicians in management (unpaid, sessional or full-time) continues to be debated.

This management input has indeed revolutionized the running of all major hospitals and their community counterparts, though not without significant difficulties. The arrival of 'management' coincided with the widely held view that the NHS was significantly underfunded. Thus management decisions and indeed legal obligations to remain within budget result in direct and indirect cuts in patient care (bed closures, waiting lists, etc.).

Management costs have inevitably risen with little new money for direct patient care yet management reform of such a huge and expensive organization was inevitable. The performance of the new NHS and its 'market' approach will be watched with great interest both here and overseas. It is hoped that an increased part of our gross national product will be directed to health care as the general public becomes more aware that the limitations in what they receive from the health service are a consequence of underfunding and not simply due to poor management.

NURSES

Nursing care in a ward for elderly people is different in that the basic premise (for many patients) is that the greatest degree of caring often lies in consciously choosing to do less rather than more for the patients, in order to help them regain independence. This can be difficult for nurses trained to do everything for their patients. Time is important, it is much easier (and quicker) to dress a patient than to wait while they take the time to dress themselves. Nurses have to allow the patient to dictate both tempo and routine.

There is emphasis on patient choice. If medication,

therapy or any other form of treatment or care is refused this rejection must be considered sympathetically. The cause for refusal should be established and discussed. Occasionally it may be necessary to accept a refusal as being absolute. The object is not to force people to do what you want but by encouragement and help achieve the goal that they want themselves. Goals should be set within the patient's capabilities.

The dignity of the patient should be considered at all times. An apparently caring attitude of leaving a toilet door open to avoid accidents may be profoundly disturbing. If surveillance is necessary the nurse should be outside, listening carefully with the patient enjoying the illusion of total privacy. Toilets and bathrooms should have call bells (clearly explained) so that a greater feeling of security is encouraged. Other important factors include drawing the curtains around when the patient is undressing, receiving treatment or being examined, and arranging for privacy when seeing relatives and friends.

Measures such as these enable the patient to maintain his or her sense of identity. This can be further fostered by encouraging patients and relatives to bring in familiar things such as family photographs. A sense of comfort and belonging follows and helps prevent the feelings of isolation. Visiting should be encouraged at all times of the day and even by special arrangement during the night. Visitors may be of all ages as none of the usual restrictions on children need apply (except in specific cases). Arrangements should be made for elderly friends to visit.

The nurse takes a great deal of responsibility and must therefore be involved in decision-making. The aims, objectives and treatments must be clearly written down. The admitting nurse will complete the nursing profile or care plan where the care is planned in detail and updated as necessary. The aim is to show at a glance the diagnosis, progressive treatment and ultimate goal (e.g. to return home). In this way both the recording nurse and other nurses involved at a later date have a clear reminder of the pattern of care decided upon and any alterations in the patient's progress.

Observers of nursing profiles within wards will have noticed marked changes. Student nurses working on the wards for long periods for part if not the majority of their pre-staff nurse education has ceased. Student nurses have more specific education courses away from the ward setting and return for specific training and experience. The work nursing skill-mix evaluation is an attempt to relieve nurses of the less complicated aspects of nursing and give these to nursing aides. Nursing expertise will then be more supervisory with practical input to these areas requiring specific expertise. The changes in training methods, the use of running aides and the decline in the applications for nursing indicate a potential area of concern.

The nursing process

This is the name given to a more personalized method of patient care. It has two main themes:

1. A nurse has overall responsibility for a particular patient and develops a specific relationship with him or her.
2. Treatment is based on individual need.

The nurse involved with admitting the patient takes a history, fills in the nursing notes and prepares the care plan or nursing profile. One nurse is then given responsibility for the care and treatment of a certain number of patients during the shift. A student will be supervised by a trained member of staff. No nurse is required to administer treatment beyond the scope of their experience but within these limitations the duties are carried out as indicated in the nursing profile. The order in which the treatments are carried out is determined as far as possible by the pattern of the patient's normal day when at home and by the availability of all members of the multidisciplinary team.

The second theme of the nursing process has four parts — assessment, planning, implementation and evaluation. Assessment includes the physical, mental and emotional state of the patient together with details of the home environment. Following this the individualized care plan is worked out based on specific needs and is then implemented. This is closely linked with the final part, evaluation, an on-going assessment from which comparisons are made based on the patient's progress. The implementation involves not only the nurse but the whole of the multidisciplinary team.

OCCUPATIONAL THERAPISTS

Occupational therapists (OTs) provide a further cornerstone in the assessment, monitoring and advising on discharge and resettlement — providing for a better quality of life for elderly patients whether short, medium or long stay. The aims of occupational therapy are:

1. The assessment, maintenance/improvement of mental and physical function to enable the person to cope with the environment and to advise on resettlement if appropriate.

2. Work with families to increase awareness of potential capabilities of the patient in hospital and in the community.
3. Liaising with the multidisciplinary team and community services.

OTs work both in the hospital setting (with outreach services) and in the community (within social services). Early referral is essential. In many departments of health care of the elderly all patients are assessed (to find previously undiagnosed problems). OTs assess in terms of level of function (eating, dressing, coping in the kitchen) and provide reports on activities of daily living (ADL), suitability for old people's homes and home visits when specifically requested.

Role of the OT

1. Assessment and grading of level of function and suitability for home, safety, etc.
2. Improving/maintaining function (and general health) using graded tasks and activities to lessen fatigue and increase range of movements.
3. Restoring local function, by use of remedial games, craftwork, etc.
4. Helping the permanently disabled achieve maximum independence within the constraints of their disability.
5. Prophylactic measures (diversional therapy). The use of activities to stimulate patients mentally and physically to maintain a sense of well-being and encourage socialization. The activities should be purposeful and enjoyable.

Activities of daily living (ADL)

These consist of the tasks undertaken daily to maintain levels of personal care. To the elderly person the ability to perform these tasks may mean the difference between returning home or not. Information obtained by questioning must be substantiated by observation (some people will exaggerate to get home and be unrealistic as to their true capabilities). Assessment includes ascertaining those activities that are deficient, evaluating the potential for improvement and deciding on a programme to achieve this potential.

Mobility

All mobility is considered and assessment of the environment (height of chairs, toilet, floor covering, tables, stairs — both in and out of hospital) is essential.

Wheelchairs need skilled assessment to suit the needs of the patient and carers.

Eating and drinking

This is probably the area in which a very handicapped patient can attain independence. Special crockery and cutlery is available as is expertise on arranging the dining area.

Toilet management

A crucial function for independence or resettlement. Practical solutions such as a handrail or raised seat can sometimes cure incontinence. Commodes at night or chemical toilets can be invaluable but need ordering well in advance of discharge.

Personal hygiene and dressing

Assessment here should be as soon as possible after admission as increasing abilities can boost a patient's morale tremendously. Severe problems are often encountered but perseverance in dressing practice, the use of aids and self-care is essential.

Communication

Liaison with the other members of the team means that patient's with communication difficulties can continue to receive therapy. Advice can be given on specific alarms or communication aids in the home.

Domestic tasks

Training must be combined with the knowledge of the patient's home circumstances. One must guard against the blanket provision of full services such as meals on wheels, home help, etc., when the patient can cook and clean. Practice may be essential in some tasks, especially in those involving the kitchen (gas, boiling water). Remember that patients usually perform better in their own home. Many activities can be encouraged to increase general and local functioning — reading newspapers, gardening, games, etc. Some activities encourage social integration and will involve other staff members.

Home visits

Visits need organization (keys, access, joint visit, relatives or carers present) and then time to implement the findings. The assessment includes:

1. the patient's ability to cope with the accommodation and its furniture; its suitability in terms of the patient's disability (long and short term);
2. what (if any) aids/adaptations have been or need to be provided — essential or just useful;
3. the patient's attitude to the home environment, their motivation and wish to return home and cope;
4. the attitude of family/neighbours and support services to the patient.

Some units provide outpatient occupational therapy. If not, and continued therapy is thought necessary, it may be possible to refer patients to a day hospital or for them to receive domiciliary therapy.

PHARMACISTS

The role of drugs in elderly people, their dosage, interactions, side-effects and administration is assuming increasing importance. The hospital pharmacist can advise on current medication and be involved in new prescribing.. Possible drug interactions and the side-effects of medication can profoundly affect the success or failure of a course of treatment or even necessitate a hospital admission. New formulations of drugs mean that more treatment options are open depending on individual circumstances. However, all these advances are reflected in cost. The pharmacist can advise on the cost–benefit ratio so that the patient and hospital receive the best possible deal.

The pharmacist can also advise on the practical aspects of drug taking, fitting regimes to individuals and assessing the likelihood of compliance with self-medication trials, or the use of dosettes (small containers with a day's or week's worth of tablets). Most hospitals now operate their own drug policy with doctors and pharmacists agreeing on a selected core of drugs for hospital use and the prescribing of drugs outside this core being by mutual agreement, with patient needs predominating.

Community pharmacists provide an advice and education service to many of their elderly customers. Surveys have shown that these pharmacists are often approached before GPs with medical problems. They often help with minor ailments and advise consultation with a doctor for the more serious complaints. They, like their hospital counterparts, can help explain treatment regimes, possible side-effects and the need for a course of drugs often in a more relaxed environment leading to a better understanding by the patient.

PHYSIOTHERAPISTS

Physiotherapy remains one of the cornerstones in the successful rehabilitation of elderly people, helping them to achieve maximum independence with minimal assistance. Most elderly people admitted to hospital are likely to need some form of physiotherapy and referral should be made at the earliest opportunity. Elderly people benefit from prophylactic physiotherapy (pre-operative breathing exercises, how to get up off the floor following a fall, etc.).

Methodology has three aspects: reviewing the past history, assessing the present problem, and planning a future programme.

Reviewing the past history often involves collating and reading the information gained from others (nurses, doctors, etc.) and asking specific therapy-orientated questions (layout of house, aids used, stairs/steps/slopes, garden, previous mobility, etc.).

Assessing the present problem involves seeing the patient at the earliest possible opportunity, often with other members of the multidisciplinary team. The assessment should begin with introductions and an explanation of the procedure involved. An experienced physiotherapist can quickly get an overall impression — the state of mood of the patient, their dress and general demeanor, communication problems, etc.

The brief physical assessment should include the abilities listed in Table 47.2.

Table 47.2 A brief physical assessment

Raise arms above head	Balance in sitting
Hand grip/release	Reaching forwards
Lift feet	Sitting/standing
Straighten knees	Use of aids
Lift knees	

Continual assessment is made throughout the person's stay in hospital and modifications are made to accommodate the variable improvement.

Fuller assessment includes the functions listed in Table 47.3.

Table 47.3 Fuller physical assessment

Range of movement of all joints
Strength of muscle groups
Functional activities, e.g. turning/moving in bed/lying/sitting over edge of bed. Bed to chair.
Dressing (liaise with OT)
Liaison with nursing staff over particular difficulties — transfers, i.e. chair to commode, sitting to standing

Following assessment, the physiotherapist will plan a treatment programme, involving carers if appropriate. Goals will be set with the patients and family and progress will be monitored. The treatments used are eclectic (e.g. heat, ice, passive and active resisted movements, hydrotherapy, Bobath technique—Table 47.4.) and there is great variation between therapists in their approaches. Increasing effort is going into testing the effects of different treatments.

Table 47.4 The Bobath technique

A bilateral technique (i.e. not compensating the unaffected side)
Uses feedback, repetition and the full use of the affected side
Sensorimotor re-education to help decrease spasticity
The aim is to decrease spasticity to get normal movement patterns

Home visits

A home visit without the patient can bring to light certain difficulties which can be simulated in hospital, e.g. different floor surfaces, deep steps, etc. On home visits with the patient the physiotherapist takes note of any difficulties that occur with furniture, doorways and passages and can then provide assistance in planning a safer room and advise on sites for rails, ramps, etc. If relatives, friends or neighbours are going to have to assist a patient then advice and technical guidance can be given to ease anxieties about lifting etc.

Future

All members of the team help in assessing and deciding when a patient has reached optimum mobility and function. This is the prime time for discharge but the physiotherapist can be of continued help. Patients can be referred to the physiotherapy department or to the day hospital for continued help in maintaining them in the community. Domiciliary physiotherapy is a treatment service available to elderly people in their own homes (including sheltered accommodation) and old people's homes. Community physiotherapy is an assessment and advisory service — treatment can be arranged at either the physiotherapy department or the day hospital.

PLACEMENT OFFICERS

A placement officer is often part of the social work team (but not usually qualified as a social worker) and is brought in to facilitate the move of an elderly person from hospital to institution. They are aware of the complex government legislation and can advise the client and carer/relatives on the total situation. This involves being part of the counselling process in making or accepting this difficult decision and then explaining the financial and day-to-day consequences. The placement officer will assist in choosing an appropriate home and environment (usually from a vast list of personal contacts). In addition they will assist in visiting to inspect the accommodation and later help in the discharge. The officer will usually accompany the social worker for the post-discharge visit or if any intervening difficulties arise.

SOCIAL WORKERS

A social worker works with and on behalf of the client/patient (advocacy role). The role is two-fold: to enable the client through counselling to cope with the problems and stress of daily living; and to enable the client to obtain those services which are appropriate to their needs.

Social workers are employees of the local authority and most are based in the community but there is an obligation to provide a hospital-based service because of the enormous needs of the clients there. Social workers mainly work in teams, often neighbourhood or 'patch' based. While the aim is to serve all client groups, the reality is an overwhelming amount of child protection work which is statutory. In many areas elderly people receive a poor, crisis service. In most large hospitals there are teams, one of which usually concentrates on the needs of the elderly and the elderly mentally ill.

In April 1993 the funding arrangements (Care in the Community) for domiciliary services and residential accommodation (local authority Part 3, private rest home and nursing home) changed. The fundholder and hence purchaser of that care became the local authority. Social workers are charged with organizing packages of care which can be simple (meals on wheels, home care) or complex (24 hour domiciliary services or placement in an institution). These packages of care must be agreed with a care manager before a client is entitled to any service. Simple packages can usually be agreed quickly after receipt of the appropriate set of forms. Complex packages may need much longer and the convening of a case conference. A nursing home placement is still paid for by the local authority but must be agreed by the health authority.

The care manager has a limited budget and many clients. All institutional care is means-tested (continuing care in hospital is not) and many authorities charge for domiciliary services. Social workers are thus part of a hospital team trying to ensure the best and safest discharge from hospital yet under the pressures of ever-present need to admit other clients. It is not surprising, therefore, that this interface can be somewhat fraught.

Referrals

Referrals should provide basic personal information on the client (including contact phone numbers of relatives, wardens and other relevant people), state the aim of the referral (service provision or counselling role) and state whether the client is aware of the referral. Written requests are less common than the more informal approach during ward rounds or ward meetings. Indeed all patients should ideally be reviewed by a social worker who in an advocacy role may highlight certain dilemmas and change practice. Social workers can only request domiciliary services, they cannot demand them; hence patients should not be given absolute assurances of a certain level of support. These decisions are made by the relevant department or agency itself (guided by the social worker but usually after independent assessment). No two local authorities offer identical services, and the availability and cost to the client vary widely. Requests for services should be made as early as possible for they are as crucial as the correct drugs and well-being of the patient if a successful discharge is the aim.

Social reports

The collation of general information on a patient's social/environmental background is not solely the responsibility of the social worker. A social report, however, is a detailed analysis of a patient's lifestyle, involving for example relationships, attitudes, experiences and expectations. It cannot be compiled quickly and should not be requested unnecessarily.

Domiciliary care

In general inner-city districts provide a higher level of resources than elsewhere (to compensate for the difficulties encountered — housing, isolation, etc.). In some areas domiciliary services will not start until a home assessment has been made (following discharge) and then the service may be limited initially. This can put a great strain on the client and carers. Home helps assist with basic household tasks. The term is gradually being replaced by home care, with some expansion of the role. Sometimes home carers provide the only source of regular social contact and hence have a major role in monitoring how the client is managing. They can inform others in the social network of circumstances that may need attention/action.

Specialist teams (e.g. family aides) exist in some areas to provide an intensive level of support to selected clients in the first few days after discharge or following a crisis. They are designed to gradually withdraw and let the usual services take over responsibility. Some districts have domiciliary sitting services to allow relatives/carers a short break.

Meals on wheels

These were originally provided by the voluntary agency WRVS (Women's Royal Voluntary Service). In some areas voluntary groups have retained control of the service but for most it is now administered by the local authority. Advantages include cost (most authorities charge clients a modest sum), the provision of one hot 'nutritious' meal a day, social contact and a basic requirement for the physically or mentally handicapped who could not prepare a meal. Disadvantages include timing (lunch may be delivered at 10.30 am with reheating problems), provision (up to five days per week may be arranged, seven days a week provision is scarce), quality ('Muck on trucks' is a verbatim quote!), and ethnic requirements (Jewish Kosher food is well established, but this is not the case for Halal meat for Moslem's and oriental tastes).

Day care

The range of social activities is designed to meet many needs, e.g. therapy, rehabilitation, assessment, stimulation and respite for family/carer.

Luncheon clubs

These are mainly used by the active elderly in their immediate neighbourhood. They provide inexpensive meals and act as social centres.

Day centres

These cater for a mixed client group but usually can manage the less active and transport is arranged. They offer a wide variety of activities hopefully catering for all tastes. The larger establishments may have a social worker, OT and physiotherapist attached part-time.

The very frail (though not in need of nursing attention) may also attend a day centre but often their day care is within a residential unit (or attached to one). Some units are open seven days a week and offer a means of assessing suitability for alternative care as well as providing rehabilitation.

Sheltered housing

This is accommodation designed specifically for elderly people, usually in the form of flats, with the added security of a warden to help in an emergency. Sheltered housing varies in its complexity from accommodation for the very frail with a warden calling twice a day, to units where tenants are expected to be virtually independent and where the warden is not 'on site' and has periods 'off' altogether. Each social service housing department should have someone informed about the local availability and provision of warden help.

Residential homes

The term 'Part 3' home arises from that numbered section of the 1948 National Assistance Act which states that it is the duty of every local authority to provide 'residential accommodation for persons who by reason of age, infirmity or other circumstances are in need of care and attention which is not otherwise available to them'. However this is qualified by the statement that such accommodation should not provide 'services of a kind normally provided only on admission to a hospital', i.e. it is not designed to offer nursing care. Residents are means-tested and if possible pay for their care at the going rate. Once resident, most of their pension is taken to offset the cost. On admission they are expected (and may be rejected if not) to be mobile with or without aids, able to attend to basic daily needs with the minimum amount of supervision (i.e. dress and be continent) and capable of adjusting to living in a communal environment. The elderly mentally infirm may be accommodated in special units (EMI homes) or placed in the ordinary units. Each local authority has its own system of either integration or separation.

Residential homes have historically been staffed at levels consistent with this concept of frail but independent. The reality of the last 10 years, however, has been that the homes are inundated with increasingly more frail people in need of higher and higher levels of care. Numerous studies have shown that in most residential homes the majority of residents are both confused and incontinent. Staffing levels are too low and morale is down, accompanied by poor pay and a distinct lack of training. Despite this, some homes are places where you would happily entrust a loved one (a good test) whilst others conform to Victorian workhouse descriptions.

Private care

The 1980s saw a government-led explosion in the private sector, both residential and nursing home. Through Department of Social Security funding, tens of thousands of people are now in private institutions. Choice was argued as a reason — to be nearer relatives, pay for added luxuries, type of home, etc. Private homes can provide a wider range of choice, from rest homes with minimal care to nursing homes with intensive nursing help. The direct DSS-funded placement scheme is now over, with all placements now agreed and funded through social services by local care managers (unless private income ensures no local authority responsibility). Clients have to spend all resources (including capital value of a dwelling) down to £8000 and then the difference in care costs will be met (to an agreed maximum). Social workers usually review clients five to six weeks after they have entered a home. The closure of hospital beds and local authority Part 3 places has increasingly forced many districts to use the private sector. Indeed some areas no longer have an NHS or local authority controlled long-stay resource. The implications of these changes alongside the other monumental changes in the health service and local authority have yet to be fully evaluated.

SPEECH THERAPISTS

Normal communication is a highly complex two-way process which involves a receptive phase (receiving and decoding information) and an expressive phase (the encoding and transmission of information in a comprehensible form). Communication can be verbal, comprising spoken and written language, or non-verbal which includes eye contact, facial expression and gesture. In everyday interactions both types of communication are used simultaneously. When dealing with a person with speech or language impairment it is obviously important to know at what point and to what extent the process has broken down. It is also essential to look at the impairment in terms of the effect it has on the individual, their family and environment.

Communication impairment

Cerebrovascular disorders (strokes) are the most common cause of specific speech or language problems in the elderly. One third of people who suffer a stroke have speech and/or language problems.

Communication problems can be considered in terms of disorders of language, articulation, voice or fluency.

Disorders of language

Dysphasia is the difficulty in encoding and decoding language and hence can be receptive (the comprehension of incoming speech is lost and may be gross or subtle) and expressive, where speech formation is impaired (words may be used repetitively or inappropriately). Receptive and expressive dysphasia often coexist. Dysphasia is usually associated with a left hemisphere lesion.

A dyspraxia is the difficulty initiating and carrying out voluntary movement (e.g. tongue) and hence can affect speech; it results from damage to the parietal lobe.

Disorders of articulation

Dysarthria is the term used to describe impaired articulation, the effects being on the rate and clarity of speech. Causes include stroke, Parkinson's disease, motor neurone disease and multiple sclerosis.

Disorders of voice

Disorders of voice include dysphonia, aphonia, laryngectomy and disorders of fluency (Table 47.5).

Table 47.5 Disorders of voice

Dysphonia (abnormal voice, e.g. hoarse)
  This can be due to anxiety, vocal abuse, disease (carcinoma of larynx, hypothyroidism) and post-surgery

Aphonia
  This can be due to neurological conditions or be psychogenic

Laryngectomy
  These patients are more commonly found in the 50+ age group and can communicate using oesophageal speech or an electronic artificial larnyx

Disorders of fluency
  Stammers are found in people of all ages. Dysfluency may follow brain trauma

Role of the speech therapist

Assessment

This involves the use of both formal standardized tests and informal procedures. The aim is to investigate:
1. the nature and extent of the communication problem;
2. the remaining intact communication skills;
3. the effect of other factors, e.g. hearing loss, hemianopia, depression;
4. all aspects of the personality and lifestyle of the patient (early contact with relatives and/or friends is therefore essential); and
5. other aspects involved, (e.g. swallowing). This may involve detailed investigations and ongoing further assessment, advice and management plans.

Treatment and management

This involves retraining and developing speech, language and communication skills using material which is relevant and of interest to the patient. It also involves introducing alternative means of communication.

1. *Communication charts* — these consist of picture words and letters and may be useful but they may be too simplistic for some and too complex for others.
2. *Sign systems* — such as Makaton are taught to some patients. It is most effective for the dysarthric or dysphasic patient with a predominantly expressive problem. A reasonable level of comprehension is needed and mobility in one arm. The people within one's environment must also be taught to use it.
3. *Communication aids* — there is a wide range of electronic or battery powered aids on the market. They come in all shapes and sizes and many are portable. They range from glorified communication charts to computers producing electronic voices (with a strong American accent!). These machines are generally more appropriate for the severely dysarthric client.

Advising staff and relatives about communication

First and most importantly, think in terms of normal everyday communication. If the patient is anxious or tired, receptive and expressive skills are likely to be affected. Ensure you can see and hear each other clearly and try to check that there is a minimum of distraction in terms of noise and activity. Allow plenty of time for information to be absorbed and for the reply. Try not to go from one subject to another too quickly. Beware of talking too slowly or too strangely or it may be you who is creating the communication barrier.

FURTHER READING

Bennett G. *Alzheimer's Disease and Other Confusional States* 2nd edn. Macdonald Optima, London, 1994.

Cartwright A, Smith C. *Elderly People, their Medicines and their Doctors*. Routledge, London, 1988.

Durnin JUGA. Nutrition. In: Brocklehurst JC (ed.), *Textbook of Geriatric Medicine and Gerontology*, 3rd edn. Churchill Livingstone, Edinburgh, 1985.

Hooker S. *Caring for Elderly People — Understanding and Practical Help*. Routledge & Kegan Paul, London, 1987.

Isaacs A, Post F (eds). *Studies in Geriatric Psychiatry*. John Wiley, Chichester, 1978.

Mace NL, Rabins PV. *The 36-Hour Day: a family guide to caring at home for people with Alzheimer's disease and other confusional illnesses*, 2nd edn. Age Concern, London, 1993.

Maczka K. *Assessing Physically Disabled People at Home*. Chapman & Hall, London, 1990.

McClymont M, Thomas S, Denham MJ. *Health Visiting and the Elderly*. Churchill Livingstone, Edinburgh, 1986.

Murphy P. *Dementia and Mental Illness in the Old*. Papermac (Macmillan), London, 1986.

Norton C. *Nursing for Continence*. Beaconsfield Publications, 1986.

O'Malley K (ed.). *Clinical Pharmacology and Drug Treatment in the Elderly*. Churchill Livingstone, Edinburgh, 1984.

Redfern SJ (ed.). *Nursing Elderly People*. Churchill Livingstone, Edinburgh, 1986.

Rowlings C. *Social Work with Elderly People*. No. 3 Studies in Personal Social Services. George Allen & Unwin, London, 1981.

Smith L. *Physiotherapy with Older People*. Chapman & Hall, London, 1989.

Squires A. *Rehabilitation of the Older Patient*. Croom Helm, London, 1990.

Thompson K. *Caring for an Elderly Relative*. Macdonald Optima, London, 1988.

Wagstaff P, Coakley D. *Physiotherapy and the Elderly Patient*. Croom Helm, London, 1988.

Willard T, Spackman T (eds.) *Occupational Therapy*, 7th edn. JB Lippincott, Philadelphia/London, 1988.

INDEX